Marsden Wagner completed his medical training at the University of California. After specialty training and practice as a paediatrician and neonatologist, he completed two further years of post graduate studies at UCLA to train in the science of medicine and public health before embarking on a career as a perinatal epidemiologist in the United States and Denmark. During 15 years as the Responsible Office for Maternal and Child Health for the European Office of WHO (32 countries) he has worked tirelessly to promote safe and effective maternity care in industrialised countries. He continues to live in Denmark, and serves as a consultant to WHO focusing particularly on the emerging countries of Central and Eastern Europe, advising on appropriate health systems for women and children.

To Robin
the
keep up
good fight
M...

PURSUING THE BIRTH MACHINE

The search for appropriate
birth technology

Marsden Wagner

ACE Graphics

Published by ACE Graphics

10 Mallett Street (PO Box 366)
Camperdown NSW 2050
Australia
Phone: +61 2 516 3077
Fax: +61 2 516 1040

First published 1994

ISBN 0 646 16837 1

Printed in Australia by Australian Print Group
Cover design by John Lee
Text design and layout by James Robertson

This book is dedicated to the memory of Galba Araújo who combined the best of the medical world with the best of the social world and showed us all how it can be done.

Acknowledgements

This book has had a long gestation. Susanne Houd and David Banta were involved in the conception as they helped to organise the three consensus conferences and then agreed that, rather than the traditional World Health Organisation conference report, a book was needed to bring the issues, approach, ideas and recommendations together in one place. Early drafts were reviewed and advice given by Ann Oakley, Elizabeth Davis, Richard Guidotti, Jose Villar, and Jo Asvall. A thorough early editing was done by Mary Stuart Burgher. I am grateful to Patricia Stephenson for her continuous support and encouragement throughout the seemingly endless revisions. Sheryl Ruzek and Andrea Robertson assisted greatly at the birth of the book during the final editing process. We are all indebted to the conference participants who worked hard generating the recommendations which are not mine but World Health Organisation consensus recommendations.

Foreword

The book 'Pursuing the Birth Machine' is a milestone in contemporary bibliography on childbirth. It clearly presents the 'medical model' with all the modern technology versus the 'social model' in which emphasis is given to psychological, emotional and social factors.

The two models are not mutually exclusive but rather complementary. In each case their adequate balance depends on the setting, and a good example of wise application is the program developed by the late Dr Galba Araújo to whom this book is dedicated.

This book is a well documented challenge to the efficacy of many modern technologies which are widely used before their efficacy and safety are scientifically established.

Childbearing, i.e. conception, pregnancy, childbirth, puerperium, lactation and childrearing are physiological events of life and not diseases. Consequently not much technology appears to be needed.

However even a healthy population of adult human beings needs activities of health promotion and protection in order to remain healthy. No-one will reasonably oppose the widespread use of vaccines: for example in pregnant women the advantage of tetanus vaccination is clear for mother and baby.

Provided that the psychological, emotional and social factors as well as the wishes of the mother and ethnic traditions are taken into account, I see no disadvantage to employing interventions and technologies when they are really needed as long as their efficacy has been proven scientifically.

I have worked within both models. From 1947 onwards, mainly doing research, I enthusiastically developed and employed aggressive technologies. Because I was present and interacted with the mother and her family during pregnancy and throughout childbirth until the infant was sucking the mother's breast, I started to pay more and more attention to what we called the 'humanised care of labour', in which a conservative, non-aggressive approach became the centre of our attention.

Having cared for the birth of my six children and twelve grandchildren, I had the opportunity of living the event, not only as a doctor, but, most importantly, as one of the family having a new member, and sharing in the family celebration.

Professional medical staff (obstetricians) are slowly accepting some changes in the care of labour. For example the participation of the husband or companion and other relatives receives better acceptance than a decade ago. A similar statement can be made in relation to the freedom of the mother to move and change posture during childbirth.

I hope that more progress can be made in this direction by multidisciplinary conferences like those successfully organised by Dr Wagner which I found very inspiring.

I fully share with Dr Marsden Wagner his admiration for our dear Brazilian friend and colleague Dr Galba Araújo, Professor and Chairman of the Department of Obstetrics and Gynaecology at the University of Ceara. He trained in the USA and married an Anglo-American nutritionist, Lorena. With her help Galba developed a realistic and pragmatic approach to improve maternal child health care in his native State of Ceara. This is one of the poorest areas of northeastern Brazil, plagued by underdevelopment, big social inequities, ignorance, illiteracy, drought and corruption.

Galba progressively organised a coherent health care system, making an intelligent use of the already existing resources. The tertiary level was at the University Maternity Hospital in the city of Fortaleza, where all modern technologies for diagnosis and therapy were available. From there the health system spread to smaller cities, towns, hamlets and to the rural areas, providing a 98% coverage in maternal, perinatal and child health care, a unique achievement in our Afro-Indo-Latin America. After 10 years of action of this program, the State of Ceara had the lowest rates of maternal, perinatal and infant mortality in Brazil.

One of the most important factors explaining the success of Galba's project was his ability to recruit the empirical midwives (traditional birth attendants) who were trained in some 'complicated' technologies such as accurately measuring blood pressure in mothers, detecting glucose and proteins in urine with reactive strips, measuring fetal heart rate with the wooden Mauriceau stethoscope, counting fetal movements per hour, measuring uterine height, etc. The empirical midwives also learned other signs of potential complications such as vaginal bleeding, fever, etc. When they suspected that the health of the mother or fetus were 'at risk' they accompanied their rural clients to the nearest health centre where, at least, a general practitioner and a nurse were available. Without the encouragement and the presence of their empirical midwives whom they trusted, mothers from rural areas would never have thought of going to a health centre. Less than 15% of mothers were referred to health centres and less than 5% needed transfer to the tertiary level.

The system organised by Galba and Lorena is an example for the whole world, particularly for the Third World but also for some regions of the United States such as the Appalachian area. I had the privilege of making several thorough visits to Galba's program and learned very much during every minute of my 7–10 days' visits. I was very happy to be present when Galba received a standing ovation at the Royal College of Obstetricians and Gynaecologists in London. I only deplore that Galba did not receive the Nobel Prize for Medicine or for Peace which he fully deserved.

As shown by my honorary academic titles I strongly belong to the medical establishment. During the last three decades, when our attention became increasingly focused on the human components of childbirth care, a few of my colleagues were somewhat disappointed. However in more recent times they progressively better understood that the 'social' and the 'medical' models complement each other in optimal birth care.

Prof. Roberto Caldeyro-Barcia, MD
FACOG (Hon) FRCOG (ad eundem) FACS (Hon) FAAP (Hon)
Past President of FIGO
(International Federation of Gynaecology and Obstetrics)

Contents

i

Preface

This book is, in a sense, a 'case study' of what's wrong with Western health care. Because clinical practitioners, using the medical approach, have controlled both how they practice and what technology is available for them to practice with, the proliferation of the technology before adequate evaluation and the cost of health care have skyrocketed. There is no better example of this than present health care before, during and following birth. A look at what has happened with this perinatal technology is therefore instructive for all concerned with improving the quality and controlling the cost of health care.

Health care reform fortunately is on the political agenda in many countries at present and needs to involve a public health approach based on combining the medical model with a social model of health. A public health approach was used in the three international consensus meetings on perinatal technology organised by the World Health Organisation and described in this book. The reader will soon discover that these meetings differed markedly from many past WHO meetings that used the medical approach — formal affairs marked more by posturing and pomposity than innovative thinking. The public health approach, involving all interested parties and perspectives, can be difficult to bring about but it is certainly not boring.

The consensus recommendations from each meeting are based both on the 20–30 scientific review papers prepared for that meeting by participants as well as the discussions at the meeting. After the three meetings it was clear that the review papers contained a wealth of information and perhaps should be published. It soon became apparent, however, that together they would make a very long, disconnected book which would tell only half the story since the essence of the discussions would be missing. It was therefore decided to publish a book summarising both the review papers and the discussions leading to the final consensus recommendations. This book also provides an introductory description of the issues and of how the World Health Organisation became involved. Since the consensus meeting approach is fairly new in the health field, the book includes descriptions of events leading to, during and follow-

3

ing the meetings. Ultimately, public understanding of the consensus approach is crucial to its success. Health care reform and control of medical technologies will require wider use of consensus conferences. To date, little is known about how they actually operate or about how their recommendations are acted on by policy makers.

The format of the book mirrors the format of the meetings themselves. Following the first three chapters which define the issues, chapter 4 describes how the meetings were set up, and chapters 5, 6 and 7 focus on the content of the three conferences including the scientific review papers and discussions leading to the final consensus recommendations. The reader may safely assume that all statements are based on the extensive literature reviews and the discussions. The final consensus recommendations are available from WHO in English, French, German, Russian and Spanish.

As the WHO staff person responsible for maternal and child health in greater Europe, I had principle responsibility for organising these meetings. As in any large organisation, there were many bureaucratic delays in preparing the book. Several years have passed since the meetings but all of the consensus recommendations are still valid and relevant. However, the text has been updated with the most recent scientific literature and in the last chapter, events since the meeting are described.

Because WHO policy prevents identifying countries by name in official publications and puts other constraints on a full description of events, I chose to publish this book independently. This allowed me greater latitude in describing certain issues. However, the consensus recommendations are indeed official WHO recommendations. It is also a logical follow up to my earlier WHO publication, *Having a Baby in Europe*.

Chapter 1
The issue

And let the angel whom thou still hast served
Tell thee,
Macduff was from his mother's womb
Untimely ripp'd.
Shakespeare, Macbeth, V, vii, 43

The global struggle for control of pregnant and birthing women can be illustrated by several recent incidents: an unmarked police car pulled up in front of a midwife's home in the United States. A plain clothes police officer and government officials searched the house, jailed the midwife on charges that she was practising independent midwifery, and separated her from her breast-feeding infant. An obstetrician in the United Kingdom fought for her professional life, contesting a suspension that resulted from a charge made by male colleagues that she made insufficient use of birth technology in the hospital where she worked. Dr. Keith Russell, former president of the American College of Obstetricians and Gynecologists publicly declared that "home birth is child abuse in its earliest form" (*Los Angeles Times* 1992). In the same year, more than one-third of all births were home births in The Netherlands, a country that has a lower rate of perinatal deaths than the United States.

Within the past few years, several events occurred which high-lighted the fact that the World Health Organisation (WHO), widely regarded as a careful, serious, scientific member of the United Nations system, was embroiled in a growing international conflict over the technology[1] used during and following pregnancy and birth. Among these telling incidents were the following: In Copen-

---

1. In this book, technology is defined as "an association of methods, techniques and equipment which, together with the people using them, can contribute significantly to solving a health problem". From Alma-Ata. Primary Health Care. Geneva, WHO 1978.

hagen the Regional Office for Europe of WHO received a call from the Department of Health of the United Kingdom, reporting that the British Royal College of Obstetricians and Gynaecologists was upset by a series of WHO recommendations on the use of technology during birth, published in a prestigious medical journal (WHO 1985). A letter of protest from the obstetricians of the Federal Republic of Germany demanded that WHO publicly retract these same recommendations. The WHO recommendation that women should participate in decision making related to their childbirth was rejected by the executive board of the Hungarian National Obstetrical Society which believes that only obstetricians are competent to make all decisions regarding birth. A major weekly television program in Austria devoted an entire show to a heated debate on the WHO recommendations.

While professional interest groups fought the WHO recommendations, they were received favourably by women worldwide. For example, they were translated by more than 20 women's organisations in Italy, printed by the thousands, and posted in health facilities. Consumer groups concerned with birth in France, the United States, Brazil, Australia, Finland, and the United Kingdom also translated, printed and distributed thousands of copies in their countries. Few official recommendations generate such grass-roots involvement.

These events are not isolated events, nor are they insignificant 'local skirmishes'. Conflict over birth technologies is a major battle in a contemporary health revolution. There are several reasons why issues related to birth and to birth technologies are among the serious challenges facing established health care systems worldwide.

One of these challenges reflects fundamental conflict over the way we conceptualise health care. The social model of health care conflicts with the medical model. The conflict is sharpest in the areas of birth and death where the social model seems to offer an important contribution to services based on the orthodox medical model, the model on which most health care systems are based.

WHO has made a major commitment to the revolution in health in the form of supporting the concept of health promotion. The health promotion paradigm questions many of the assumptions underlying present health services and works to add the social to the medical model of health care. Examining health services for birth has propelled WHO into the conflict between medical and social models of health.

Another challenge to current health care systems is to bring health technology under control and ensure that it is effective and appropriate (Reiser 1978). The necessity for state control of pharmaceuticals distribution and consumption is well established. Only the United States has begun to use technology assessment methods and regulatory policy to attempt to control medical procedures, devices and equipment. Technological innovation appears to follow a well defined process, moving from experimental and local use, through adoption by powerful interest groups, to widespread public acceptance and routine use (McKinlay 1981). It usually takes more than a decade after the technology is introduced for scepticism to arise, owing chiefly to the lack of systematic evaluation. Technology passes very quickly from experimental status to routine use, at which point withholding it during a clinical trial becomes unethical. This short interval for proper evaluation is a considerable problem for all medical technology and for the whole of society because new procedures, drugs and equipment for use in health services are developed almost daily. Once manufactured, they are aggressively promoted to physicians, especially at medical meetings. Increasingly they are marketed to hospitals and health provider groups such as managed-care organisations. The technologies are made to be appealing to the buyer — the hospital or the physician, not the patient. Many technologies that are in widespread use have not been systematically assessed by researchers with no vested interest in their success.

Governments have begun to recognise that health technology needs regulation if the public is to be protected and the costs of health care contained. WHO is working actively with governments to promote the development of systems to monitor and control health technology and insure that the technology is appropriate to the needs of the public rather than the personal interests of health professionals. Inevitably, as this effort grows, conflicts develop over such issues as who is to assess, approve and distribute technology. These issues are not merely technical. They raise intense ethical and political controversy when matters of access and allocation arise. No country in the world is rich enough to replace every failing heart or kidney or provide in-vitro fertilisation for every infertile couple. At the end of the day the issue becomes a choice of who shall be born, live and die (Fuchs 1975). These matters are far too important to be decided by vested interests in the health and medical care systems. They require serious public debate and the involvement of many diverse groups.

This book is concerned with debate over one such matter — the *birth machine*: a wide array of medical interventions, often of a technical nature, used before, during and following birth. Chapters 2 through 4 provide the historical context for understanding controversies over the current state of perinatal technology and WHO's role in this area of health promotion. Subsequent chapters discuss the debates and resulting WHO consensus meeting recommendations related to prenatal, birth and postnatal care. The concluding chapter discusses the dissemination of the recommendations, focusing on the considerable obstacles that still block their adoption. The birth machine has become a centre of controversy because it unites two key issues in the revolution in health care: birth as a health promoting act and the role of technology in appropriate health care. In telling the story of technology development for pregnancy and birth, as well as WHO's pursuit of this birth machine, I have several goals. I hope to help break the cycle of information hoarding and arbitrary decision making on the part of physicians and policy makers. I also hope to prompt the involvement of non-medical groups in society in defining the key issues and deciding how to provide birth care. These deliberations are certain to be applicable to other areas of health and health policy-making. Learning how policy is made, adopted and rejected is important, because sound health policy making is crucial to making improvements in health care.

References

Fuchs V. 1975, *Who Shall Live?* Basic Books, New York.

Los Angeles Times 1992, 'Midwifery', April 28, p. E1.

McKinlay J. 1981, 'From "promising report" to "standard procedure", seven stages in the career of a medical innovation', *Milbank Memorial Fund Quarterly*, vol. 59, no. 3, pp. 374–409.

Reiser S. J. 1978, *Medicine and the Reign of Technology* Cambridge University Press, Cambridge.

World Health Organisation 1985, 'Appropriate technology for birth', *Lancet* vol. 2, pp. 436–7.

Chapter 2
Building the birth machine

The difference between men and boys
is the price of their toys.

Anonymous

The roots of modern, high technology, western birth care can be traced to the seventeenth century, when men began to use both surgery and forceps to extract babies from women. These men were not physicians, but barbers, tailors or butchers who called themselves barber-surgeons. Their first priority was the woman's life. In obstructed labour, their job was to save the life of the woman even if this meant, as it sometimes did, the destruction of the fetus. The early users of surgical birth technology created a great deal of mystique to surround their practice. They refused, for example, to allow anyone to look at their instruments and delivered babies under sheets. An eighteenth-century practitioner William Smellie, used to go to births dressed as a woman with the forceps hidden beneath his long skirt.

The vast majority of women, however, did not use such men's services. They gave birth in their homes with the help of experienced women from the local community. Physicians described pregnancy and birth as natural conditions in which the job of the physician was to give women advice in accordance with this view.

A body of Western, scientific knowledge on pregnancy and birth was slow to develop. Although a description of the fetal heart was first written about in 1818, in the 1830s one famous physician objected that applying a fetal stethoscope to the "naked belly of a woman would be indignantly rejected by every practitioner of reputed respectability" (Radcliffe 1967). On the other hand, the medical textbooks of the eighteenth and nineteenth centuries contained the rather modern notion that pregnancy is not a disease, merely a "temporary alteration in the condition of particular functions" (Montgomery 1856).

The development of scientific knowledge about pregnancy and birth, however, was a precondition for the more extensive use of technology. Until well into the twentieth century, no one knew when in the menstrual cycle conception occurred, where menstrual blood came from, how long an average pregnancy lasted or how to diagnose the condition of pregnancy (the birth of a baby was not unreasonably considered the only sure sign). Until the end of the nineteenth century, few women had the money or the inclination to seek medical supervision for their pregnancy. Those who did were likely to encounter the hazardous remedy of blood-letting.

Hospital birth and prenatal care

The first signs of a radical change in birth care appeared about 100 years ago, with two major steps in the evolution of the birth machine: the legitimation of hospital birth and the beginning of prenatal care. While providing free hospital births for poor women was a well established practice, bringing women of all social classes to give birth in hospitals was the consequence of the emergence of a group of physicians with a special interest in birth. The hospital served the new profession of obstetrics by: restricting competition from female midwives; establishing the principle of medical control over patients; and enabling the teaching of the new clinical expertise (the patients acting as teaching objects for medical students). The growth of hospital care at the beginning of this century helped redefine pregnancy and birth as medical problems rather than natural phenomena.

The establishment of prenatal care appears to have resulted from quite different forces. Until the beginning of the twentieth century, the concept of prenatal care did not exist in any country in the world. Neither the providers of health care, nor pregnant women, considered routine medical supervision necessary. No clinics or hospitals were set aside for that purpose, nor was there a systematic body of knowledge or available technology to provide the rationale for medical supervision during pregnancy. How did routine prenatal care, the first mass screening program in the history of health care, come about?

In the late 1890s and early 1900s, high infant and maternal mortality rates persisted, while birth rates actually fell. Because of the state's interest in the size and vitality of the population, there was some concern about what to do. During these years, a new concept of health and the responsibility for health was formulated in many industrialised countries, positing that the health of the adult depended on the health of the child, and that the health of the child depended on its mother. How, then, should the state assist in improving the health of the child and its mother? Even then, evidence showed that both environmental factors such as poor housing and inadequate food on the one hand and on the other, personal health factors such as untreated disease and alcoholism, were to blame. The state chose to address individual rather than environmental factors for complex reasons, which include the politically more acceptable approach of blaming the victims (the poor) rather than the state. In addition, physicians urged that the individual approach be taken, under their control, and they had some experience to back up their position. Experiments with the institutional prenatal care of poor unmarried women suggested the value of the individual approach. Whatever the reasons, the industrialised countries chose this approach and prenatal care was born.

The choice of the individual approach set the pattern of health services for children and their mothers in the twentieth century. In 1901, the first hospital bed allocated specifically to pregnant women was established in the United Kingdom, and the first routine prenatal visit was made in the United States. By the First World War, most industrialised countries had established a wide variety of official regulations and institutions to provide routine health care during pregnancy, birth and the first year of life. The profession of obstetrics flourished, and by 1930 many obstetrical societies had been established. The profession of midwifery was brought into the official care system and regulated, except in Canada and most of the United States, where it was outlawed. By 1929 the basic structure of today's prenatal care had been set up: monthly visits for about 30 weeks of pregnancy, then fortnightly visits to about 36 weeks and weekly visits thereafter. This practice was not based on any scientific work, but was simply the pattern that most clinics had evolved.

Technology, in the form of new monitoring techniques, also appeared on the scene during these years (Reisner 1978). X-rays were used more and more during pregnancy and by the 1920s someone suggested them for all pregnant women. The note of caution sounded by a few as to the hazardous effects of x-rays was disregarded until a study published in 1956, many decades after the practice began, demonstrated an increase in cancer among children x-rayed in utero (Stewart et al. 1956).

An enthusiastic appraisal in the early twentieth century of obstetrical technology — as the answer to all the problems of childbearing — changed into disillusionment by the late 1930s. Part of the reason was the failure of obstetrical intervention to affect the maternal mortality rate, but some practitioners and policy-makers also voiced scepticism about the new technology. Although rare, some analyses of technology were performed. These showed that the use of birth technology, such as induction of labour and caesarean section, varied widely among hospitals.

Nobody seemed to know the reason for this variation or for the rapid increase in the use of technology in the 1930s. Increasing prenatal care and the battle among different professional groups for the control of birth, however, were clearly involved. This battle had progressed to the point at which, in general, normal pregnancy and birth were the province of midwifery and abnormality was obstetrical territory. This division started the trend towards categorising pregnant women.

The Second World War gave a salutary message to the debate on the effectiveness of birth technology. At this time, when less specialist care was available and the birth machine nearly ground to a halt, all obstetric mortality rates fell to an unprecedented degree. This phenomenon, almost worldwide has never been adequately explained. Theories attributed the improvement in pregnancy outcome to decreases in parity (the number of children borne by a woman), improvements in health from one generation to the next and to the redistribution of income and resources, from the rich to the poor, and from men to women, brought about by governments' wartime social and economic policies.

The 1950s and 1960s, however, could well be described as the reign of technology. By the end of the 1940s nearly all pregnant women in most industrialised countries received prenatal care. This provided a captive population of pregnant women on whom developing prenatal technology could be used. Further, the trend towards hospital birth now accelerated rapidly, providing captive populations of labouring women and infants on whom birth and neonatal (newborn) technology, respectively, could be used.

A brief look at trends in the place of birth since the Second World War is instructive. In the United States in 1940, 44% of all births were outside hospitals. By 1970 this proportion had dropped to less than 1% (US Vital Statistics 1985). In Great Britain out-of-hospital birth declined at a slightly slower rate, decreasing from over 50% in the 1940s to 35% in 1960, and to less than 10% in 1970 (United Kingdom Department of Health and Social Services 1970). Among the industrialised countries, The Netherlands has had the slowest decline. In 1963, planned home births represented 70% of all births; the figure decreased to its lowest level of 32% in 1982 and gradually increased to 35% in 1990 (The Netherlands Ministry of Public Health and Environmental Hygiene 1990).

The reasons behind the trend to hospital birth are complex. The role played by professional organisations and government agencies can be documented in the United Kingdom, where a national health service was in place. In 1956 a government report recommended 50% hospital birth but the Royal College of Obstetricians and Gynaecologists (RCOG) recommended 100% (Department of Health and Social Services (DHSS) 1956). In 1959 another government report recommended 70% hospital birth. Again the RCOG recommended 100% hospital births but both the Royal College of Midwives and the British Medical Association emphasised the importance of women having the option of home birth (DHSS 1959). By 1970 a government report recommended 100% hospital birth (DHSS 1970).

In the 1980s, however, the scientific justification for this trend to hospital birth was questioned. It was shown that out-of-hospital births are heterogeneous, including planned and unplanned home births, and therefore the poor outcomes reported are biased against planned home birth (Murphy et al. 1984). The National Perinatal Epidemiology Unit in Oxford, England evaluated the statistics and arguments that provided the basis for obstetrical recommendations and government policy. They conclude "Perhaps the most persistent and striking feature of the debate about where to be born, however, is the way policy has been formed with very little reference to the evidence" (Campbell & MacFarlane 1987). Recent research in several developed countries has repeatedly shown the safety of home birth: from the United Kingdom (Campbell et al. 1984; Ford et al. 1991); from The Netherlands (Damstra-Wijmenga 1984; Buitendijk 1993); from the United States (Schramm et al. 1987; Durand 1992).

Recent research also has shown the safety of another out-of-hospital birth option, the freestanding birth centre. In a pioneering research study, it was found that for over 10,000 women giving birth in over 80 freestanding birth centres in the United States, the outcome was just as safe as a matched group of low risk hospital births (Rooks et al. 1990). At the present time a randomised controlled study of maternity care at a birth centre or standard hospital obstetric service is taking place in Sweden (Waldenstrom & Nilsson 1993). This and other studies have shown significantly less obstetrical interventions in these birth centres (Feldman & Hurst 1987; Baruffi et al. 1990).

The trend to hospital birth has been accompanied by a trend to close maternity units in small hospitals (WHO 1985, p. 23) with the justification that larger hospitals, where obstetricians and technology are in place, are safer. However, research in Finland (Hemminki 1985), New Zealand (Rosenblatt et al. 1985) and Australia (Lumley 1988) contradicts this argument; all showed that "normal infants fared worse in larger hospitals" (Lumley 1988). As with home birth, the trend to birth in larger hospitals is not justified by the scientific evidence.

The growing scientific literature on the safety of birth outside big hospitals, as just reviewed, is at least partly responsible for a most recent counter-trend encouraging births at home, in free standing birth centres and in smaller hospitals, all associated with less use of high technology. Thus in a WHO publication (WHO 1985, pp. 86–87) are the statements: "It is important to remember that it has never been scientifically proven that the hospital is a safer place than the home for a woman who has had an uncomplicated pregnancy to have her baby. Studies of planned home birth in developed countries with women who have had uncomplicated pregnancies have shown morbidity and mortality rates for mother and baby equal to or better than hospital birth statistics for women with uncomplicated pregnancies. These studies have also found significantly fewer interventions used in home births than in hospital births".

"Discussions of home birth usually generate much more heat than light, especially among health professionals. Clearly, some women need the specialised care of the hospital. Equally clearly, some women could just as well, or better, have their babies at home."

Similarly, in the United Kingdom, the latest government report rejects the earlier recommendation of 100% hospital birth. In spite of the continuing insistence by the RCOG that there should be 100% hospital birth, the House of Commons Health Committee strongly recommends free choice of place of birth, including home birth, with adequate encouragement and backup by the National Health Service (House of Commons 1992). A wide number of groups, including the Royal College of Midwives and many consumer organisations urged such a recommendation, based on the scientific research of the past 10 years.

The importance of hospital birth and routine prenatal care in fuelling the birth machine would be difficult to overestimate. The extraordinary proliferation of obstetrical technology in the 25 years following the Second World War is well known. Although the search for a means to know and control what goes on inside the uterus received a set-back with the documentation of the hazards of prenatal x-rays in 1956 (Stewart et al. 1956) only two years later the application of ultrasonic imaging techniques to pregnant women was suggested. Although there was some early caution expressed over this innovation, it was quickly overridden and by the late 1960s it was obviously becoming popular. While ultrasound is clearly valuable in selected complications, by the mid-1970s, statements about the value of ultrasound in the *routine* surveillance of pregnant women — similar to those on routine x-rays — were being made. The long list of other new types of obstetrical technology that rapidly gained widespread use during this reign of technology includes fetoscopy, amnioscopy, amniocentesis, electronic fetal monitoring and chorionic villus sampling.

The birth machine in operation

By the early 1970s, the birth machine was humming at full throttle in the developed countries. Physicians sat in the driver's seat, helping to design the technology, creating demand for it and using it. Midwives and nurses might occasionally use some technologies, but they were under the direct supervision of physicians in almost all cases. The possibility that the woman herself might use technology was unheard of.

Designed in part by physicians for physicians' use, the machinery and the users were found in the same places: hospitals and clinics. This fact produced procedures and machines that function properly only in these settings. Technology for home use was not developed until the 1980s, when the first major effort, the home uterine activity monitor, was developed but ran into great difficulty. The technology of this period tended to be mechanical, complex, electrical, and difficult to maintain. The result was elegant, impressive looking and very expensive machinery.

The development of the birth chair illustrates all the qualities of birth machinery. When some obstetricians realised that a horizontal position was detrimental to women giving birth, they set about designing a variety of birth chairs. All were mechanical and made of metal, many were quite complex, allowing for a number of different positions and looked rather like the chair in a dentist's office. Most were expensive, sometimes costing thousands of dollars. Midwives in several countries, on the other hand, brought bean-bag birth chairs into hospitals. These fabric sacks, filled with beans or similar kinds of stuffing, cost a few dollars and required no maintenance. A labouring woman could sit on the bag and hold any position with excellent support.

Another technology illustrates the dehumanising approach to birth care and the lengths to which the medical-industrial complex will go to mechanise human functions (and create a market). When oxytocin, the drug used to stimulate uterine contractions during labour, was found to have side effects and complications, it was suggested that the drug might be replaced in some cases with a non-invasive method of stimulating the uterus indirectly by means of nipple stimulation. For centuries midwives had relied on the woman's partner, a midwife, or the woman herself as the nipple stimulator in situations requiring uterine stimulation. In 1990 a commercial firm applied to the US Food and Drug Administration (FDA) advisory panel on obstetrics and gynaecology for approval of a nipple stimulation device that used an electrical pump and a 'suction hood' to fit over the nipple. The panel rejected the application (FDA 1990).

The birth machine was on the road but the operator required no licence. Governments did not attempt to regulate the manufacture, distribution or use of technology. Any physician or member of hospital staff could use technology without prior training or certification of competence. There was also little or no attempt to control the distribution of technology according to proven need.

The United States is an exception but problems abound. For some years not only drugs, but many devices, procedures and systems required approval by the Federal Food and Drug Administration (FDA). This effort, however, has been sporadic, modest and "consistently troublesome" (Foote 1987). Although the law requires manufacturers to demonstrate that new products are efficacious and safe, neither term is defined. At what level of efficacy does benefit occur? How safe is safe enough? Moreover, the FDA relies heavily on data collected by manufacturers. Although a Code details the types of scientific evidence considered acceptable, "manufacturers have enormous leeway in what they choose to study" (Ruzek 1993). The results of this attempt to regulate medical devices in the United States, while highly commendable and an important pioneering effort, can sometimes fail to protect the public. A case in point is the FDA's withdrawal of blanket approval for breast implants after it was discovered that the manufacturers had not released all of their data on risks and side effects. Other countries would do well to start similar efforts at regulation but should take care to learn from the experience of the United States.

Free of constraint, the birth machine was commercialised, and, in the western industrialised countries at least, competing manufacturers promoted an extraordinary variety of products. This in turn led to physicians working closely with industry. The positive effect of this collaboration was the development of new or better technology; even in positive cases, however, there was the possibility for the negative effect of conflicting interests for physicians.

These conflicts of interest can be economic and professional. The economic conflict is illustrated by a meeting organised by the International Federation of Gynaecology and Obstetrics (FIGO) to develop guidelines for the use of electronic fetal monitors. The WHO participant learned on arrival that most of the cost of the meeting was borne by the manufacturers of the monitors to be evaluated and that participants had to pass through a manufacturers' display of monitors to get to the room in which the value of the monitors was to be discussed. The professional conflict of interest is illustrated by the activities of another international organisation: composed of physicians who use ultrasound, this group has assumed the role of watch-dog, monitoring all scientific reports for the possible hazards of ultrasound. At the same time, however, the professional advancement of most members of this organisation is tied to the continuing and expanding use of ultrasound technology in medical care. The potential for bias from conflict of interest in such situations is a serious concern.

Sources of birth technology development

The history of the birth machine highlights the lesson that the nature of birth technology used is not determined solely by the health needs of women and babies. While a physician, midwife or nurse decides on the care of a woman or baby, the diagnostic and therapeutic options available and the attitudes of the people making the choices are determined by factors external to the woman or baby. Thus, there is an urgent need to discover just how birth technologies are adopted, since clearly no rational system prevails. Some observers explain the process of adopting new medical technologies as a progression through predictable stages (McKinlay 1981) or as a process specific to the interaction of various groups (scientists, clinicians, industry, government, consumer groups) at a given time (Bell 1986). Some believe that the interactive model is particularly apt for birth technologies (Ruzek 1991), but the need to examine how birth technologies become 'standard procedure' so quickly is important.

Understanding the birth machine — and eventually attempting to change its nature — means that we cannot be limited to the clinical medical approach of examining individual cases. While attending medical conferences or planning meetings of national or local public health authorities, WHO staff members frequently hear proposals for the purchase of more technology defended on the basis of 'horror stories' that describe individual medical cases in which a mother or baby died, supposedly because the particular technology was absent. According to the Director of Maternal and Child Health for the City of Vienna, a doctor demanded that she use her limited budget to buy his hospital an expensive new technology. When she hesitated, he claimed that a patient's recent death could have been prevented by this technology and he would hold the Director responsible for the next such death.

Conversely, at birth conferences attended by women's groups, WHO staff also hear many horror stories about a woman or baby harmed by the use of a particular kind of technology. Such stories, however tragic they may be on an individual level, cannot form the basis of the rational planning of appropriate health technology for an entire community.

If they do not develop from health needs or from some pure spirit of scientific endeavour, where do new technological procedures come from? A profession's desire for technical expertise and credibility is one source. In the nineteenth century, and well into the twentieth, the people who helped women to give birth had to rely on the women's knowledge and ability to assess her situation (concerning the stage of her pregnancy, for example) — a profound disadvantage for professional groups who need to make persuasive claims of expert techniques and successful births. The need to make such claims seems to explain the insistence that x-rays and ultrasound have greater reliability than a woman's memory of her last menstrual period or a midwife's examination in determining pregnancy length; to date, no scientific data supports the superiority of these technologies (see chapter 5).

The way professions define their mandate is another spur for the development of technology. For example, as newer technologies have enabled the observation, diagnosis and, in some cases, treatment of the fetus before birth, the idea that the fetus is now a patient (Gallagher 1987) who needs medical care has precipitated a host of new technologies.

Related to definition is control — for example, through the designation of who may use specific technologies. In many countries, midwives, general practitioners and obstetricians have been struggling for control of perinatal health services for many years. Some procedures are normally restricted to physicians and a midwife's access to them varies from country to country. Generally, midwives use less technology, so that the number of practising midwives and their degree of independence in their practice affects the prevalence of technological interventions.

Along with the proliferation of technologies there is a deluge of scientific information, but doctors and midwives are poorly trained to evaluate research reports. Few countries have assigned the responsibility for tracking the evidence on the safety and efficacy of existing technologies; consequently practitioners are vulnerable to the claims made in manufacturer's advertising. Fortunately, review articles on a given procedure are becoming increasingly common in professional journals. One organisation, Midwives Information and Resource Service (MIDIRS), publishes reports summarising the scientific literature for practising midwives. Other organisations would do well to use this model (MIDIRS 1993) yet, as discussed above, many of the most prestigious and influential bodies are heavily involved in the use of technology and have a stake in seeing its widespread use. How well will they be able to assess risks and benefits?

Industrialised countries typically support scientific research and development, and over the long term, funding priorities will influence the availability of particular types of technology. In addition, the state's concern for its present and future citizens strongly influences health policy, which in turn influences the development of health technology. Political decisions, such as policies to promote higher birth rates or expand prenatal care also have implications for the development of technology. The relationship of such policy to the growth of birth technology is not sufficiently documented or appreciated. Similarly, commercialisation is well recognised as a factor that determines the nature of the birth machine in many countries, but there is very little real information on how economic factors operate in the private and public sectors. Every hospital and clinic, private or public, purchases technology, and someone decides what to buy and from whom. These decisions undoubtedly play a role in setting development agendas for health technology but the linkages are still poorly understood.

Private sector research and development is largely driven by economic considerations and is conducted without public accountability. As mentioned earlier, commercial interests are also largely in control of birth technology assessment since assessment procedures are designed by the manufacturers and carried out by doctors connected in one way or another to the manufacturers. When the results are published in journals these connections and potential conflicts of interest are not mentioned; one result is that the medical literature "is biased in the direction of assessing capital intensive products over labour intensive approaches to solving birth outcome problems" (Ruzek 1993). In other words, commercial interests realise substantially greater profits from solutions that rely on machines rather than people.

Thus, scientific evaluation of birth technology has come as an afterthought, not a prerequisite for its application. Although a randomised controlled trial is indisputably the most reliable scientific means of assessing the benefits and hazards of a new technology, few such trials have been conducted. A number of excuses are given for this, many going beyond the reasonable complaints about the difficulty and often considerable expense of mounting these trials. For example, applications for research money to assess a new technology have been denied on the grounds that no one yet knew what benefits or hazards to seek. In another instance, negative results from a randomised controlled trial of a rapidly developing and spreading device or procedure have been dismissed with the explanation that due to its increasing use, physicians now have greater proficiency in using it, so the trial results are out of date. In fact, the opposite state of affairs may often exist. A trial may be performed by the most proficient users; many such trials are conducted in university hospitals whose staffs have much more proficiency and experience with the new machine than the vast majority of subsequent users. The rush to use new technology can impede assessment. When the assessment goals are clear and reasonable proficiency has been achieved, it is too late for a randomised controlled trial because physicians feel it is unethical to withdraw a practice that many people believe is valuable from routine use (Banta & Thacker 1979). The result is a 'Catch–22' dilemma. If doctors refuse to participate in random control trials which will deny some of their patients what they consider the 'best' care and if by definition whatever is newest is best, then "we never will be able to research the safety and efficacy of birth technology adequately and thus we never in fact will know what is best" (Ruzek 1991, p. 79). A concrete example of this dilemma regarding epidural anaesthesia is described in chapter 8.

Behind all explanations for the lack of systematic experimental assessment of health technology lies the basic reality that, except for the United States, no system exists to ensure such assessment. Equally important, in every country, including the United States, few people are trained and experienced in performing such assessment. The little training that physicians receive in research focuses on clinical assessment, not epidemiological methods that are used in randomised controlled clinical trials. Technology is assessed only when people decide to undertake it. The medical literature on technology is full of clinical reports that are descriptive, not analytical. Little research is truly experimental. Paper after paper given at scientific meetings reveals severe methodological weaknesses and unjustified conclusions even in the relatively few randomised controlled clinical trials that are conducted. Clinical case studies may generate hypotheses, but they do not provide results on which policies or practice should be based.

All interventions used in maternity care, social as well as medical, should be scientifically evaluated. It is important to avoid a double standard which insists on scientific assessment of medical interventions but not social interventions. There may, however, be more urgency in assessing medical interventions. Medical interventions usually carry more potential harm to women and babies: for example, pain management by epidural anaesthesia is riskier than the presence of a supportive person during labour. Secondly, medical interventions usually interfere more with the preservation of birth as a personal and family event. In setting priorities for scientific research on obstetrical interventions, potential harmful side effects and interference with the positive, health promoting nature of pregnancy and birth must be considered.

Nevertheless, the history of birth and other kinds of medical technology is studded with the often unarticulated assumption that things get better for mothers and babies because of technology. Such a claim obscures the influential role of social and environmental determinants of health and disease. The converse of this view also prevails: when things get worse, there may be a demand for more technology. Social and environmental policies to improve health might be more appropriate responses. Thus rather than allocate funds to research new technologies (in essence the research agenda of the manufacturers), we need to increase efforts to identify the needs of groups that have the poorest birth outcomes, so that scarce resources can be used to solve problems cost-effectively and in keeping with the social and cultural values of women who actually give birth (Ruzek 1993). The issue of relating indicators of health to levels of technology is a serious one that merits further discussion.

The emergence of the birth machine has had a subtle influence on the perception of new babies and of women who are pregnant or giving birth. The struggle for the control of birth first resulted in the division of women and babies into the categories of normal and abnormal, an uncertain dichotomy at best; later, the normal category was subdivided into those likely to remain normal (low-risk) and those likely to become abnormal (high-risk). This process of categorisation has continued. Divisions within medicine — reflected in specialties such as obstetrics, obstetrical anaesthesia, gynaecology, paediatrics, neonatology, fetal medicine and reproductive medicine — have undoubtedly segmented both the treatment of women's bodies and the social process of reproduction and family life into competing charters and domains of medical work.

One consequence of the changing perception is the dehumanisation of women and babies suggested by a recent international symposium in Hungary on 'The Pregnant Uterus' as well as by commonly used expressions in maternity care, such as 'the incompetent cervix' and 'the active management of labour' where 'active' refers not to the woman but to the manager-doctor.

A final theme from the historical review of the birth machine is — who is in the driver's seat? Modern birth technology has not evolved with the active participation and consultation of all (in addition to the medical profession) who have a legitimate role to play. Midwives, nurses, social scientists, economists, epidemiologists, health administrators, politicians and, most important, the women on whom the technology is used, are interested parties. How all these interested parties might be given some control of the birth machine is an important issue.

References

Banta H. D. & Thacker S. 1979, 'Costs and benefits of electronic fetal monitoring', *Dept. of Health, Education and Welfare Publ. 79–3245*, Hyattsville, Maryland, US National Centre for Health Services Research.

Baruffi G., Strobino D. M. & Paine L. L. 1990, 'Investigation of institutional differences in primary cesarean birth rates', *J Nurse Midwifery*, vol. 35, no. 5, pp. 274–281.

Bell S. E. 1986, 'A new model of medical technology development: a case study of DES'. *Research in the Sociology of Health Care*, no. 4, pp. 1–32.

Buitendijk S. 1993, 'How safe are Dutch home births?', in *Successful Home Birth and Midwifery: the Dutch Model*, ed. E. Abrahams, Bergin & Garvey (Greenwood Publ.), Westport, Connecticut (in press).

Campbell R. & McFarlane A. 1987, *Where to be born: the debate and the evidence*, National Perinatal Epidemiology Unit, Oxford.

Campbell R., Davies I. M. & Macfarlane A. 1984, 'Home birth in England and Wales, perinatal mortality according to intended place of birth', *British Medical Journal*, vol. 289, pp. 721–24.

Damstra-Wijmenga S. 1984, 'Home confinement: the positive results in Holland', *J Royal College of General Practitioners*, vol. 34, 425–430.

Department of Health and Social Services (DHSS), United Kingdom 1956, *Enquiry into the cost of the National Health Service*, Her Majesty's Stationery Office (HMSO), London.

—— 1959, *Report of the Committee on Maternity Services*, HMSO, London.

—— 1970, *Domiciliary Midwifery and Maternity bed needs*, HMSO, London.

Durand A. M. 1992, 'The safety of home birth: the Farm study', *American J Public Health*, vol. 82, no. 3, pp. 450–3.

Feldman E. & Hurst M. 1987, 'Outcomes and procedures in low risk birth: a comparison of hospital and birth centre settings', *Birth & Family Journal* vol. 14, no. 1.

Food and Drug Administration, United States 1990, *Advisory Panel on obstetrics and gynaecology minutes*, April 4.

Foote S. B. 1987, 'Assessing medical technology assessment: past, present, future'. *Milbank Memorial Fund Quarterly*, vol. 65, no. 59-80, p. 60.

Ford C., Iliffe S. & Franklin O. 1991, 'Outcome of planned home birth in an inner city practice', *British Medical Journal*, vol. 303, pp. 1517–19..

Gallagher J. 1987, 'Fetus as patient', presented at the Rutgers University Forum on Reproductive Laws for the 1980s, New York.

Hemminki E. 1985, 'Perinatal mortality distributed by type of hospital', *Scand J Soc Med*, vol. 13, pp. 113–118.

House of Commons, United Kingdom 1992, *Health Committee Second Report on Maternity Services*, HMSO, London.

Lumley J. 1988, 'The safety of small maternity hospitals in Victoria 1982–1984', *Community Health Studies*, vol. 12, no. 4.

McKinlay, J. 1981, 'From "promising report" to "standard procedure", seven stages in the career of a medical innovation', *Milbank Memorial Fund Quarterly*, vol. 59, no. 3, pp. 374–409.

Midwives Information and Resource Service 1992, *MIDIRS Midwifery Digest*, vol. 2, no. 1, March, 9 Elmdale Road, Clifton Hill, Bristol BS8 1SL, England.

Montgomery W. 1856, *An exposition of the signs and symptoms of pregnancy*, Longman, Brown, Green, Longmans & Roberts, London.

Murphy J. F., Dauncey, Gray O. P. & Chalmers I. 1984, 'Planned and unplanned deliveries at home', *British Medical Journal*, vol. 288, no. 12, pp. 1429–1432.

Netherlands Ministry of Public Health and Environmental Hygiene 1990, *Annual Reports*, Staatsuitgeverij, The Hague.

Radcliffe W. 1967, *Milestones in midwifery*, John Wright & Sons, Bristol.

Reiser S. J. *1978, Medicine and the Reign of Technology*, Cambridge University Press, Cambridge.

Rooks J. P., Weatherby N. L., Ernst E. K., Stapleton S., Rosen D. & Rosenfield A. 1990, 'Outcomes of care in birth centres: The national birth centre study'. *New England Journal of Medicine*, vol. 321, no. 26, pp. 1804–1811.

Rosenblatt R. A., Reinken J. & Showmack P. 1985, 'Is obstetrics safe in small hospitals?', *Lancet*, vol. 2, pp. 429–432.

Ruzek S. 1991, 'Women's reproductive rights: the impact of technology', in *Women and New Reproductive Technologies: Medical, Psychosocial, Legal, and Ethical Dilemmas*, eds J. Rodin & A. Collins, Hillsdale, New Jersey, US, Lawrence Erlbaum Assoc..

—— 1993, 'Defining reducible risk: social dimensions of assessing birth technologies', *Human Nature*, vol. 4, no. 4 (in press).

Schramm W. F., Barnes D. E. & Bakewell J. M. 1987, 'Neonatal mortality in Missouri home births, 1978–1984', *Amer. J Public Health*, vol. 77, no. 8, pp. 930–35.

Stewart A., Webb J., Giles D. & Hewitt D. 1956, 'Malignant disease in childhood and diagnostic irradiation in utero', *Lancet*, vol. 2, p. 447.

United States Vital Statistics 1981, *Vol 1 Natality, 1981*, Dept of Health and Human Services Pub. No. (PHS) 85-1113, Wash. DC, GPO.

Waldenstrom U. & Nilsson C. 1993, 'Women's satisfaction with birth centre care: a randomised controlled study', *Birth: Issues in Perinatal Care*, vol. 20, no. 1, pp. 3–13.

World Health Organisation 1985, *Having a Baby in Europe, Public Health in Europe No 26*, Copenhagen.

Chapter 3

Medical and social views of the birth machine

The greatest danger arises from ruthless application of partial knowledge on a vast scale.

E. F. Schumacher

The birth machine is the creation of the orthodox medical establishment. Behind this creation lies a set of assumptions, ideas and ways of thinking called the medical model of health. Here we analyse these assumptions and compare them with those underlying a social model of health. Our purpose is not to label one model right and the other wrong, but to explore how to combine them by identifying the elements in each that might be effective in addressing specific health issues.

The conflict between the two models arose from the view of the world that originated in ancient Greek philosophy and is deeply ingrained in current Western thought. In this dichotomised world view, science and art are antithetical (as are objectivity, logic, masculinity and emphasis on quantity on the one hand and subjectivity, intuition, femininity and emphasis on quality on the other).

art	science
subjective	objective
feminine	masculine
intuition	logic
quality	quantity

At the beginning of the modern era, Descartes argued persuasively for science as the only path to knowledge and for the control of the artistic impulse. About a hundred years ago, the profession of medicine aligned itself with science and classical, mechanical physics, applying them to the body, its functions and its disease processes: this was the basis for the medical model of health (Wagner 1982). As pregnancy and birth were brought into the domain of the medical profession, this view was applied to birth and birth technology.

Before the modern era, however, health and birth were clearly placed on the artistic side of the dichotomy. The view and management of health and birth reflected the subjective and intuitive side of life, which is the basis for the social model of health and birth and birth technology. Although the medical profession transferred birth from art to science, the profession of midwifery did not, nor did most women, at least until quite recently. Accordingly, two views can be taken of health, birth and birth technology.

Health as a problem

According to the medical model, life is a problem, as it is full of risk and in almost constant danger — an assumption easily accepted if one's professional career is spent surrounded by pathology, suffering and death. The body is seen as imperfect or even corrupt, and health is obtained only with help from the outside. Health is the success of external agents (treatments) over nature in temporarily eliminating disease or other pathological conditions from the body. Nevertheless, the risk, whether high or low, of disease or death remains. Disease results from the failure of the external agents and, therefore, the failure of the individual and the medical care system. The ultimate failure of the individual and the physician is death: the greatest enemy, against which an all-out struggle must be waged.

The best weapons in the struggle against disease and death, according to the medical model, result from the use of the power of science to create the necessary interventions and to determine when and on whom to use them. This approach is based on contact between the physician and the person who is, or may become, ill rather than on efforts to change the environment. The imperfections of the patient's body must be located and correctly understood; accurate diagnosis requires that the body be reduced to smaller and smaller units — from organs to cells to molecules — and that the imperfection be quantified. Then the correct external agent must be scientifically selected and applied in the most effective way to the corrupt place in the body. If this is not possible, the corrupt place must be surgically removed. Further, all these tasks require an objective, scientific physician to control, and ideally to quantify, each step in the process.

Implicit here is the assumption that any kind of health deviance, illness or disability should be corrected. The medical system spends almost all of its energies in this effort. The focus is on the problem, which is used to define the person who has it. When physicians walk down the hospital corridor, they may describe the person they see as a diabetic, not as Mr. Hansen who has diabetes.

Health as a solution

According to the social model, life is a solution, not a problem. The most important health statistic in the world is the worldwide mortality rate — 100%. Since everyone dies, what is important is how people live. Thus, life and health are solutions — positive forces to assist the pursuit of fulfilment. It is normal to feel good and disease or disability is often a temporary alteration in this state.

Rather than focusing only on correcting or getting rid of a person's health problem, the social model suggests beginning with a focus on the part of the person that is normal. Regardless of the nature of the problem, in most cases it is only a small part of the human being which is not normal. Attention can next be given to the disease or disability, not just to eliminate or avoid it but in some cases even to redefine it as something that can be useful (Wagner 1991).

Adherents of the social model assume that the best approach to disease is to rely on people to heal themselves. Medical care should help them in this task, respecting their integrity and supporting them with the least intervention necessary. The person is seen as a kind of ecological system that is not yet well understood. This system includes the body, mind and spirit, each of which is involved in health and disease. Psychological and social factors (such as love and social support or the lack of them) are emphasised in curing as well as producing illness. The importance of the environment in health and disease is also emphasised, and ecological solutions are urged that imply changing the environment and the structures of society.

Medicine has become a major institution of social control, in which physicians act as the new repository of truth (Stephenson & Wagner 1993). In this role, physicians believe they are capable of making absolute judgements, as morally neutral and objective experts, about people's lives and the form health services should take. According to the social model, physicians in their vain attempt to be completely objective, have professionalised care-giving and have forgotten that health service means serving others.

Views of birth

The views of birth held by the medical and social models follow from their assumptions about health (Davis-Floyd 1992). According to the medical model, birth is a medical problem. Many kinds of disability originate in the period before, during and after birth. This perinatal period clearly carries a high risk of pathology, disability and death. For about half of the time, it is impossible to discover which women will develop complications leading to disability or death for themselves or their babies. The only reasonable assumption on which to proceed, therefore, is that all pregnancies and births are potentially pathological until proved otherwise (in retrospect). Adherents of the medical model see birth as a bodily function with anatomical, physiological and biochemical components. The woman's body is a complex machine that can only be understood through a scientific approach that separates the parts of the process for study. Because of the imperfections of the body and the complexity of the machinery of birth, the process malfunctions easily, particularly when the patient abuses the delicate machine. Nature is indeed a bad obstetrician; medical intervention is absolutely necessary. It consists of the careful scientific evaluation of an individual patient for problems, followed by scientifically controlled correction of the bodily imperfections or malfunctions of the birth process.

The medical approach to pregnancy, birth and the aftermath may employ more prevention than any other in medical care. The reasons are probably partly historical. In general, two of the greatest previous killers of women during pregnancy and birth were conquered in industrialised countries only when preventive measures were applied. Proper washing of birth attendants' hands eliminated childbed fever, and early diagnosis followed by proper diet and rest eliminated most toxaemia of pregnancy.

Pregnancy is thus seen as a time for close medical control of each woman, with preventative examinations and special care for patients who may be at high risk. Labour is a time for even closer medical control, to provide quick assistance when trouble develops and before things get out of hand. Every physician using these methods has seen them save women's and babies' lives, and truly believes that this approach works.

From this world view, safety — a healthy woman and baby — can only be guaranteed by such a system, in which the doctor objectively chooses the best course. The woman is viewed as subjective, and unable to comprehend the medical and scientific intricacies involved in the decisions. It is best, of course, if the woman feels good and is satisfied with the care she receives during pregnancy and birth, but her feelings are regarded as less important than her safety and that of the baby.

According to the medical approach, obstetrics is unique in having two patients to care for simultaneously. The obstetrician must have equal concern for both; this has raised a new dilemma. In the past the physician's allegiance was always to the patient: the woman. Some physicians today feel that the interests of the woman and the fetus or baby may conflict. In such cases, physicians have become the defenders of the rights of the unborn or just born. This suggests an allegiance to their profession and to society that supersedes their allegiance to the individual woman patient. Some doctors demand that pregnant and birthing women "be subjected to physical regulation, forced surgery, detention, and to criminal and civil punishment for behaviour deemed dangerous to the fetus" (Ruzek 1991).

The dual patient dilemma is further complicated because obstetricians now often have to share patients with neonatologists and the two can become adversaries rather than collaborators. This can be clearly seen in a country like Romania where neonatology is beginning to be established as a specialty and the chief of obstetrics in every hospital is still in charge of all newborn infants, well or sick. The often adversarial nature of the obstetrician/neonatologist relationship is still out in the open.

In the framework of the social model, reproduction is neither medical nor a problem: pregnancy is not an illness, birth is not necessarily a medical or surgical procedure, the pregnant and birthing woman is not necessarily a patient. Birth is seen as a biosocial process that is part of daily life. Advocates of the social model believe that in the endless debate and dissection in the academic and scientific press, as well as in television and other public media, birth has been removed from the natural world and turned into a mystery requiring expert control. In the professionalisation of birth, people have lost sight of the fact that birth — like death — is something that happens to everyone. Yet personal experience has been separated from professional expertise.

The concept of birth as a biosocial process is basic to the social model. Birth is a biological — anatomical, physiological and biochemical — event integrated with mental and spiritual components (Gaskin 1978). Basic to this view is that birth is also by nature feminine, intuitive, sexual and spiritual — qualities not found in the medical model.

The second half of the word biosocial shows the greatest divergence from the medical model. Birth involves society as well as the person who may be subject to medical control. Thus the management of birth has important implications for society as a whole: for its view of reproduction, the position of women, family relationships and the socialisation of children and the construction of the adult personality. Birth may say more than any other life event, and at least as much as mating and death, about the status of women and the place of the family in a culture. It is far more telling than legal or education systems. Although an examination of women's reproductive status and history in a culture is necessary for a full understanding of the context of birth, such a task is beyond the scope of this book.

The social model of health draws on anthropology to point out that religious belief systems are integral to or underlie fundamental practices in all cultures, particularly the practices dealing with mating, birth and death. According to the social model, modern medicine (including obstetrics) has emerged as a new and competing belief system with its own set of taboos, rituals and mysteries, which is the hallmark of religion (Davis-Floyd 1992).

The social model goes beyond defining birth in its social context. It also lays great emphasis on the importance of social factors on the outcome of any pregnancy. There are considerable data to show that many social factors have a harmful impact on pregnancy and birth, including poverty, bad housing, poor diet, stressful life events, lack of social support, smoking and the abuse of alcohol and drugs. People subscribing to this view use the phenomenon of low birth weight as a case in point. In the more developed countries, the factor most commonly associated with the death of the baby around the time of birth (perinatal mortality) is low birth weight (less than 2500 g). There is no really effective medical intervention to prevent low birth weight. The only factors proven to be associated with low birth weight are social: stress and anxiety (Pagel 1990), lack of social and emotional support (Oakley 1985a; Oakley 1985b), smoking and substance abuse (Kleinman 1988).

A recent survey of all births in Greece showed this country to have one of the lowest rates of low birth weight in the world — lower than those of many more affluent countries (Tzoumaka-Bakoula 1990). Since this rate is known to be much higher in poorer areas, this finding is surprising. A plausible hypothesis is that the effects of the poverty found in Greece are outweighed by those of the extraordinary social and psychological support given to pregnant women. The extended family is still common in this country, and nothing is too good for pregnant women, who receive the best of the available food and other resources, along with a lot of attention and love (Draganos 1992). Does the solution to low birth weight, then, really lie in more and more medical intervention, as often urged by physicians?

Subscribers to the social model of birth contend that the social and psychological results are as important as the biological ones. The woman's satisfaction with her condition and her care is not a nice bonus; it is of central importance to her and her family and should be so to those serving her.

How different are these models regarding reliance on technology? Intervention during pregnancy and birth is not simply accepted in the medical approach and rejected in the social approach. It is more complicated than that. Birth can never be natural, because to be human is to be social, and birth is not treated only as a physiological function in any known society. Society sees birth as a time of vulnerability and uncertainty. Every culture in the world, regardless of level of development, has a system of birth practices that are adhered to in a way that gives them the appearance of moral necessity (Oakley 1987). They are felt to be the only right way for a mother to bring her child into the world.

All birth practices are interventions, of course, but the assumptions and ideas behind the interventions endorsed by the social model differ markedly from those of the medical model. Medical (biological) intervention or treatments are seen as necessary and important, but are preferably non-invasive. The real difference lies in the way technologies are used in the larger context of birth. The social model is a holistic, as opposed to a reductionist, approach and includes the social, psychological and spiritual components of technologies. The relationship between the woman and the care giver is considered an integral part of the intervention, nearly as important as the nature of the treatment itself. Inherent dangers are seen in putting women and babies into categories such as 'high risk'. Such categorisation is artificial and unreliable, and has detrimental psychological and social consequences for the woman and her family. Further, when women are labelled abnormal or at high risk and come into contact with the birth machine, the increased level of intervention used tends to remove them from their social support systems at a time when such support is urgently needed.

According to the social model, social intervention in pregnancy and birth and following birth equals or even surpasses biological intervention in importance. Social intervention is of two types: directed towards individuals and directed towards the environment, including the structures of society. The first type includes: providing social support networks and self-help groups to help make up for the loss of the extended family structure (Oakley 1985b), help with the control of substance abuse (Banta and Houd 1985), and maternity benefits (WHO 1985). The second type of intervention takes a variety of forms, such as: the reduction of environmental hazards known to be particularly dangerous to fetuses and pregnant women, especially where women work; special support programs for vulnerable groups such as adolescent, migrant and poor women, all of whom are known to have greater difficulties in pregnancy and birth and following birth. Here it is relevant to recall the extraordinary improvement in the health of women and their infants during the

Second World War, which may have resulted from such general social intervention.

In countries where such data is collected, for example in the United States and the United Kingdom, perinatal mortality is higher in the lower socioeconomic groups (Oakley 1985a). The social interventions mentioned above are of particular importance to poor families. In contrast, there is a tendency for the obstetrical interventions to be used less on the poor in spite of their increased risk and need. Studies in the United States show significantly more caesarean section births on well-to-do private patients than on poor women in public hospitals (Gould 1989; Haynes 1986; Stafford 1990).

Views of birth technology

As might be expected, supporters of the two models hold widely different views of birth technology. In the medical model, a reliance on technology is the natural outgrowth of the mechanistic view of the body. The body is a complex, rather imperfect machine whose efficiency can be improved by other machinery. It is important to react to signals from or information about the body, but those reported by the patient are subjective and qualitative. Machines, which relay quantitative and objective information directly from the body, are more reliable.

This reliance on birth technology is part of the larger reliance on health technology. Today's technological revolution is the outgrowth of the industrial and scientific revolutions. According to the technological imperative of modern science, the advantages of development and the better standard of living in the industrialised countries are largely the result of technology. Thus technology is the hope for a better world. The computer, for example, is the elegant extension of the imperfect human brain, and has opened up amazing new possibilities. As part of this technological revolution, the adherents to the medical model see medical technology as responsible for wonder drugs, the reduction of disease and the extension of life expectancy. In addition, they see the birth machine as having saved women from dying in childbirth and babies from dying around the time of birth. According to this view, technological solutions are not only appropriate but necessary for addressing many of the problems of childbirth and not to use these opportunities would be to retreat into the Dark Ages.

Working in Eastern Europe since the recent political changes, I have had to confront the power of the medical model approach to birth. The maternal and perinatal mortality rates in Eastern Europe are significantly higher than Western Europe. Most physicians in Eastern Europe believe this gap is the result of their lack of new, sophisticated birth technology. A Minister of Health in Romania pushed WHO to use most of the funds given by the United Kingdom for Romanian children to buy high technology equipment for ten neonatal intensive care units in spite of the fact that most prenatal clinics had no stethoscopes or blood pressure apparatus and most maternity hospitals had no basic, simple newborn resuscitation equipment. In Eastern Europe extensive medical care systems were in place (although poorly equipped), but no social care systems existed for pregnant women and families. The poverty and poor nutrition that led to health problems in pregnant and birthing women were not ameliorated, even in simple ways. Instead, doctors have tried to combat problems with narrowly focused orthodox medical treatments despite the futility of such an approach, particularly when low-technology equipment and supplies were often passed over in favour of costly equipment that had low marginal utility.

According to the social model, a crucial ethical and practical dilemma at present is uncertainty about the nature of technology, its real benefits and hazards, and the extent to which people are able to make informed choices about how and where technology may influence or dominate the structure of everyday life.

This dilemma is exacerbated by several widespread myths (Oakley 1987). The first myth is that value equals evaluation. In other words, because technology is valued, it need not be evaluated. A second myth is that technical innovation is synonymous with progress. Evaluation, however, is necessary to test the truth of this assertion in each case. A third myth is that new and newly fashionable technology is the outcome of democratic choice. Democratic choice exists, but most of what is seen as choice is really the limited outcome of power relationships. Finally, problems in and with technology are believed to require technological solutions. This idea is based on the inevitable but usually unarticulated assumption that all human problems are essentially technological in nature (Oakley 1987).

While these criticisms leave supporters of the social model suspicious of technology in general, they do not necessarily lead to the rejection of birth technology. Technology has always been used to assist in birth. Whether labour is accelerated, for example, by a midwife's empirical use of herbal medicines or an obstetrician's intravenous infusion of drugs, the purpose is the same: to control birth. The social differs from the medical model in the approach taken to the technology used at birth. In general, the body is assumed to be competent and trustworthy until proven otherwise whereas technology, on the other hand, is assumed to be untrustworthy until proven otherwise. These two assumptions are the polar opposite of the medical model which posits that birth is dangerous until proven safe and that technology is safe until proven dangerous.

The social approach to technology is to focus on making it appropriate, recognising that the people who define appropriateness control the technology. In general, what is defined as appropriate in a social model is birth technology that is simple, inexpensive, can be used in the clinic or home, is preferably non-invasive and is always socially and psychologically acceptable to women and their families. A fundamental principle underlying this definition of appropriate use of technology is first to do no harm — one of the ancient cornerstones of physicians' practice.

In considering whether technology is appropriate, it is imperative to make a distinction between facts and value judgements. Efficacy and risk are facts — probabilities which can be measured. Benefit and safety are value judgements about the acceptability of those probabilities (Lowrance 1976). To be appropriate, both the benefit and the safety of technology must be assessed by those on whom it is used. Scientists can measure the efficacy (the chance a *desired* outcome will occur), and the risks (the chance an *undesired* outcome will occur), but the person taking these chances (the patient) is the only one who can legitimately decide whether one chance outweighs the other. It is thus inappropriate and dangerous for a doctor to tell a patient that something is 'safe'. Rather, the doctor's role is limited to explaining the level of risk that is involved.

Just as subscribers to the medical model, in distrusting the body, demand more evaluation (diagnostic tests) of it, so users of the social model, in distrusting technology, demand more examination of technology. Both epidemiology and the social sciences are increasingly employed for this purpose. Although the rapid development of technology for birth coincided with the fall in perinatal and maternal mortality there is no scientific proof that the first event caused the second. The Irish playwright George Bernard Shaw wrote "to advertise any remedy or operation, you have only to pick out all the most reassuring advances made by civilisation, and boldly present the two in relation of cause and effect: the public will swallow the fallacy without a wry face. It has no idea of the need for what is called a controlled experiment" (Oakley 1987).

The evidence suggests that although the birth machine has indeed saved the lives of many women and babies, the most important causes of the falling perinatal and maternal mortality rates are not medical but social (Richmond 1990). These causes include: better nutrition, better general health for women, better housing, and changes in fertility patterns. Improved birth outcomes are linked to reductions in: the number of children for each woman; births to very young and very old women and to women who do not want them. Access to contraception and abortion are essential to give women the means to control their fertility which is critical to improving not only perinatal mortality and morbidity, but child survival as well. Thus overall, the contribution of birth technologies per se to women's and children's health are overstated. The claims of the proponents of the medical model for the success of the birth machine have convinced the public and its representatives to continue pouring more and more resources into medical technologies for infants and women during pregnancy and birth, at the expense of more important health and social services. Unfortunately, this tendency to develop and support systems of care for birth based on the unquestioning acceptance of advice from the medical profession, is nothing new. Careful historical examination of the changing definitions of standard practice has shown the absence of any kind of scientific foundation for a variety of types of birth management.

One classic example of this is the management of the pregnant woman's increase in weight. During the 1950s and 1960s the generally agreed standard of obstetrical practice was to limit maternal weight gain to under 10 kg, preferably under 8 kg, using restrictive diets if necessary. Then in the 1970s and 1980s controlled trials showed that restrictive diets during pregnancy had the undesirable effect of significantly reducing birth weight (Campbell 1983; Campbell & Brown 1983). Even at 4 to 6 years of age, children born to women who had been on restrictive diets were still smaller. Gradually, restrictive diets during pregnancy have gone out of obstetrical fashion. How many of the other practices that we view as 'scientific' are in fact simply fads and fashions?

Conclusion

Despite the differences in the medical and social models of technology and birth, the two approaches share certain areas of agreement. Why, then, do they arouse such heated debate in many countries? Primarily, the models are rooted in different world views, reflecting the dichotomy that we began to explore in this chapter. These views naturally lead to conflicting views of birth and technology.

Considering the fundamental beliefs involved, it is ironic that medical practice, perceived as grounded in medical science, is still mostly art while the social approach, associated with humanistic and holistic health, urges the wider application of controlled scientific research to better assess the actual outcomes of medical technological interventions.

The different world views naturally generate different professional views. The medical model when applied to birth, is represented by much of the obstetrical profession, along with the rest of the medical profession and medical schools. The social model, on the other hand, is represented by a much more diverse and splintered group, which includes the midwifery and public health professions (somewhat split at present), epidemiologists, social scientists and, most important, women's organisations. All these groups are vying for control of the definition of birth and birth management. It is another irony that all the opponents have the same goal — a healthy mother and baby — and they honestly believe that their approaches are most likely to achieve this end. Physicians tell how they have seen women's and babies' lives saved. They have faith in the birth machine because, in their view, they have seen it prove its worth again and again. Further, they can cite hard data in support of their view; autopsies on babies and careful analysis of cases show specific causes of perinatal death, such as atelectasis (collapsed lungs) for which there are proven methods of prevention or treatment. Physicians believe that most women are satisfied with the services they receive because they have experienced the result: a beautiful, healthy baby to take home. Physicians believe that objections come only from a small fringe minority of radical women, mostly feminists, who cannot comprehend the complexities of clinical work. Physicians believe that they are contributing to the advancement of the modern world and that proponents of the social model are impeding medical progress.

Midwives, epidemiologists, social scientists and women's organisations express different beliefs. They say that they have studied the medical literature and find the value of the birth machine inflated far beyond its scientific basis. They cite hard data to support this assertion. In many countries, for example, the perinatal mortality rate is twice as high in the lowest socioeconomic groups than in the highest (Oakley 1985a). They ask "Might large scale feeding programs and income redistribution make greater contributions to improving birth outcomes than expensive medical machines and procedures?" (Ruzek 1991). They say they have personally experienced birth with the birth machine and have found it a dehumanising process in which they lost control of their bodies, and their wishes and goals were disregarded. Their objections fall on deaf ears because challenging physicians' demands is tantamount to challenging the foundation of society; at present, the dream of progress for almost all people on earth includes access to the magic and power of modern medicine. Women have been assigned the role of observing and maintaining cultural values, and the failure to conform to cultural requirements at birth is seen as flagrantly deviant. Social scientists point out that deviants in society are punished by a variety of means, including invalidation, coercion, ostracism, abandonment or, in extreme cases, death. Groups who are actively involved in promoting a social model of birth report how all of these pressures are used against them, giving examples from many countries (see chapter 1).

In 1979 the WHO Regional Office for Europe first became involved in the conflict between proponents of the medical and social models with respect to the birth machine: the remaining chapters of this book are concerned with the specifics of that involvement.

References

Banta H. D. & Houd S. 1985, 'Health education by professionals during pregnancy: assessing needs and effectiveness', *International Journal of Technology Assessment in Health Care*, vol. 1, no. 4, pp. 855–862.

Campbell D. M. 1983, 'Dietary restrictions and its effect on neonatal outcomes', in *Nutrition in Pregnancy*, eds D. M. Campbell & M. D. G. Gilmer, Proceedings of the Tenth Study Group of the Royal College of Obstetricians and Gynaecologists, pp. 243–250.

Campbell D. M. & Brown M. 1983, 'Protein energy supplements in primigravid women at risk of low birthweight', in *Nutrition in Pregnancy*, eds D. M. Campbell & M. D. G. Gillmer, Proceedings of the Tenth Study Group of the Royal College of Obstetricians and Gynaecologists.

Davis-Floyd, R. 1992, *Birth as an American Rite of Passage*, University of California Press.

Draganos T. 1992, personal communication.

Gaskin, I. 1978, *Spiritual Midwifery*, Summertown, Tn., USA, The Farm Book Press.

Gould J. B., Davey B. & Stafford R. S. 1989, 'Socioeconomic differences in rates of caesarean section', *N Engl J Med*, vol. 321, pp. 233–9.

Haynes deRegt R. 1986, 'Relation of private and clinic care to the caesarean birth rate', *N Engl J Med*, vol. 315, pp. 619–24.

Kleinman J., Pierre M. B., Madans J. H., Land G. H. & Schramm W. F. 1988, 'The effects of maternal smoking on fetal and infant mortality', *Am J Epidemiology*, vol. 127, no. 2, pp. 274–82.

Lowrance W. 1976, *Of Acceptable Risk, Science and the Determination of Safety*, Willliam Kaufman, Inc., Los Altos, California.

Oakley A. 1985b, 'Social support in pregnancy: the "soft" way to increase birthweight?', *Soc Sci Med*, vol. 21, no. 11, pp. 1259–68.

—— 1985a, 'Social support and perinatal outcome', *Inter J Technology Assessment in Health Care*, vol. 1, no. 4, pp. 843–54.

—— 1987, 'Consequences of obstetric technologies: social, psychological and medical', paper given at International Conference on Childbearing and Perinatal Care, Jerusalem, Israel, March 1987.

Pagel M., Smilkstein G., Regen H. & Montano D. 1990, 'Psychosocial influences on newborn outcomes: a controlled prospective study', *Soc Sci Med*, vol. 30, no. 5, pp. 597–604.

Richmond J. 1990, Keynote address, American Academy of Pediatrics Conference on Cross-national Comparisons of Child Health, Washington DC, March 1990.

Ruzek S. 1990, 'Defining risk: the assessment of new birth technologies', presented at the NICHD-SSRC Conference on Birth Management, West Virginia, USA, May 1990.

—— 1991, 'Women's reproductive rights: the impact of technology', in *Women and New Reproductive Technologies: Medical, Psychosocial, Legal, Ethical Dilemmas*, eds J. Rodin & A. Collins, Lawrence Erlbaum Assoc., Hillsdale, New Jersey, USA.

Stafford R. S. 1990, 'Caesarean section use and source of payment: an analysis of California hospital discharge abstracts', *Am J Publ Health*, vol. 80, pp. 313–15.

Stephenson P. & Wagner M. 1993, 'Reproductive rights and the medical care system: a plea for rational health policy', *Journal of Public Health Policy*, vol. 14, no. 1, 174–182.

Tzoumaka-Bakoula C., Lekea-KIaranika V., Matsaniotis N. S., McCarthy B. J. & Golding J. 1990, 'Birthweight specific perinatal mortality in Greece', *Acta Pediatrica Scandinavia*, vol. 79, pp. 47–51.

Wagner M. 1982, 'Getting the health out of people's daily lives', *Lancet*, vol. 2, pp. 1207–8.

—— 1991, 'Does he take sugar?', *World Health Forum*, vol. 12, no. 1, pp. 87–89.

World Health Organisation 1985, *Having a Baby in Europe, Public Health in Europe Series No. 26*, Copenhagen.

Chapter 4

Building consensus around perinatal health policy

If the Lord Almighty had consulted me before embarking upon the Creation, I would have recommended something simpler.

Alfonso X of Castile

Evolving role of WHO

WHO began in 1948 as a specialised agency in the new United Nations family, with the hope of separating international health policy making and action from political conflicts. Essentially every country in the world, even those not belonging to the United Nations, belongs to WHO — a testimony to the universal understanding that germs do not honour national borders and that health for all can only be achieved if all work together. The first two decades of WHO's life saw no significant conflicts, political or otherwise, within the Organisation or between the Organisation and countries. Everyone agreed on common enemies, such as the malaria mosquito and the smallpox virus. During what might be called the honeymoon period in WHO's history, great achievements were made. They were easy to measure and politically safe; malaria was significantly reduced in many countries and smallpox was completely eradicated from the globe.

In the past two decades came a series of dawning realisations about health: that it is a social process, profoundly influenced by culture and political realities. For example, serious inequities in access to health services are often related to race and social and economic status. Further, health care is expensive and countries have finite and often shrinking resources. These new ideas were, of course, the result of bringing the social model of health alongside the medical model.

Gradually WHO's role began to shift to one of attempting to influence national health policy by bringing these new perspectives on health and health care to all countries. Since most technical staff in WHO have always been physicians, this new role involved finding new enemies — themselves. Specialist medical care in hospitals (called tertiary health care), for example, was taking most of the money and benefiting only a few people, but this is the most prestigious work for physicians. WHO acted more and more as a conscience, helping governments to confront these issues which often brought them into conflict with their medical establishment. The honeymoon was definitely over. WHO strongly favoured countries putting most of their health resources (financial and human) into local, community-based and community-controlled primary health care — not a universally popular approach. WHO is more fortunate than government health agencies, both in having access to international data and in not having to worry about inappropriate influence from national or local pressure groups such as professional organisations and commercial interests. WHO is like a consulting firm with the responsibility to gather and report information to countries. Sometimes this information has not been really welcome, and countries must decide what action to take and how to deal with the consequences of following courses of action that contradict WHO policy recommendations.

WHO and policies on perinatal care

Government policy-makers formulating national and local policy on perinatal care know too little about pregnant women, birth, newborn babies and health care to be able to make decisions without help. They usually organise some kind of expert advisory committee by turning to a university medical school and perhaps obstetrical and paediatric organisations. The expert committee thus formed usually consists of several professors of obstetrics and paediatrics and possibly one or two public health physicians. As a result, the advice they give (usually behind closed doors) is based only on the medical model. The policy-makers assume that these physicians know best and in general do not question the advice. They are unaware of the need to conduct systematic review of the relevant scientific literature or to get the advice of other parties, such as epidemiologists, midwives, nurses, social scientists and the users of services, who have great interest and expertise in perinatal care.

The policy formulated by this method, not surprisingly, focuses on the role of physicians, medicine and high technology — the birth machine. In nearly every country, the emphasis is on medical prenatal care, hospital-based high-technology birth care and more and more medical intensive care for a small number of newborn infants. This type of policy rapidly escalates costs; policy-makers may then turn to WHO for advice on how to control those costs.

Advising countries on perinatal care policy is a delicate task. If WHO advice contradicts the medical advice in a country, policy-makers do not know whom to believe. Since the medical advice is closer to home, and the policy-makers may not wish to create political problems, they tend to go along with the local advice, which in turn tends to propose clinical solutions involving physicians, machines and hospitals. These solutions are not only politically safe but also immediately visible and therefore attractive to politicians. In contrast, WHO advice requires finding ways to combine key elements of the social and medical models of health. Increasingly this advice stresses the need to address social and economic issues to solve health problems. For example, policy-makers seldom welcome the view that the most urgent priority for improving the outcomes of pregnancy and birth is to do something about poverty. Such a solution is politically unsafe, and action on it does not give easy, quick and highly visible results. Similarly, advice to shift routine birth management away from obstetricians to midwives creates political dilemmas.

An example of this dilemma is the result of my visit as a WHO staff person to Austria several years ago. Asked by the Minister of Health to give advice on routine ultrasound screening for *all* pregnant women, I pointed out that the medical literature made it clear that there was no scientific justification for such a measure (see chapter 5). Further, such screening is very expensive and I suggested that money could perhaps be spent more wisely on other services, such as programs to help pregnant women stop smoking. The Minister explained that the country's obstetricians advised two routine ultrasound scans of *all* pregnant women. He requested that I send him and his staff all relevant scientific articles on the topic. This was done, but two months later a policy was established for ultrasound scans for all pregnant women in Austria.

The countries belonging to the WHO European Region asked for consultation on their perinatal health services. Each year, representatives of these 32 countries meet and, as the Regional Committee for Europe, review and make suggestions on the work of the Regional Office. As 1979 was the United Nations International Year of the Child, the regional program on maternal and child health was reviewed and discussed at length by the Regional Committee. Representatives of country after country rose to express concern about perinatal services. They had many complaints.

Countries were becoming aware of the rapidly expanding technology for birth and were beginning to question its necessity and high cost. Some countries expressed alarm about rates of caesarean section, which had doubled or even tripled in the 1970s, and the possibility that the rise was partly the result of the sudden, widespread use of electronic fetal monitoring during labour (Lomas & Enkin 1991; Banta & Thacker 1979). Consumers were becoming more vociferous in questioning the type of birth services available. The women's movement combined forces with the consumer movement to demand that there be more choice and a more humanistic approach. Action groups were formed in a number of Western European countries including, for example, the Association for Improvements in the Maternity Services in the United Kingdom, Femme Sage Femme in France, Forældre og Fødsel in Denmark. The rising demands of these women for more control of their own bodies and more humane birth practices were being heard. Finally, countries were at a loss to explain satisfactorily to their people why the number of babies dying around birth (the perinatal mortality rate) was greater among the poor, greater in some regions of the country and, frequently, greater in some countries than in neighbouring countries of equal socioeconomic development.

One reason for this questioning of the birth machine can be found in the health care sector. By the mid-1970s the uncritical acceptance of health technology was over. The extent of iatrogenic disorders (disorders directly attributable to medical or surgical procedures) was well publicised. Scientists demonstrated that modern medical care has only a marginal effect on the level of health of the people. Two new fields of science — clinical epidemiology and, later, social epidemiology — began generating data on the lack of efficacy or questionable safety of certain types of health technology. The new field of health services research made it possible to evaluate scientifically the value of particular health service activities. All of this work came to the attention of countries' health authorities, and sparked a disillusionment with simply maintaining the same types of health care and technology. Disillusionment with perinatal services was particularly strong because of the explosive expansion of the birth machine and its inconsistent impact on the health of women and babies.

Nevertheless, the reasons undoubtedly extend beyond events in health care. The worldwide economic recession of the 1970s required governments to be very careful with expenditure on health and welfare services. Meanwhile, the health care system ate up more and more of the gross national product, and the expanding birth machine helped inflate health care costs. One of the European countries, the United Kingdom, pointed this out in a report in 1976 concerning maternity services (DHSS 1976). Between 1970 and 1973, the total number of births fell by 5.0% per year, the number of maternity hospital in-patients fell by an average of 1.6% per year and the number of outpatient attendances by 2.6% per year. The number of maternity beds fell marginally, and the average length of inpatient stay also decreased. Nevertheless, the cost of maternity services rose by about 4% per year (see figure 1).

Further the new profession of health economics began to publish reports questioning the efficiency of various health services, as measured by cost-effectiveness and cost-benefit analyses. The building of too many expensive hospitals in almost every developed country became evident. Books such as *Who Shall Live* (Fuchs 1975) began to point out that no country in the world could afford to buy all the technology that physicians might want and that many of these costly technologies have marginal utility.

These events were part of a larger questioning of all technology. The concern with the negative side of technological development, including the environmental and psychological hazards, increased worldwide. It could be that the reaction that occurred in the 1970s was part of the swinging of an historical pendulum in the public's attitudes towards health and social services and technological advances. A similar dissatisfaction arose in the 1930s, after about 30

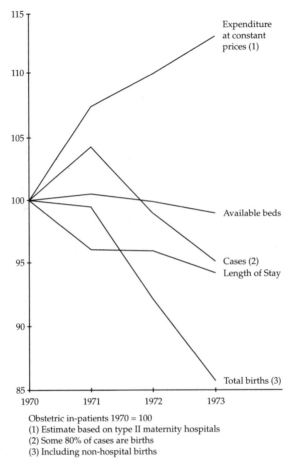

Figure 1: *Maternity services (England 1970–73).*

years of expanding obstetrical services for women during pregnancy and birth and during a decade of economic recession. For all these reasons, in 1979 the 32 countries of the European Region, while attending the annual Regional Committee meeting, unanimously passed a resolution challenging WHO to examine maternity and perinatal services and suggest improvements.

The WHO Perinatal Study Group

To meet this challenge, the European Regional Office of WHO selected members for a Perinatal Study Group to give advice on how to proceed. The Group drew its 15 members from 10 countries and 10 professional disciplines: economics, epidemiology, health administration, midwifery, nursing, obstetrics, paediatrics, psychology, sociology and statistics (see appendix for members). For five years the Group conducted surveys, reviewed the literature and brought the members' personal and professional experience to discussions of perinatal health services for women and their babies.

The conflict and heated debate in this field were quickly found. The Group recognised that there were two distinct approaches to birth and gradually sorted out the supporters of each. An amazing range of services outside or at the fringes of the official services — called alternative perinatal services — was also discovered. The official services followed the medical model of birth and technology while the alternative services followed the social model. Finally, the Group came to understand that the struggles between health professions and over the setting for birth were firmly rooted in the philosophical and empirical split between the two models as well as in vested interests.

The members of the Perinatal Study Group were disconcerted by two additional discoveries: that they were the first to collect data on rates of obstetrical intervention at the international level; that these data showed a fourfold variation in the rates (among countries where such data were available), with little or no correlation with pregnancy and birth outcomes (Bergjso 1983). Further, birth technology was expanding geometrically, with little effort on the part of any government to conduct careful scientific evaluation of outcomes. The Group had stumbled into the path of the birth machine and began to see its international character and impetus.

The Group presented its findings in a published report, *Having a Baby in Europe* (WHO 1985). This report provides considerable information on perinatal services in the European Region, both official and alternative, and analyses present trends and future needs. The policy recommendations adopted are based on all the information available to the Group.

The Group's first recommendation was to unite the medical approach and the social approach in the further development of perinatal services. Second, careful scientific evaluations should be made of all levels and types of services, particularly those involving birth technology. These were fine words. But in view of the heated debate in this field, how could such recommendations be implemented, particularly when the recommended action involved bringing the two hostile sides together, and slowing down the birth machine long enough to take it apart and look at it? How could WHO get the medical establishments worldwide to reconsider the path they were on? As described here, the Group found innovative ways to bring the message to countries, often almost accidentally stumbling on approaches quite new to WHO. These strategies for stimulating policy debate in contested arenas are important to examine, because they provide insight into a process that must take place throughout the health and medical care systems worldwide. Thus the process that WHO went through to promote re-evaluation of the birth machine is a microcosm of what will be entailed in bringing about medical care reform that is needed to improve the health of populations of every country in the world.

Building consensus

The beginning was modest. A WHO consultant, a midwife from Denmark, decided to try to gather representatives of the midwives, obstetricians and consumer groups of this small country to discuss the Perinatal Study Group's recommendations and their implications for birth and birth services. The result was the first national birth conference organised in collaboration with WHO's Regional Office for Europe. The conference received wide media coverage and prompted considerable nationwide debate. Eventually it became part of a process resulting in new national guidelines for perinatal services in Denmark. Getting the opponents to sit down together and come to agreement on some issues was clearly productive.

Because some WHO staff had been in China, where the birth machine was not yet fully developed, it was decided to hold a similar meeting to discuss the European experience with birth and its possible relevance to 2000 million Chinese. The resulting meeting was a breakthrough, not only because of moving from a small country to the biggest in the world, but also because it was the first chance to confront a new issue — the development of the birth machine in the more developing countries. China was opening up rapidly to the rest of the world and wanted to incorporate new technology. The meeting of about 50 physicians from all over China and about 15 Europeans and WHO staff, focused on the dynamics of the birth machine and possible ways to harness it appropriately in countries with different levels of development. This meeting prompted others in China to address these issues.

One of the Directors of the WHO Regional Office for the Americas was present at the initial meeting in China. As a result, discussions began between the Regional Offices for Europe and the Americas to find ways to encourage countries to combine the best of the medical and social approaches, particularly with regard to birth technology. These discussions led to three WHO consensus meetings, each lasting five days and bringing together disparate groups of people from North and South America and Europe, to reach consensus and make recommendations on appropriate prenatal, birth and postnatal technology.

Organising these innovative events proved to be a delicate task and holding them was an extraordinary adventure. Bringing their messages back to the countries has been difficult and rewarding and always exciting. The first paragraphs of this book briefly describe the widely varying reactions of groups of obstetricians and users of services in a number of countries to the publication of the recommendations from just one of these meetings. This chapter describes how the meetings were organised and carried out. Subsequent chapters include the results of each of these consensus events.

The consensus approach was tried to help WHO staff in both of the Regions advise countries more effectively on policy on perinatal care. The consensus approach is a kind of 'science court' in which the available scientific evidence is weighed by a jury of all interested parties and, when all can reach agreement (consensus), recommendations are given to practitioners. Pioneered in the United States (Jacoby 1985), it begins with organising a group that includes all parties interested in the issue at hand. After reviewing the relevant scientific literature, the group attempts to reach consensus through discussion and debate. So that the group could follow this method, the participants at all three of the WHO consensus meetings were asked to write and circulate scientific review papers.

If a consensus building conference is successful, the group makes recommendations that are later presented at public meetings for open debate. In the case of building consensus over how to harness the birth machine, this method would have to include subscribers to both the medical and the social approach in the consensus process. Scientific evidence must be reviewed carefully because it must lie at the heart of the official recommendations and subsequent policy. The consensus report must be written so that it will serve as the basis for national and local birth conferences at which the applicability of the recommendations to the local situation can be openly debated. In general, these were new qualities and new desired outcomes for WHO meetings. Would the strategy work?

Consensus meeting on Appropriate Technology for Prenatal Care

The first meeting was held at the Regional Office for the Americas in Washington DC, to provide a neutral meeting ground. This Regional Office was chosen because it is located in a country known for its highly developed birth technology while most of the Member States of the same Region have difficulties in providing any kind of health service to large numbers of pregnant women. Since the meeting involved both Europe and the Americas, both English and Spanish were spoken, with simultaneous translation.

Choosing the participants was complicated, as many criteria had to be met. Balance had to be maintained:

- between medical and social orientation;
- in geographic representation (Eastern and Western Europe, North and South America);
- between highly industrialised and developing countries;
- between all the interested parties (midwives, nurses, obstetricians, epidemiologists, health administrators, sociologists,

anthropologists, economists, psychologists and users of services);
- between women and men;
- between younger and older people.

The 52 participants included 10 epidemiologists, 8 health administrators, 2 medical engineers, 4 midwives, 1 nurse, 14 obstetricians, 4 paediatricians, 6 social scientists (representing anthropology, economics, psychology and sociology) and 3 users of health services. While it would be fair to say that all of the obstetricians present adhered to the medical model, and all social scientists and users of the health services to the social model, the other groups were divided in their adherence to the medical or social models, leaving a reasonable balance between these two perspectives. In spite of efforts to secure a balance, there were twice as many men (35) as women (17) and the women who came were disproportionately adherents of the social model of birth. Geographically, 34 participants came from North or South America while 8 came from Europe; an additional 10 were WHO staff members. The participants were evenly divided between industrialised and developing countries (26 each). The invitations to the participants explained that they would be expected only to represent themselves, not their professions, countries or anything else. The meeting was designed to be just 52 people from very divergent backgrounds trying to reach agreement on how to get good birth outcomes for women and babies (see appendix A for a list of participants).

The organisers of the meeting wanted it to have a format that would combine the medical and social approaches. Both the running of the meeting and the working methods of the participants had to explicitly illustrate this combination. Methods were chosen and gradually refined; they were felt to be entirely successful by the third meeting.

Scientific and medical meetings are usually organised around the presentation of a long line-up of papers. Each takes about 20–30 minutes to deliver and only a few minutes are scheduled for questions or discussion afterwards. This format is tedious and does not encourage the wide-ranging discussions that WHO staff believed would be necessary to build consensus between people from different backgrounds. To begin with some kind of draft proposal — a format frequently used in WHO meetings — was felt to be too confining.

All participants had to have a chance to present their views. The organisers wanted all 52 people to meet at least some of the time, to build a feeling of solidarity and to debate key issues; they also knew that discussion in small groups of about 15 people was a good way to build consensus. As a result, each participant was asked to prepare a paper reviewing the scientific evidence on a subject relevant to the issues of the meeting. This paper had to be submitted in one of the working languages; then it was translated into the other and distributed to all participants long enough in advance of the meeting to be read before the meeting was convened.

Each day the meeting focused on one or two major themes. In each of the morning sessions for all participants, everyone who had written a paper relevant to the theme of the day was given a maximum of five minutes in which to summarise the scientific evidence and the main points of the paper. These presentations took up only half of the morning; the other half was devoted to an open discussion of the papers and the themes. The six main themes were: prenatal care, social factors during pregnancy, human resources in prenatal care, methods of surveillance, research, and appropriate technology. In the afternoons the participants formed three groups of about 17 people each, in which the balance between the key characteristics of the participants was maintained. The groups were asked to try to reach consensus and draft recommendations on the issues discussed in the morning. Each group had a rapporteur. Each evening the rapporteurs met to combine the draft recommendations. During the fourth evening the rapporteurs put together a final draft of the recommendations. The fifth and last day was given over entirely to a general discussion by the entire group and to hammering out consensus on every recommendation.

Built into this format was information given to all participants before the meeting. The subject was defined to create a minimum fund of common information and definitions of the topics to be discussed. For this reason, staff from the Regional Office for Europe wrote a working paper summarising the main findings of the five years of work of the European Perinatal Study Group, including those findings that addressed the main characteristics and problems of services and technology for pregnant women in Europe. Staff from the Regional Office for the Americas prepared a similar working paper on the Americas. In view of the meeting's title, it was important to have a common definition of technology. It was broadly defined as knowledge applied to specific purposes, thus comprising not only machines and clinical techniques but also the people giving and receiving care, in order to cover the educational and social aspects of care. This was a large topic for five days of work, even when limited to care during pregnancy.

As the participants drifted into the meeting room on the first morning, a strange mixture of excitement and anxiety filled the air and people spoke in whispers. Most of the participants had just arrived in Washington DC, having travelled long distances, and most were strangers. Everyone felt uneasy. The room — very large, formal and elegant, with a huge circular table with a name card, microphone and earphones at each place — increased this feeling. Despite efforts to minimize formality (by means such as omitting titles from the name cards), the cultural, linguistic, professional and other differences clearly separated the participants.

There were two chairpersons, one from each Region, to stress the inter-regional nature of the meeting and to alternate the two working languages in the chair. For symbolic reasons, both chairpersons were women: one a health service provider with a medical orientation and the other a user of health services with a social orientation. Through luck or foresight, the European chairperson, a lay person from a consumer group called the Association for Improvements in the Maternity Services, was asked to chair the first session. She was able to set just the right tone as the meeting got started.

WHO meetings begin with a rather formal greeting from a senior WHO staff member: in this case, the Regional Director for the Americas. When he marched into the conference room, followed by his entourage of assistants, all of the participants rushed to find their seats. The Regional Director's speech underlined the importance of the task and left everyone feeling serious and important. When the chairperson took over, however, her calm and sense of humour helped the Group enthusiastically take up its task and avoid a common pitfalls of such meetings — feelings of excessive seriousness and self-importance that interfere with open exchange of ideas.

The individual presentations soon showed the difficulty for many people of limiting themselves to five minutes. Rather than giving a brief summary, some tried to cover their whole papers by the simple expedient of talking twice as fast as normal — a disaster in such a meeting. Fortunately, the European chairperson set an important precedent; she was gentle but very tough and held each presentation to the allotted time. Gradually the presentations improved. They revealed widely divergent viewpoints, and the morning plenary sessions evolved as times for defining issues and differences. Consensus and solutions were found in the smaller groups in the afternoons. The membership of the subgroups remained constant, and people began to get to know each other and work well together. Slowly a feeling emerged that consensus could indeed be reached. On the fourth day, the women participants decided to organise their own informal caucus. This separate meeting produced a set of recommendations that supplemented, rather than contradicted, the final recommendations. By the end of the fifth day, consensus was reached (after considerable debate, often somewhat heated) on all recommendations.

Consensus meeting on Appropriate Technology for Birth

The second consensus meeting, on Appropriate Technology for Birth, was held in Fortaleza, a city in north-eastern Brazil. It was important to hold this meeting in Latin America, and Brazil was chosen because of the extreme contrasts in birth care found within the country. In some private hospitals in Sao Paulo and Rio de Janeiro, the birth machine has developed to such an extraordinary degree that 80–90% of all births are by caesarean section (Instituto Brasileno de Geografia Estadistica 1981). In other parts of Brazil, most women received no health care during pregnancy and gave birth at home, possibly with an empirical midwife (this term is preferred to equivalents such as lay midwife, traditional midwife and traditional birth attendant) to assist. Fortaleza is located in one of the poorest regions of Brazil, whose rural areas have little or no official birth care.

The organisers believed that this second meeting, focusing on birth itself, would be more contentious than the first. There was already general agreement worldwide that routine prenatal care was desirable: the issue was the kind of care to be given. But with birth and birth care, this kind of agreement seemed to be totally absent. The issues included: where birth should take place, who should be the principal birth attendant, how to monitor the progress of a birth and when to intervene. The appropriate use of a number of types of technology during birth was also hotly debated. National and local policy on perinatal care needed to include recommendations on birth technology. It was hoped that this second meeting could reach consensus and give policy-makers a place to start.

Although the format of the meeting remained essentially the same, panel discussions on each major issue replaced the five-minute presentation of papers. As before, all the participants prepared scientific review papers, but were also asked to include a final section on how to implement change. Further, members of each panel met the night before their discussion, to plan debates that would go beyond summaries of individual papers. This allowed the group to focus on how to implement the changes recommended. This method was used to increase the emphasis on how to change policy and practice. Each day, all participants were given a list of the working papers to be covered in the next day's discussion, so that they could review the papers that evening, or read them if they had not already done so. The meeting addressed six themes: present characteristics of birth care in Latin America, North America and Europe; birth as a normal process; social factors in birth care; the use of human resources for birth care; assessment and appropriate use of birth technology; and how to implement change. The only other major departure from the earlier format was a field visit on the second day that is described below.

In general, the same criteria were used for selecting participants as before, except that more health administrators and policy-makers were sought. The 62 members included 1 educator, 8 epidemiologists, 11 health administrators and policy-makers, 1 medical engineer, 7 midwives, 2 nurses, 16 obstetricians, 3 paediatricians, 10 social scientists (3 anthropologists, 2 economists, 2 psychologists and 3 sociologists) and 3 service users. The Group proved to have a good mixture of the medical and social perspectives. It also had a better gender balance: 34 men and 28 women. Twenty people came from industrialised countries and 42 from developing countries (see appendix A for a list of participants).

After breakfast on the second day, the participants boarded buses for a day's field trip in the countryside. The Director of Obstetrics at the university hospital in Fortaleza, Dr Galba Araújo, had developed a highly innovative maternity outreach program in the nearby rural areas. The first level of care was given by empirical midwives, who practised in their own villages and had been trained through apprenticeship to more experienced midwives. They received further training from a team sent out from the Fortaleza hospital. Small, very simple birth centres were built in each village, in which the local empirical midwife provided prenatal and postnatal care and the women of the village gave birth. Women with complications during pregnancy and birth were referred to the small rural district hospitals. The Fortaleza team advised these rural hospitals, from which cases could be referred to the hospital in Fortaleza.

The participants visited village birth centres and a district hospital and talked with midwives and hospital staff and pregnant women. Everyone was impressed with the commitment of the care givers and the quality of the care. The program clearly combined the social and medical approaches to perinatal care in a way that respected the local culture and the key role of local women. There were many examples of appropriate technology, such as home-made birth chairs. It was encouraging that this program was the brainchild of Dr Araújo, a male Brazilian professor of obstetrics, trained in the United States. A participant of the first meeting, Dr Araújo died just before the second, which met in Fortaleza in part to honour his work. The field trip inspired the Group in its efforts to reach consensus.

Consensus meeting on Appropriate Technology following Birth

The original topic of the third inter-regional meeting, held in Trieste, Italy, was neonatal technology. Then the organisers realised that we were making a common error: focusing on the newborn infant and neglecting the woman who has just given birth. We reminded ourselves that women are not just ambulatory incubators and intermittent milk factories, and renamed the meeting Appropriate

Technology Following Birth, vowing to give the woman her rightful place in the discussions.

The third meeting was held in Europe, because the first two meetings were held in North and South America. Trieste was chosen because a group of enthusiastic and broad-minded neonatologists was located there, and women in northern Italy were working hard to improve their lot in life, including childbirth and motherhood. The meetings had demonstrated both the feasibility of mixing the medical and social perspectives and the importance of including all interested parties. Thus, the same criteria were used to select participants, except that there were fewer obstetricians and more neonatologists. The 43 participants included 1 economist, 6 epidemiologists, 5 health administrators and policy-makers, 1 journalist (an important interested party which we had not invited to the first two meetings), 3 midwives, 12 neonatologists, 1 nurse, 6 obstetricians, 2 psychologists, 3 sociologists and 3 service users. A real gender balance was still a problem; there were 27 men and 16 women. In addition to 7 WHO staff members, 22 participants came from Europe and 14 from the Americas. Reflecting the characteristics of the European Region, twenty-nine people came from industrialised countries and the remaining 14 from developing countries (see appendix A for a list of participants).

Because of the success of the Fortaleza meeting, the same format was used for this meeting. The panels covered four main issues. Each participant prepared a paper reviewing the scientific literature on and current situation of some aspect of: the care of the normal and the abnormal newborn infant; the health of the woman following birth; research on newborn infants; the economics of the care of newborn infants; professional and non-professional human resources for care of the woman and baby. The papers were translated and distributed to participants before the meeting.

One departure from the format of the two earlier meetings was almost accidental, but played an important role in this meeting. The panel discussions in Brazil, while making for reasonably effective and stimulating plenary sessions, were quite formal; each panel member briefly presented material and took part in the discussion. The night before the Trieste meeting began, however, the group assigned to the first panel met to decide how to handle the theme "the first month following birth — a normal process" during the allotted 30 minutes. The group agreed to a member's suggestion that each person be given five minutes not to present a paper or give scientific data but to tell a story from personal experience about the first month following birth. The group hoped that these personal stories would illustrate some of the issues.

As the stories unfolded the next morning, the participants found them riveting. Widely varying experiences were described. The last panel member, the Regional Director for Europe of the World Health Organisation, gave an open and honest description of how his first child was born dead and how the health care system failed to give him and his wife any support during this crisis. They had not even been allowed to see their baby. The panel presentation was an effective spark to active participation in the plenary discussions that followed and the meeting as a whole. The stories showed the participants that they could combine the scientific with the personal, and the medical with the social, in searching for consensus on appropriate technology following birth.

Telling personal stories had the effect of defining the participants not only as thoughtful, rational scientists but also as human beings who had experienced in their personal lives the very issues to be discussed. It reinforced that birth is something we all experience in daily life and that it is not the exclusive domain of scientists and health professionals. Suddenly the issues were not just theoretical but were real. They drew the participants together as human beings in a way which motivated and allowed them to compromise with each other during the subsequent struggles to reach consensus. While 'anecdotal evidence' has fallen into disfavour, and certainly should not be the only basis on which to set policy, it has a real place in professional education and in consensus building. Perhaps this human dimension in policy-making deserves greater attention.

Conclusion

The experience in Washington, Fortaleza and Trieste suggests that at least four elements are important in building consensus. First, it is essential to begin with a firm synthesis of the scientific facts. The consensus meeting is an attempt to begin the process of formulating or re-evaluating policy; all too often, scientific synthesis is lacking from this process.

The second essential element in the consensus process is also frequently neglected in policy formation: a healthy, direct confrontation between differing points of view. For example, there was real struggle and conflict early in the Fortaleza meeting. After reviewing the scientific evidence, a group in Fortaleza drafted a recommendation that no country should have a caesarean section rate over 10%. A heated debate followed in the plenary session with several obstetricians insisting that such a recommendation, while ideal and scientifically justified, at this moment in time was not practical and had the potential danger of being rejected out of hand by obstetricians. The obstetricians argued that to help the implementation of the recommendation, it should rather be 15%. A consensus was achieved only when the recommendation was changed to 10–15% caesarean section rate. Although many people fear such conflict, the open challenging of assumptions in the debate was instrumental in moving participants away from fixed convictions to more open minds.

Another element was the use of successful models of birth care. Coming to recognise the extent of the differences between the social and medical approaches to perinatal care can be quite discouraging. But seeing how Dr Araújo, for example, had been able to combine the best of both in the area around Fortaleza prevented discouragement that can lead to inertia or policy-paralysis. Being able to see a positive model motivated the participants to try to do the same with their recommendations.

The fourth element contributing to a successful consensus process is the least tangible and most elusive but perhaps most important: the development of the recognition among those involved that everyone wants the same thing, healthy women and babies. When conflict was rampant and could help or harm the consensus process, reminders of the common goal — such as Dr Araújo's life work — are necessary. Informal discussions in the evenings also served this purpose. What makes a hard-working collection of people begin to coalesce into a group is hard to say. Nevertheless, this delicate process was completed at least partly because the discussions in the plenary sessions, in the smaller groups, over dinner, in the hallways and in the streets gradually revealed that everyone cared — even the people who had been considered the enemy. The results were not only final recommendations that everyone could endorse. The meetings also facilitated the emergence of a set of people who were more open to change and more committed to using the recommendations to work than is usual as the result of WHO meetings. In fact, the participants did go on to interact with relevant groups in their countries to find ways to put the birth machine to the most appropriate uses. As in other situations, the resolution of conflict by people who share a common goal forges ownership and commitment to find ways to achieve their aims. This approach is very different from the approach to policy-setting that is based on limiting participation to those who will not differ in their views.

References

Banta H. D. & Thacker S. 1979, 'Assessing the costs and benefits of electronic fetal monitoring', *Obstet & Gynecol Survey*, vol. 35, pp. 627–642.

Bergsjo P., Schmidt E. & Pusch D. 1983, 'Differences in the reported frequencies of some obstetrical interventions in Europe', *Br J Obstet Gynaecol*, vol. 90, pp. 629–632.

Department of Health and Social Services, United Kingdom 1976, *Annual Report on National Health Service*, no. 30, figure 5, Her Majesty's Stationary Office, London.

Fuchs V. 1975, *Who Shall Live?*, Basic Books, New York.

Instituto Brasileno de Geografia Estadistica 1981, 'Encuesta Nacional de Domicilios', as reported in Faundes et al., *Caesarean Section, When is it appropriate?*, presented at the Consensus Meeting on Appropriate Technology for Birth, WHO, Brazil, 1985.

Jacoby I. 1985, 'The consensus development program of the National Institutes of Health', *Int J Tech Assess Health Care*, vol. 1, pp. 420–432.

Lomas J. & Enkin M. 1989, 'Variations in operative delivery rates' in *Effective Care in Pregnancy and Childbirth*, eds I. Chalmers, M. Enkin & M. Kierse, Oxford University Press, Oxford, pp. 1182–1195.

World Health Organisation 1985, *Having a Baby in Europe*, WHO Regional Office for Europe, Copenhagen.

Chapter 5

The first step: a consensus meeting on technology for prenatal care

A tool exploited for its own sake is no better than a saw given to a small boy for cutting wood who must presently look around the home for suitable objects of furniture wanting amputation.

Ian Donald (discoverer of obstetrical ultrasound) 1980

Introduction

The methods used to organise the three WHO consensus meetings on perinatal technology have already been discussed. This chapter and the two that follow describe the results of these meetings. Both the description of the issues and the recommendations were based on careful reviews of all the relevant scientific literature: the participants' review papers. In addition, the issues and recommendations have been updated with scientific documentation which has appeared since the meetings.

The meeting on Appropriate Technology for Prenatal Care struggled to reach consensus in generating recommendations on policy on care for pregnant women. A key issue, and the major element in present health services for pregnant women was routine prenatal visits. A number of questions faced the participants. Why should women make routine prenatal visits? What should they include? Who should provide the care? How should the services be delivered?

Discussion on this topic was originally contentious. The Latin American participants emphasised offering better access to prenatal care. As stated in a background paper: "The general solution to perinatal problems in Latin America must start with increasing coverage of expectant mothers. Approximately 50% of pregnant women in Latin America have access to organised health care services when they are pregnant" (Schwarcz 1985, p. 803). This is also a serious problem even in the United States: "Between 1979 and 1985, the percentage of women obtaining late or no prenatal care increased throughout the US" (Ruzek 1990, p. 19). In Washington DC, for example, the number increased 43% (Brown 1988). The European participants, on the other hand, argued that their experience showed that consideration should first be given to what routine prenatal visits should include. In addition, some participants gave regular medical supervision during pregnancy the highest priority, while others gave social support equal importance. A single fact on which everyone could agree gradually emerged from the presentations of relevant scientific literature and from discussions, and brought about consensus on the issue: no one knows what makes prenatal care effective.

Content and effects of prenatal care

Very little is known about the content of routine prenatal care and its impact on the health of the woman and her baby. This understanding helped the participants resolve a number of questions on prenatal care.

First, does a system of routine visits to health care providers during pregnancy improve the chances for a live, healthy baby and mother? The papers presented reviewed hundreds of articles in the medical literature on this question. It is interesting that while most studies of effectiveness of medical care focus on the actions of the providers, studies of prenatal care focus on client behaviour — when did the pregnant woman initiate care and how many visits did she make (Brown 1988, p. 27). By the time of the consensus meeting, no well controlled experimental studies of routine prenatal care had been found. Nevertheless, the available evidence indicated that routine prenatal care probably has an overall beneficial effect of some sort for at least some pregnancies. Many statistical studies have demonstrated a relationship between routine prenatal care and both higher birth weight and lower perinatal mortality, although other studies have failed to find such a relationship.

In debating these findings, the members of the consensus meeting came to recognise the basic problem, that this research attempted to measure the value of unknowns. Systems for routine prenatal check-ups vary in what is recommended, as the recommendations are based on clinical practice, not on controlled scientific data, and there are gaps between what is recommended and what actually takes place in each pregnancy and routine check-up. In addition, a visit includes many medical, psychological and social elements. As a result, the true nature of the care any pregnant woman receives is unknown. Variations in routine prenatal visits thus involve not only the content but also the care provider, timing, frequency, setting and duration. The usual medical record for prenatal visits does not adequately document the full nature of this care. It is no wonder that the results of statistical studies have also varied.

Another factor that hinders the assessment of the effectiveness of prenatal care is the balance between the benefit and harm caused. Some beneficial and harmful effects neutralise each other, confounding the overall assessment. Because the harmful effects of prenatal care are often overlooked, several examples follow. Some practices routinely used in prenatal care have subsequently been abandoned as harmful. In the 1940s and early 1950s x-ray examination of all pregnant women was recommended until a report demonstrated a link to childhood cancer (Stewart 1956, p. 40) and more recently a possible link to mental retardation (*British Medical Journal* 1988). As mentioned in chapter 3, in the 1950s and 1960s, pregnant women were strongly advised to limit food intake and weight gain, and diuretics were widely used. These practices have now been shown to be harmful. "Dietary restriction can cause markedly decreased birth weight. During famine mean birth weight can be depressed by as much as 550 g. Iatrogenic dietary manipulation and restriction can have almost as serious an effect" (Rush 1991, p. 277).

In the 1960s, 1970s and 1980s glucose tolerance testing of pregnant women became widespread as did the diagnosis of gestational diabetes. After a thorough review of the scientific literature, Hunter and Kierse nicely summarise how this practice can be harmful:

"The diagnosis of gestational diabetes, as currently defined, is based on an abnormal glucose tolerance test. This test is not reproducible at least 50–70% of the time and the increased risk of perinatal mortality and morbidity said to be associated with the 'condition' has been considerably over-emphasized. No clear improvement in perinatal mortality has been demonstrated with insulin treatment for gestational diabetes, and screening of the pregnant population with glucose tolerance testing is unlikely to make a significant impact on perinatal mortality. An abnormal glucose tolerance test is associated with a two- to threefold increase in the incidence of macrosomia, but the majority of macrosomic infants will be born to mothers with a normal glucose tolerance test. Thus far, no improvement in neonatal outcome has been demonstrated from insulin treatment for gestational diabetes, nor has there been any demonstrated benefit to the mother or infant from reducing the incidence of macrosomia by insulin therapy. There is, however, a great potential to do more harm than good. A positive test labels the woman as having some kind of diabetes. This is an unpleasant label to have under any circumstances, particularly when repeat testing will not confirm the diagnosis in up to 70% of cases. Pregnancy is likely to be transformed into a high risk situation, invoking an extensive and expensive program of tests and interventions of unproven benefit. Women who had a less than perfect outcome of pregnancy and who had not been screened for gestational diabetes, may unfairly accuse their physicians of negligence, while the large amount of money and resources that are tied up in diagnosing and treating this 'condition' could be diverted to areas where they might be more effective. A negative glucose tolerance test, on the other hand, also has a potential for harm by falsely reassuring the physician and the woman that the risk, engendered by the indication for the test, has been removed. Except for research purposes, all forms of glucose tolerance testing should be stopped" (Hunter & Keirse 1991, p. 409).

One other potentially harmful effect of prenatal care is utilisation of drugs. Although considerable attention has been given recently to illegal drug use during pregnancy, too little attention is given to what is discussed here, legal drug use. Increasing the number of prenatal visits increases the number of drugs pregnant women consume. "Most medicines taken by or administered to pregnant women cross the placenta and enter the bloodstream of the fetus. Thus, when a pregnant woman takes a medicine, she not only gives medicine to herself but she is also giving the same medicine to her unborn baby. Since the not-fully-developed body systems of the fetus cannot process medicines as the mother's systems do, and since some medicines may affect normal development of the fetus, medicines that cross the placenta may have negative effects on the fetus or newborn. One only has to remember the thalidomide disaster to recognise the possible extent of the potential problems" (UNICEF 1992).

To what extent are pregnant women taking medicines? WHO has completed an international survey on drug utilisation during pregnancy involving 14,778 pregnant women from 22 countries on 4 continents. Eighty six percent of these women took medication during pregnancy (before coming to the hospital for birth), receiving an average of 2.9 (range 1–15) prescriptions. Of the total 37,309 prescriptions, 73% were given by the obstetrician, 12% by the general practitioner, and only 5% by the midwife. This extremely high drug utilisation rate during pregnancy is then elevated by drug utilisation during birth: the survey found that during the intrapartum period 79% of the women received an average of 3.3 drugs. Wide intra- and inter-country differences were found in habits and drug utilisation profiles. The survey concludes:

"There can be no doubt that at present some drugs are often more widely used in pregnancy than is justified by the knowledge available. . . This may be one aspect of the medicalisation of pregnancy, a process in which the use of a series of techniques and drugs is associated even with normal pregnancies, the employment of one technique or drug readily leading to the use of another. It would seem that whereas pregnancy is usually regarded as dangerous until proven safe, drugs may be regarded as safe in pregnancy provided they have not been proven dangerous, views which are often almost diametrically opposed to reality" (Collaborative Group on Drug Use in Pregnancy 1991, 1992).

What is the effect of all this medication on the fetus? Far too little is known about this: "Because of ethical, technical and financial reasons, few experiments are being implemented on pregnant women before drugs are put on the market. Therefore, knowledge on the effects of these drugs is limited and grows slowly" (UNICEF 1992). Ironically, even medications given to the pregnant woman for the sake of the fetus may be harmful. After reviewing the literature on hormone administration for the maintenance of pregnancy, Goldsteir et al. conclude: "In spite of the fact that progestagens continue to be prescribed on a wide scale, there is no good evidence that they are either effective or safe" (Goldstein et al. 1991, p. 620). When a number of newer and widely used diagnostic measures and medications used in prenatal care (such as routine ultrasound scanning, and prenatal fetal heartrate monitoring) are adequately evaluated, they may be added to the list of procedures abandoned because of possible harm.

Balancing social and medical care

A second question was the priority to be given to social and medical care during pregnancy. The members of the consensus meeting tried not to exclude either approach but to find the best balance between the two. The proponents of the medical model pointed out that the essentially medical routine prenatal surveillance applied in most countries identified many serious medical conditions, such as diabetes and toxaemia of pregnancy. Prompt medical management of these and other conditions had saved the lives of many mothers and babies and reduced the maternal and perinatal mortality rates. These participants felt strongly that medical prenatal services must remain the base on which social services might be added.

Those participants who favoured a higher priority for social services during pregnancy agreed that some kind of surveillance of the physical health of women and the progress of their pregnancies was desirable. They also felt that the contribution of the psychological and social components of prenatal services had been seriously underestimated. Reviews of a number of social intervention programs aimed at pregnant women were presented to the consensus meeting. These programs had significantly improved birth weight and reduced medical complications of pregnancy and birth.

In developed countries, the most important goal in pregnancy care is the prevention of low birth weight, as this is the factor most strongly associated with perinatal mortality. Furthermore, low birthweight infants are five times more likely than normal weight infants to die later in the first year and those who survive are more likely to have neurodevelopmental handicaps (Wallace 1988). To date medical interventions have had little or no success in preventing low birth weight or preterm birth. The efficacy of drugs in this regard is described as follows:

> "The introduction of beta-adrenergic drugs as tocolytic agents two or three decades ago led to widespread optimism that the problem of spontaneous preterm delivery could be overcome. A meta-analysis of many of the trials revealed that these agents can delay delivery for at least 48 hours and can slightly reduce the incidence of preterm delivery. The same analysis, however, showed no decrease in perinatal mortality or serious morbidity associated with preterm delivery. The absence of a positive effect may be due in part to errors in diagnosis and to patients' being too advanced in preterm labour for tocolysis to be successful" (Creasy 1991, p. 727).

The same author summarised the medical effort to prevent low birth weight:

> "Effective preventive measures are essentially unavailable, largely because we do not know how to predict the problem with enough certainty to warrant enrolling patients in a trial of preventive approaches. Such preventive methods have been tried mainly in multiple pregnancies, and even the time honoured approach of bed rest in pregnancies with twins has recently been shown in controlled trials to be of little value" (Creasy 1991).

Several kinds of social interventions, on the other hand, have had some success in increasing birth weight. For many, it might seem rather far fetched to think that social interventions could impact on something as biological as birth weight. Oakley clarified this relationship in a conference background paper: "Western systems of medical care have been preoccupied with medicine rather than with health. They have tended to view human beings as machines which break down from time to time and can be repaired mechanically, that is, by means of surgery and drug therapy. This same mechanical model of the human body has been applied to pregnancy. But neither in the case of pregnancy nor in the case of health generally is the model appropriate, because bodies are joined to minds and emotions, and human beings live in an intimate relationship with their social and cultural environments. The way bodies behave is thus affected by peoples' mental and emotional condition and both physical and emotional states are profoundly affected by environmental factors" (Oakley 1985a, p. 852).

One social variable found to be associated with birthweight is stress. Reporting on a controlled prospective study, Pagel et al. conclude: "Life events stress accounted for significant variation in birthweight, and social supports and anxiety were associated with the two paediatric Apgar scores. Gestational age bore a simple relationship to anxiety with higher anxiety predictive of lower gestational age" (Pagel et al. 1990, p. 597). Social intervention programs aimed at lowering stress and increasing social support have shown that this 'soft' approach can affect 'hard' outcomes: "There is considerable evidence to suggest that intervention programs aimed at improving the 'social' side of antenatal care are capable of affecting birthweight and other 'hard' measures of pregnancy outcome. Traditional professional approaches to pregnancy which divide the medical from the social perspective, have acted to prevent recognition of this evidence and its relevance to maternity care policy" (Oakley 1985b, p. 1259).

Another social variable which has been repeatedly correlated scientifically with birthweight is smoking. A report in 1986 found that women smoking more than 20 cigarettes a day during pregnancy had a 60% increase in births before 33 weeks compared to non-smokers (Shiono 1986). The largest data base ever available (360,000 births, 2500 fetal deaths, 3800 infants deaths) to assess the impact of smoking on fetal and infant mortality found:

"Compared with non-smoking women having their first birth, women who smoked less than one pack of cigarettes per day had a 25% greater risk of (fetal and infant) mortality, and those who smoked one or more packs per day had a 56% greater risk. Among women having their second or higher birth, smokers experienced 30% greater (fetal and infant) mortality than non-smokers, but there was no difference by amount smoked. The prevalence of smoking in this population was 30%. It was estimated that if all pregnant women stopped smoking, the number of fetal and infants deaths would be reduced by approximately 10%" (Kleinman 1988).

Further studies show the feasibility of smoking cessation programs during pregnancy. As an example, one random control trial of a smoking cessation program reported a significant increase in birthweight in the experimental group (Sexton & Hebel 1984). Another randomised controlled trial showed the smoking cessation group 2.5 times more likely than controls to stop smoking and their newborns weighed on average 57 g more at birth. They were 45% less likely to have a premature birth or low birth weight baby (Ershoff et al. 1990). Despite all the evidence, medically oriented prenatal care is not focusing on how to help women stop smoking: "Clinicians do not appear to worry about being sued for failing to refer women for smoking cessation treatment. In a recent study of pregnant smokers, Miller (1989) found that over 30% of clinic patients reported that neither a doctor or nurse had ever mentioned stopping smoking to them" (Ruzek 1990, p. 20).

Another social variable linked to low birth weight is nutrition during pregnancy. While earlier attempts by doctors to restrict dietary intake during pregnancy (see earlier in this chapter) fortunately have been abandoned for the most part, efforts to improve nutrition through counselling and food supplementation are sporadic. It is difficult to find reliable data on the efficacy of nutrition programs as they are usually part of a prenatal package of services. In the United States there is a nationwide program for poor pregnant women, the special supplemental food program for women, infants and children (WIC). Several studies have shown better birth outcomes of those participating in this program. In one study in which 4,126 pregnant women in the WIC program were compared to a matched control group of non WIC participants, WIC participants had: lower incidence of low birth weight; lower neonatal mortality; increased gestational age (Kotelchuck et al. 1984).

The supporters of the social approach pointed out that in many countries systems for identifying high-risk pregnancies placed increasing emphasis on social factors. Yet when a woman is put in a high-risk category because of previous or current social problems, the result is usually more medical attention. The available data on the content of prenatal care suggest that screening for medical problems (including biological indicators such as the results of laboratory tests and physical measurements) has received the most emphasis. At the same time a scientific double standard tends to be applied to the 'soft' interventions compared with 'hard' technological interventions: "It is striking to see how far more evidence of both efficacy and cost-effectiveness are demanded of prenatal care than of electronic fetal monitoring, caesarean section and other interventions which carry known risks and high costs and potentially benefit only a tiny proportion of births" (Ruzek 1990, p. 21). Studies show that the average prenatal visit with a doctor lasts about ten minutes, and expert recommendations from obstetrical organisations, public health organisations and medical textbooks offer detailed recommendations for medical screening but little guidance for providing health education, counselling and social support. Although an earlier set of recommendations from the American College of Obstetricians and Gynecologists (ACOG) advised prenatal counselling for nutrition, exercise, rest, anxiety and sexual relationships (ACOG 1965), a more recent version, except for nutrition, has dropped this advice (ACOG 1982). After analysing these recommendations, 3 participants at the conference wrote: "There is no mention (in the ACOG recommendations) of social supports. In short, the recommendations focus on biological interventions that have not generally been shown to be of value. What is needed are assessments of the biological interventions currently used, and of educational and social interventions that are candidates for inclusion in prenatal care" (Banta et al. 1985, p. 785). Thus it is not surprising that the prenatal care provided by physicians retains a medical orientation, regardless of the social or psychological conditions present. The proponents of the social model of pregnancy also pointed out that most prenatal health education and counselling followed the medical model, focusing on the individual in trying to eliminate certain kinds of behaviour and encouraging compliance with medical advice. In contrast, the social model of pregnancy uses a health promotion approach, which emphasises self-reliance and aims to link behaviour with the conditions of daily life.

After intense discussion of the question of medical and social priorities in prenatal care, the participants agreed that the medical component of prenatal care is essential and is in place almost everywhere that this care is offered. The consensus was that the social (and psychological) component of prenatal care should have equal importance. Because this component is not part of prenatal care in most places, the final recommendation stressed the need for countries to design strategies to ensure its inclusion. Social factors and strategies to evaluate them are culture-specific, and the debates in the consensus meeting between people of different countries and views provided ample proof that each country must develop its own strategies and prenatal programs to address social factors. As an example, it is gratifying to note that the recommendations of the US Institute of Medicine in 1988 give emphasis to the social and behavioural management of pregnancy, including smoking reduction, better nutrition and stress alleviation (Brown 1988). If these recommendations are heeded in the United States, it might start to correct a scandalous situation in that country: "The United States is virtually unique among its peer countries in failing to provide family allowances and in regarding many child health and welfare services — which consensus considers basic to life in a complex industrial society — as amenities to be purchased only by those who can afford to do so. Instead of squarely facing the issue of government responsibilities to support a floor of equity in access to essential services, we seem to need other reasons before taking action. Paradoxically, our generosity of heart relative to very costly services is the reverse of our position in relation to basic and less costly services" (Yankauer 1984, p. 1148).

The debates also demonstrated the difficulties to be surmounted in integrating social elements into prenatal care. For example, the importance of social factors was frequently dismissed because it depended on what were pejoratively described as soft data. Some participants from poorer countries with very limited resources felt that they had to choose medical over social care, although a number of review papers had made it clear that poverty is the primary killer of babies and the unborn.

The damage done by poverty to pregnancy and birth must be countered by social and financial solutions and not more medical attention. When the city of Indianapolis in the United States discovered it has one of the highest infant mortality rates in the industrialised world, the response was to buy a mobile van equipped with ultrasound and send it into the ghetto. Routine prenatal ultrasound scans will not counteract the effects of chronic malnutrition; social solutions, such as ensuring a good system of emotional support from relatives and friends to pregnant women, may soften some of the impact of poverty. As mentioned earlier, the reduced number of low birth weight babies born in Greece may be due in part to the intense support still offered by the extended family (Tzoumaka–Bakoula 1990).

Need for objectives

Because of the pervasive assumption that prenatal care, as now constituted, is a good thing, attempts at systematically planning and evaluating services have been few. Although any evaluation must begin with a clear set of objectives, this is difficult to find for prenatal care. The members of the consensus meeting agreed that lowering the perinatal mortality rate and decreasing the number of low birth weight babies, while worthy goals, are far too narrow and medical to be the sole objectives. Nevertheless, most studies of prenatal care use only one of these goals to measure effectiveness. Before deciding on policy on perinatal care, each country and community must determine its own objectives for prenatal care. More social objectives can be incorporated such as continuity of care, uptake of social services when recommended, smoking and other substance abuse reduction. Armed with a set of clear objectives for prenatal care, a country or community can take a more rational approach to evaluating its prenatal care and then to improving policy in this field.

Access to and continuity of care

Providing prenatal care to all pregnant women is an urgent issue in both North and South America and for special groups in Europe such as migrants, immigrants, gypsies, ethnic minorities. Most countries are following WHO's lead in formulating health policy that emphasises primary health care in the local neighbourhood rather than specialist care in hospitals as the basis for all health care. Ironically, in these same countries prenatal care is moving in the opposite direction, from midwife or general practitioner to obstetrical specialist and from the home or neighbourhood health centre to the hospital. A study in Finland documented this trend:

> "Traditionally, the Finnish prenatal care system has been based on special maternity centres outside hospitals. In recent years, however, the use of hospital outpatient clinics has increased. The purpose of this study was to describe the use of the clinics and to see whether clinics serve as an addition or as an alternative to maternity centres. [We found that] the content of care and means of care delivery differ between clinics and maternity centres. Clinics are technologically and provider-oriented without continuity of care. Clinics are not just referral centres for high-risk mothers; at least half of pregnant women visit them. Ultrasound screening is an important reason for use of the clinic. . . Hospital clinic care now seems to replace care in maternity centres" (Hemminki et al. 1990, p. 221).

Increasingly, the location at which prenatal care is provided is determined by the technology involved. For example, a routine ultrasound scan is most often done in a hospital because both the machine and the obstetrician to carry out the procedure are found there. The members of the consensus meeting agreed that this trend must be reversed and that countries should develop strategies to incorporate prenatal care (whatever its nature) into primary health care systems. Only in this way can countries begin successfully to address the issue of lack of access by pregnant women to prenatal care.

Current prenatal care is designed for the convenience of the people who provide it. The best proof of this assertion is the lack of continuity in the care given during pregnancy, birth and following birth. These three periods see frequent changes of the provider of and in the setting for care, and even in the records kept. Recently the home based (woman held) maternity record is gaining popularity as one attempt to provide at least a small degree of continuity:

"The issue of medical records is related to that of information giving. The usual procedure, in which women leave their records in the hands of the caregivers after consultations, often results in them being asked the same questions by several different caregivers (Macintyre 1981), as well as leaving them frustrated by their own lack of information. Giving the woman a summarised 'co-operation card' does not really solve the problem. Women have difficulty in reading the abbreviated notes on their summarised record. Two experimental comparisons of programs in which women held their own obstetric records with the conventional systems (Elbourne et al. 1987; Lovell et al. 1987) showed that women who held their own record felt in control of their antenatal care, more able to communicate effectively with their caregivers, and would want to hold their maternity record in another pregnancy. The authors also estimate that fewer records were lost or unavailable when required in the experimental (women-held) groups" (Reid & Garcia 1991, p. 133).

Lack of continuity in care is an important source of complaints from women during pregnancy and giving birth (Oakley 1979). For the most part they have gone unheeded, perhaps because to provide real continuity would require major alterations in the system of services for pregnancy and birth and possibly major inconvenience for some service providers. Nevertheless, the participants agreed that continuity of care should be encouraged.

Strategies for improvement

How can continuity of care be encouraged? How can social factors be incorporated into care? Considerable discussion focused on how the clinical model of prenatal care, little changed since its development decades ago, hampers some of the suggested improvements. The one-to-one relationship between the pregnant woman and a midwife or physician, the setting of a clinic or hospital, and the focus on events inside the pregnant woman's body to the exclusion of those in her mind, family or community hinder significant innovation in prenatal care. Consequently, alternative methods for providing prenatal care were discussed and encouraged. For example, the possibility of using the self-help or mutual aid group to provide prenatal care (including its medical component) was proposed. A small group of pregnant women, with the assistance of a midwife (as a consultant), would learn how to take each other's blood pressure, test each other's urine and measure each other's uterine growth. Rather than attending prenatal classes with a set curriculum, the group would make its own choices for prenatal education. The midwife would either provide this education herself or find someone who could. Such an alternative method could fit into the orthodox system, as each woman could still have an initial visit to a physician and special tests, procedures or referrals as indicated. Such an approach might help to demystify and demedicalise pregnancy and empower these women to better know and believe in their bodies and gain control over their reproductive lives. The members of the consensus meeting believed that the planning, mounting and evaluating of alternative methods, regardless of their nature, is important in improving prenatal care.

The central role of women

In searching for strategies to improve prenatal care, the participants again and again raised another issue that eventually became crucial: the centrality of women to all aspects of prenatal care, including participation in the planning, conduct and evaluation of care. The difference in the way women view and experience reproduction demands the significant, if not dominant, involvement of women in health care policy on human reproduction. While more women are found in obstetrics and paediatrics than in other medical specialties, and in maternal and child health than in other public health specialties, health policy-making, even for these specialties, is dominated by men. Men dominate policy-making on perinatal care at the international level (in organisations such as WHO, the International Federation of Gynaecology and Obstetrics (FIGO) and the International Paediatric Association), at the national level (in ministries of health and national institutes of obstetrics, paediatrics, maternal health and child health), and at the regional and local levels (in hospitals and institutes).

It was interesting to see how the 17 women members of the consensus meeting came together, despite their different countries, races, cultures, professional disciplines and views of pregnancy and birth. In spite of these differences, the women decided to form a caucus. This move precipitated an argument in plenary involving all 52 participants — the men insisting that such a caucus was divisive and the women insisting it was the only way they could get their views across. Following intense discussion, the move was approved.

The consensus meeting's recommendations stressed the central role of the pregnant woman in her own care because this care cannot be isolated from the social environment and the woman's goals for her pregnancy. This need to consider the living situation and other social conditions of the pregnant woman as well as her own wishes is clearly illustrated by the issue of hospitalisation during pregnancy. In many places, routine hospitalisation of pregnant women for a variety of conditions is practised in spite of lack of scientific evidence of efficacy and the hardship it may cause the family.

> "Hospitalisation during pregnancy is costly and disruptive for many families. It is surprising, therefore, that its use has been the subject of such a small amount of well-controlled research (*Lancet* editorial 1981). There are circumstances in which discussion with individual women who have one of the conditions we have reviewed will make it clear that a prescription for rest, either at home or in hospital, would be welcome. As there is no strong evidence that this is likely to have harmful effects, such women's views should be taken into account in deciding which form of care is appropriate. By the same token, however, women with either bleeding in early pregnancy, uncomplicated multiple pregnancy, or non-albuminuric hypertension should not be coerced into resting at home or in hospital, against their better judgement. There is currently no good evidence to support such recommendations" (Crowther & Chalmers 1991, p. 631).

The issue of the medical profession's control of the pregnant woman often results in paternalistic attitudes towards pregnant women. The necessity of bringing a woman to a physician or a clinic could in itself lead to her loss of control over her pregnancy and may sometimes result in an increased risk of perceived complications and a decreased quality of life.

Informed choice

Informed choice is an important method of ensuring that the woman controls her pregnancy. This means giving the woman complete information on the reasons for, and the potential benefits and hazards associated with, all examinations or procedures proposed by the health professionals. The woman is also told of all the options or alternatives available and then chooses her response to the proposal, rather than merely consenting to it. The European participants, through the WHO Perinatal Study Group surveys, were able to document the lack of informed choice in many countries (see chapter 6).

The nature and content of the information on which the choice is based were crucial. The issue of informed choice was considered so important that it was the subject of the first of the meeting's recommendations from the final consensus.

The next recommendation goes beyond the role of the woman in her care to her role and that of others in all pregnancy care: the planning, the giving and the evaluation of prenatal care should involve at all levels the pregnant woman, companions including family, as well as the community. This is community participation, which is difficult to achieve. One way towards this goal is through consumer groups, particularly women's groups actively interested in improving prenatal care. There is a tradition for such groups to start spontaneously at grass roots level in North America and Western Europe where they have played a role in maternity services. For example, the debate in the United Kingdom over the efficacy and safety of ultrasound, and the potential risks of its routine use during pregnancy, was recognised as the result of advocacy by consumers. In Eastern Europe and Latin America such groups are much less likely to develop spontaneously in the community and may need encouragement from the official sector. Thus universities and governments can set up model programs for community participation in perinatal care; such programs were described at the meeting by participants from Chile and Cuba. The national and local birth conferences that WHO promoted as follow-up to the three consensus meetings are other examples of community participation. They bring a wide variety of community groups together with the mass media and the government to discuss the meetings' recommendations in the light of local conditions (see chapter 8).

Research

Research is urgently needed to focus not just on morbidity and mortality but also on the development of measures of quality of life of the mother and child during pregnancy and birth and following birth. The members of the consensus meeting agreed that most of the information provided to women during prenatal care, and most of the medical activities of prenatal visits are not based on sound scientific evidence. Clearly, research that focuses on the quality of life during pregnancy needs to involve women who are or have been pregnant. Such women have always been the subjects of research, but now must become involved in its planning and evaluation. There has been little experience with involving the users of a health service in its evaluation, and much needs to be learned about how to do this effectively. The Latin American participants were particularly concerned about how to involve women outside health care in research, as there was no precedent for or experience with this approach to research in their countries. A handful of European research efforts were relevant here. The National Perinatal Epidemiology Unit in Oxford, England involves consumers in planning and evaluating their research projects. The former Director, Iain Chalmers, reports that this practice increases the acceptability of the research by the research subjects (Chalmers, personal communication, 1992). The WHO European's perinatal study group, by having consumer members, insured at least some community input to its research studies.

Technology assessment

One of the central issues discussed at the consensus meeting, the evaluation of technology used during pregnancy is an urgent matter in both industrialised and developing countries. In Europe and North America, pregnancy care is characterised by the widespread use of technology that has not been scientifically evaluated. A WHO study found that approximately 10% of routine obstetrical procedures had been adequately scientifically evaluated (Fraser 1983). In Latin America, there is little or no care for poor women and rapid increases in the use of expensive technology for women who have money (their own or from health insurance) to pay for it. Policy-makers in industrialised countries are concerned about the cost, efficacy and possible lack of safety of prenatal technology. Policy-makers in developing countries are concerned about the dumping of drugs and machines that have either been widely used without adequate evaluation, or found to be unacceptable in North America and Europe. To discuss the issue, the consensus meeting focused on a few examples of technology used in prenatal care. The first was ultrasound scanning during pregnancy.

Ultrasound scanning

The ultrasound story begins in July 1955 when an obstetrician in Scotland, Ian Donald, borrowed an industrial ultrasound machine used to detect flaws in metal and tried it out on some tumours which he had removed previously, using a beefsteak as the control. He discovered that he got different echoes from different tumours. As he himself has written "So, I lost no time in applying it to my patients". (Oakley 1984) Soon, Donald was using ultrasound not only for abdominal tumours in women, but also on pregnant women. Articles began to appear in the medical literature and its use quickly spread throughout the world.

> "It was really not very long ago that the first ultrasound images of the fetus were obtained. Yet in many places ultrasound visualization of the fetus is now performed, not only routinely, but often repeatedly, in pregnancy. Despite the British Medical Research Council's design of a large randomised trial to assess the long-term effects (if any) of fetal exposure to ultrasound, this and similar research was not mounted and, like many technologies in obstetrics, widespread dissemination has preceded proper evaluation. Anxiety about this situation has been expressed publicly in several countries" (Inch et al. 1986, p. 3).

The dissemination of ultrasound into clinical obstetrics is reflected in inappropriate statements made in the obstetrical literature regarding its appropriate use. Oakley illustrates this when writing:

"One of the lessons of history is, of course, that it repeats itself. The development of obstetric ultrasound thus mirrors the application to human pregnancy of diagnostic x-rays. Both, within a few years of discovery, were being used to diagnose pregnancy and to measure the growth and normality of the fetus. In 1935 it was said that 'antenatal work without the routine use of x-rays is no more justifiable than would be the treatment of fractures' (Reece 1935) In 1978: 'It can be stated without qualification that modern obstetrics and gynaecology cannot be practised without the use of diagnostic ultrasound' (Hassani 1978). Two years later, it was said that 'ultrasound is now no longer a diagnostic test applied to a few pregnancies regarded on clinical grounds as being at risk. It can now be used to screen all pregnancies and should be regarded as an integral part of antenatal care' (Campbell & Little 1980). On neither of these dates did evidence qualify the speakers to make these assertions. As sociologist J. B. McKinlay said, 'it is reasonable then to argue that the success of an innovation has little to do with its intrinsic worth (whether it is measurably effective, as determined by controlled experimentation) but is dependent upon the power of the interests that sponsor and maintain it, despite the absence or inadequacy of empirical support' (McKinlay 1981)". (Oakley 1986, p. 7).

It is not only doctors who have tried to promote ultrasound with statements which go beyond the scientific data. Commercial interests also have been actively promoting ultrasound, not only to doctors and hospitals, but also to the general public. As an example, an advertisement in a widely read Sunday newspaper (*The Times*, London) claimed: "Toshiba decided to design a diagnostic piece of equipment that would be absolutely safe. . . The answer turned out to be very high frequency sound waves. . . The name Ultrasound." A consumer organisation in Britain complained to the Advertising Standards Authority that Toshiba was making an untrue claim and the complaint was upheld (Beech & Robinson 1993). In many countries the commercial application of ultrasound scanning during pregnancy is widespread, offering 'baby look' and 'fun-ultrasound' in order to 'meet your baby' with photographs and home videos.

The extent to which medical practitioners nevertheless followed such scientifically unjustified advice, and how this technology proliferated can be illustrated by giving recent data from three countries. In France in one year, 3 million ultrasound examinations were done on 700,000 pregnant women — an average of more than four scans per pregnancy. These examinations cost French taxpayers more than all other therapeutic and diagnostic procedures done on these pregnant women. In Australia where the health service pays for 4 routine scans, in one recent year billing for obstetrical ultrasound was 60 million Australian dollars while billing for all prenatal, intrapartum and postpartum care of the same women was 50 million Australian dollars (Newnham 1992). An editorial in a leading United States newspaper in 1993 makes the following statement: "Baby's first picture — a $200 sonogram shot in the womb — is a nice addition to any family album. But are sonograms medically worth $1 billion of the nation's scarce health-care dollars? That's the question raised by a United States study released this week. It found the sonograms that doctors routinely perform on healthy pregnant women don't make any difference in the health of their babies" (*USA Today* 1993).

After a technology has spread widely in clinical practice, the next step is for health policy makers to accept it as standard care financed by the official health sector. Several European countries now have official policy for one or more routine ultrasound scans during pregnancy. For example, in 1980 the Maternity Care Guidelines in West Germany stated the right of each pregnant woman to be offered at least two ultrasound scans during pregnancy (*Lancet* 1984). Austria quickly followed suit approving two routine scans (see chapter 4). Do the scientific data justify such widespread use and great cost of ultrasound scanning?

The first issue, efficacy, must be seen as the central issue because, cost aside, no amount of risk is so small as to justify using something in the absence of proved efficacy. In assessing the efficacy of ultrasound in pregnancy it is essential to make the distinction between its selective use for specific indications and its routine use as a screening procedure. With regard to the former:

"The contribution of ultrasonography in specific clinical situations has not, in general, been quantified systematically. Nevertheless, the available information suggests that it can be valuable in a number of specific situations in which the diagnosis remains uncertain after clinical history has been ascertained and a physical examination has been performed" (Neilson & Grant 1991, p. 435).

With regard to routine use, on the other hand, Neilson and Grant state:

"The greatest controversy surrounding obstetric ultrasound has been whether there are benefits outweighing the costs of extending its use from specific indications to either early (usually 16–19 weeks, but sometimes earlier) or late (usually 32–36 weeks) routine screening of all pregnant women. Most claims of benefit for routine scanning are based on the assumption that clinical action taken on the results of the examination improve clinical outcome. These assumptions can only be tested adequately by randomised controlled trials, but few of these have been conducted. The six trials that have been conducted are of varying design and quality, have assessed a variety of scanning regimens, and not all have used the same measures of outcome. Nevertheless, they provide the best evidence that is currently available" (Neilson & Grant 1991, p. 424).

Following an exhaustive review of these trials, the authors conclude:

"The available information does not provide a basis for recommending routine use of ultrasonography for screening in either early or late pregnancy" (Neilson & Grant 1991, p. 435).

Doppler ultrasound is a variation on this technology which measures fetal heart pulsation and assesses blood flow. Although its popularity is increasing, Neilson and Grant, after once again carefully reviewing the scientific literature conclude:

"the available evidence does not, at the present time, support the use of Doppler ultrasound in clinical obstetric practice" (Neilson & Grant 1991, p. 430).

One of the most common justifications given today for routine ultrasound scanning in pregnancy is to detect intrauterine growth retardation (IUGR). Many clinicians insist that ultrasound is the best
method for the identification of this condition. A review of 83 scientific articles on this topic was presented to the consensus meeting
(Villar & Belizan 1986). Rigorous scientific criteria were applied to
all 83 reports. The review concluded that "for intrauterine growth
retardation detection, ultrasound should be performed only in a
high risk population". In other words, an experienced midwife's
hands feeling a pregnant woman's abdomen are as accurate as the
ultrasound machine for detecting intrauterine growth retardation.
This same conclusion was reached by a study in Sweden comparing
repeated measurement of fundal height by a midwife with repeated
ultrasonic measurements of biparietal diameter in 581 pregnancies.
The report concludes: "Measurements of the fundal height are more
effective than ultrasonic measurements for the antenatal diagnosis
of intrauterine growth retardation" (Cnattingius 1984).

If clinicians continue to use ultrasound to try to detect IUGR with
ultrasound, the result will be high false positive rates:

> "The precision of a screening or diagnostic test can be meas-
> ured by its sensitivity (i.e., the ability to detect abnormality)
> and its specificity (i.e., the ability to identify normality). One
> randomised controlled trial showed that, under ideal cir-
> cumstances, and with application of devices and measure-
> ments not in widespread use, the sensitivity and specificity
> of ultrasound imaging in the detection of intrauterine
> growth retardation were 94% and 92%, respectively (Neilson
> et al. 1984). If the rates of intrauterine growth retardation
> were 50–100 in every 1000 pregnancies, 43–62% of positive
> tests would lead to incorrect classification. If the rate of intra-
> uterine growth retardation in a population were as low as 20
> in every 1000 pregnancies, the false-positive rate would be
> over 80%" (*Lancet* 1984, p. 202).

In other words, even under ideal conditions such as do not exist in
most settings, it is likely that over half of the time a positive IUGR
screening test using ultrasound is returned, the test is false and the
pregnancy is in fact normal. The implications of this are great for
producing anxiety in the woman and the likelihood of further
unnecessary interventions.

There is another problem in screening for IUGR. One of the basic principles of screening is to screen only for conditions for which you can do something. At present, there is no treatment for IUGR, no way to slow up or stop the process of too slow growth and return it to normal. So it is hard to see how screening for IUGR could be expected to improve pregnancy outcome. "We are not aware of any controlled study to evaluate the effect of ultrasonography on the outcome of pregnancies at high risk of fetal growth retardation" (Neilson & Grant 1991, p. 423).

Furthermore, even if a screening test for IUGR using ultrasound is positive, there is no way to determine later if the test was valid: "There is no absolute postnatal judgement of growth retardation that can be used to assess the validity of the 'test'" (Altman & Hytten 1991, p. 413).

We are left with the conclusion that, with IUGR, we can only prevent a small amount of it using social interventions (nutrition and substance abuse programs), are very inaccurate at diagnosing it, and have no treatment for it. If this is the present state of the art, there is no justification for clinicians using routine ultrasound during pregnancy for the management of IUGR. Its use should be limited to research on IUGR. This is why, after a thorough review of the literature, Altman and Hytten conclude: "It is particularly crucial that some sound measures of outcome should be defined. Intervention based on assessments of size and growth should be evaluated in randomised trials before they are implemented in general obstetric practice" (Altman & Hytten 1991, p. 417).

Is ultrasound scanning during pregnancy safe? Once again it is interesting to look at what happened with the issue of safety of x-rays during pregnancy. X-rays were used on pregnant women for almost 50 years and assumed to be safe. In 1937 a standard textbook on antenatal care stated: "It has been frequently asked whether there is any danger to the life of the child by the passage of x-rays through it; it can be said at once there is none if the examination is carried out by a competent radiologist or radiographer" (Salmond 1937). A later edition of the same textbook stated: "It is now known that the unrestricted use of x-rays may be harmful to mother and child" (Chassar Moir 1960). The reason for this change was the report in 1956 on fetal x-rays and childhood cancer (Stewart et al. 1956). This story illustrates the danger of assuming safety. In this regard, a statement from a 1978 textbook is relevant: "One of the great virtues of diagnostic ultrasound has been its apparent safety. At present energy levels, diagnostic ultrasound appears to be without any injurious effect. . . all the available evidence suggests that it is a very safe modality" (Hassani 1978). Ann Oakley draws attention to the leap from 'appears to be' to 'is' in this passage (Oakley 1986).

Far too little has been done to determine the safety (or danger) of ultrasound during pregnancy. A professional organisation of clinicians who use ultrasound has established a system to monitor the international literature for any reports of possible harm from ultrasound during pregnancy. Such a watchdog surveillance system is worthwhile but cannot possible be seen as a scientific approach to the evaluation of safety. It is not assessment before, or even during use, but after use. It is a passive system of waiting for someone to discover harm rather than an active scientific pursuit of the issue of safety. Several years ago, as a WHO staff person, I approached this organisation to see if a prospective multi-centre controlled trial looking at safety could be started but nothing came of my suggestion.

That ultrasound during pregnancy cannot be simply assumed to be harmless is suggested by good scientific work in Norway. By following up children at age 8 or 9 born of mothers who had taken part in two controlled trials of routine ultrasound during pregnancy, they were able to show that routine ultrasonography was associated with a higher frequency of non-right-handedness, a symptom of possible neurological problems (Salvesen et al. 1993).

With regard to the active scientific pursuit of safety, an editorial in *Lancet* says:

"Published work on the biological effects of ultrasound imaging is surprisingly thin. There have been some reports of adverse effects in fetal animals and damage to cells in culture, but the data are seriously deficient and many questions have simply not been addressed. There have been no randomised controlled trials of adequate size to assess whether there are adverse effects on growth and development of children exposed in utero to ultrasound. Indeed, the necessary studies to ascertain safety may never be done, because of lack of interest in such research" (*Lancet* 1984, p. 202).

The safety issue is made more complicated by the problem of exposure conditions. Clearly any bio-effects which might occur as a result of ultrasound would be contingent on the dose of ultrasound received by the fetus or woman. But there are no national or international standards for the output characteristics of ultrasound equipment. The result is the shocking situation described in a Commentary in the *British Journal of Obstetrics and Gynaecology*:

> "It is staggering to discover that the range of spatial peak temporal average powers (of ultrasound equipment) has a ratio of 5285 to 1 in a sample of 12 instruments and the same machines show a ratio of 3055 to 1 between the highest and lowest pulse average powers. It is inconceivable that such a huge range of output powers is either necessary or acceptable. If the machines with the lowest powers have been shown to be diagnostically adequate how can one possibly justify exposing the patient to a dose 5000 times greater, even if at this level no definite adverse effects have yet been shown to occur? There is no evidence that the machines with greatest power output produce better quality images, indeed they probably require higher powers in order to compensate for poor system sensitivity" (Meire 1987, p. 1121).

The commentary goes on to urge government guidelines on the output of ultrasound equipment and for legislation making it mandatory for equipment manufacturers to state the output characteristics. As far as is known, this has not yet been done in any country.

Safety is also clearly related to the skill of the operator. "At the present time there is no recognised structured training or certification for the medical users of ultrasound apparatus in the United Kingdom and . . . no attempt is made to examine candidates in their ability to perform and interpret an examination" (Meire 1987, p. 1121). It might be added that there is no known training or certification in any other country. Once more the birth machine has no driver's licence. No one can scientifically state that ultrasound scanning during pregnancy is either safe or unsafe.

It is important to make two short comments about the psychological and social aspects of ultrasound use during pregnancy. First is the necessity of communication with the woman: "Women's views about the indications for ultrasound during pregnancy vary, and it is important that ultrasonographers take this variation into account in their dealings with individual women. The value of good communication, with 'high feedback' of the results of the examination, has been demonstrated in a number of controlled trials" (Neilson & Grant 1991, p. 435).

The second comment has to do with the idea, pushed by some ultrasonographers, that women should have a scan during pregnancy because it helps them to 'bond' with their baby. Here the words of the sociologist Oakley are most relevant:

> "It has been claimed that ultrasound in pregnancy now enables obstetricians to 'introduce' mothers to their fetuses and facilitates a new phenomenon called prenatal bonding in exactly the same way that the medical innovation of hospital delivery enabled paediatricians to discover the phenomenon of postnatal bonding. I would suggest that this is just rediscovering-the-wheel activity of a most primitive kind. Mothers and newborns bonded before in-hospital delivery disturbed the natural process. Mothers and babies are in a relationship with one another before they meet on the ultrasound screen" (Oakley 1986, p. 9).

Although ultrasound is expensive, routine scanning is of doubtful efficacy and the procedure has not yet been proved to be safe, this technology is widely used and its use is increasing rapidly, without control. Nevertheless, health policy is slow to develop. No country is known to have developed policies with regard to standards for the machines nor for training and certification of the operators. A few industrialised countries have begun to respond to the data showing lack of efficacy for routine scanning of all pregnant women. In the United States, for example, a consensus conference on diagnostic ultrasound imaging in pregnancy concluded that:

> "The data on clinical efficacy and safety do not allow recommendation for routine screening at this time; there is a need for multidisciplinary randomised controlled clinical trials for an adequate assessment" (National Institutes of Health 1984).

Denmark, Sweden and the United Kingdom have made similar statements against routine screening (*Lancet* editorial 1984). WHO, in an attempt to stimulate governments to develop policy on this issue, published the following statement:

"The World Health Organisation stresses that health technologies should be thoroughly evaluated prior to their widespread use. Ultrasound screening during pregnancy is now in widespread use without sufficient evaluation. Research has demonstrated its efficacy for certain complications of pregnancy but the published material does not justify the routine use of ultrasound in pregnant women. There is also insufficient information with regard to the safety of ultrasound use during pregnancy. There is as yet no comprehensive, multidisciplinary assessment of ultrasound use during pregnancy including: clinical efficacy, psychosocial effects, ethical considerations, legal implications, cost benefit and safety.

"This lack of information makes decision-making and priority setting with regard to ultrasound use during pregnancy difficult. A relevant document which provides guidance and policy in this matter is the US Consensus statement, Diagnostic Ultrasound Imaging in Pregnancy, published by the National Institutes of Health in 1984. WHO can in principle support this statement including their views that the data on clinical efficacy and safety do not allow a recommendation for routine screening at this time; there is a need for multidisciplinary randomised controlled clinical trials for an adequate assessment.

"WHO strongly endorses the principle of informed choice with regard to technology use. The health care providers have the moral responsibility: fully to inform the public about what is known and not known about ultrasound scanning during pregnancy; and fully to inform each woman prior to an ultrasound examination as to the clinical indication for ultrasound, its hoped for benefit, its potential risk, and alternative available, if any" (WHO 1984a).

This statement by WHO, sadly, is just as relevant today (Beech & Robinson 1993). The entire issue has been summarised nicely in one sentence by a consultant radiologist in the United Kingdom:

"The casual observer might be forgiven for wondering why the medical profession is now involved in the wholesale examination of pregnant patients with machines emanating vastly different powers of energy which is not proven to be harmless to obtain information which is not proven to be of any clinical value by operators who are not certified as competent to perform the examinations" (Meire 1987, p. 1122).

A postscript to this discussion of ultrasound during pregnancy is necessary. As is clear from the above, during the 1980s and early 1990s a number of us were raising questions about both the efficacy and safety of fetal scanning. Our voice of caution, however, was like a cry in the wilderness as the technology proliferated. Then during the course of one month in late 1993, as this book was going to press, two landmark scientific papers were published.

The first paper, a large randomised trial of the efficacy of routine pre-natal ultrasound screening, studied the perinatal outcome of over 15,000 pregnant women who either received two routine scans at 15–22 weeks and 31–35 weeks, or were scanned only for medical indications. Results showed that the mean number of sonograms in the ultrasound group was 2.2 and in the control group (on indication only) was 0.6. The rate of adverse perinatal outcome (fetal death, neonatal death, neonatal morbidity), as well at the rate of pre-term delivery and the distribution of birth weights was the same for both groups. In addition, in the authors' words: "The ultrasonic detection of congenital abnormalities has no effect on perinatal outcome. There were no significant differences between the groups in perinatal outcome in the subgroups of women with post-date pregnancies, multiple-gestation pregnancies, or infants who were small for gestational age." The authors conclude: "Screening ultrasonography did not improve perinatal outcome as compared with elective ultrasonography on the basis of clinician judgement" (Ewigman et al. 1993). At last we have a randomised clinical trial of sufficient size to conclude that there is no efficacy to routine scanning during pregnancy.

The second landmark paper, also a randomised controlled trial, looked at the safety of repeated prenatal ultrasound imaging (Newnham et al. 1993). While the original purpose of the trial was hopefully to demonstrate the safety of repeated scanning, the results were the opposite. From 2834 pregnant women, 1415 received ultrasound imaging and continuous-wave doppler flow studies at 18, 24, 28 34 and 38 weeks gestation (intensive group) while the other 1419 received single ultrasound imaging at 18 weeks (regular group). The only difference between the two groups was significantly higher (one third more) intrauterine growth retardation (IUGR) in the intensive group. This important and serious finding prompted the authors to state: "It would seem prudent to limit ultrasound examinations of the fetus to those cases in which the information is likely to be of clinical importance" (Newnham et al. 1993, p. 890). It is ironic that it is now likely that ultrasound scanning may lead to the very condition, IUGR, that it has for so long claimed to be effective in detecting.

Although we now have sufficient scientific data to be able to say that routine prenatal ultrasound scanning has no efficacy and may very well carry risks, it would be naive to think that routine use will not continue. As this book goes to press, it has been only a month since these two scientific papers have appeared, and yet the medical reaction has already consistently found reasons to reject the findings. In Australia, when asked about the new findings "A leading Sydney authority on ultrasound said that most women required only one ultrasound, at about 18 weeks, to ensure that the foetus was developing normally" (*Sydney Morning Herald*, October 9 1993, p. 1). In Denmark, when a leading newspaper asked the doctor in charge of ultrasound scanning at the University Hospital in Copenhagen about the new findings, he said that the findings gave him no cause for concern, and will not influence their routine scanning (*Politikin* October 17 1993, p. 4). In the same newspaper article, this doctor elaborated that: the American study was irrelevant to Denmark because abortion policy in the United States does not allow therapeutic abortion for fetal abnormalities (not true); the Australian findings do not show anything reliable because the finding of a risk was a by-product in a study with a different purpose (not true, and revealing a lack of understanding of scientific methodology).

During the past month, in meeting in Luxemburg and France where I presented the findings of the two studies, I have been told that: the studies are not rigorous since they do not report on the power used in the scan (both trials used the most rigorous methodology possible); there are thousands of published papers showing the value of ultrasound scanning (lack of understanding of the difference in

validity between observational case series and randomised controlled trials); since pregnancy suspected of intrauterine growth retardation are referred for ultrasound, of course there is more
intrauterine growth retardardation in the group with more ultrasound (lack of understanding of randomisation). Unfortunately, discussions of research reports quickly reveals the inadequate
education of medical doctors in the basics of scientific method. It
will be a struggle to close the gap between this new scientific data
and clinical practice.

Other screening of the fetus

A second example of technology assessment discussed by the members of the consensus meeting was screening of the condition of the
fetus, using either fetal heart-rate testing or fetal movement monitoring. A review was presented of over 600 books and articles on
this prenatal technology. Careful scientific criteria were used in the
evaluation of this literature. These two current methods of fetal surveillance have been shown to give inaccurate results. Data from controlled clinical trials give no evidence of efficacy in predicting
morbidity or mortality. Further, the tests are expensive, with direct
annual costs of at least US$200 million in the United States alone.
For these reasons, they should not be used as the sole indications for
induction of labour or caesarean section. The wide diffusion of this
technology seemed premature and large randomised controlled trials were recommended.

In the early 1980s another example of prenatal screening technology
was introduced, chorionic villus sampling (CVS) in which a needle is
inserted into the uterus and a biopsy taken of a part of the placenta.
Because perinatal technology assessment usually comes after widespread diffusion, WHO staff decided to seize the opportunity to try
to assess this promising but invasive new technology as it developed and spread. This is at least one step in the direction of the ultimate goal — assessment before proliferation. So WHO organised a
meeting to develop a system of collaborative monitoring and assessment using a network of centres from a number of countries (WHO
1984b). The network has a CVS register which collects data and dis-
seminates it through a newsletter. As of February 1992, 78,000 cases
are included in the register. This is about half of the estimated
150,000 cases globally (WHO 1992). The CVS register has allowed for

important findings during the development of CVS. First, CVS is not without risk. The fetal loss rate following the procedure, among cytologically normal pregnancies intended to continue, has been about 4%, ranging among centres from 2% to 7%. There is clear evidence of inter-centre variation, with fetal loss rate lowest at centres with the largest experience (WHO 1992).

Another issue is whether the risks associated with CVS exceed the risks of the less invasive amniocentesis. The 5 reports comparing CVS with amniocentesis have varying results (Crane et al. 1988; Lippman et al. 1992; Rhoads et al. 1989; MRC Working party 1991; Schmidt-Larsen 1992). There is a trend toward an excess fetal losses with CVS but this reached statistical significance only in one study (MRC) where there was a 4.4% excess loss rate with CVS over amniocentesis. The simplest explanation for the discrepancy in these 5 studies is centre-to-centre differences in the safety of CVS.

The international CVS register also sheds light on the risk of transcervical versus transabdominal CVS. While data from several studies (Brambati 1990; Jackson 1990; Schmidt-Larsen 1992) suggested lower fetal loss rates with the transabdominal route, careful analysis suggests that the two routes can be equivalent if the operators have sufficient experience.

The value of an international CVS register has been clearly demonstrated by the alarm over a number of recent reports of clusters of infants born with limb defects following CVS (Firth et al. 1991; Burton et al. 1992; Hsieh et al. 1991; Monni et al. 1991; Mahoney et al. 1991; Jackson et al. 1991; Miny et al. 1991; Mastroiacovo and Cavalcanti 1991; EUROCAT 1992; Froster-Tskenius & Baird 1989; Shepard et al. 1991). The Regional Office for Europe of WHO called a meeting of members of the international network in May 1992 to analyse these reports using the register data and make recommendations (WHO 1992). Careful analysis of all international data by this meeting brought out 3 important findings:

1. The reported clusters of limb defects do not show a statistically significant increased frequency of these abnormalities over the background level but this could be the result of considerable statistical problems when comparing very large numbers with very small numbers.

2. The clusters were reported by centres with relatively small experience.
3. The cases of limb defects followed CVS done before the 8th completed week of gestation. Accordingly the WHO report concludes:

> "The global ten year experience of CVS now extends to over 150,000 cases. The technique is helpful for women at increased genetic risk, and when practised by an expert and performed between 9 and 12 weeks gestation has an acceptably low rate of complications and fetal loss. An increased incidence of limb reduction defects has been reported in some centres, but the absolute number of cases involved is very small. There is no evidence to suggest any increased risk of congenital malformation when CVS is performed after the 8th completed week. The overall incidence of limb reduction defects following CVS, including the reported clusters, is as rare (5.89 per 10,000) as in the general population (5.97 per 10,000). However, as the present evidence is consistent with an association of very early sampling (at or before 8 weeks) with some fetal limb malformations, CVS should be performed at 9–12 weeks from the last menstrual period (after the 8th completed week).

> "Considerable variation is known to exist between centres in the risk of fetal loss associated with CVS, which makes it reasonable to think that a similar variation may apply for risk of fetal malformation. CVS and in fact other fetal sampling techniques should therefore be performed only at centres having a high level of expertise and experience, capable of applying any sampling approach as appropriate, and of meeting certain standards. Training can be suitably performed in both experimental and diagnostic cases under direct supervision of a senior expert operator. Expertise in ultrasonography of the first trimester and skill in amniocentesis and/or fetal blood sampling are the main prerequisites for training" (WHO 1992).

The report goes on to detail the criteria for centres and then finishes with the following:

"Finally, it is essential that women offered CVS be given full information of the risks before giving their consent" (WHO 1992).

This experience with global monitoring of a new perinatal technology, in this case CVS, clearly demonstrates the importance of this approach. Important, practical recommendations are now possible. The recommendation to limit CVS to 9–12 weeks gestation should not be difficult to implement. On the other hand, the suspicion long held by many that the risk of a technology is to some extent related to the skill and experience of the operator has now been clearly shown and is much harder to implement. Training standards are required with the force of sanctions behind them. As stated earlier, it is necessary to require a driver's licence for the birth machine. And it is equally important that women offered CVS be fully informed of all the risks discussed here.

After reviewing examples of prenatal technology, the members of the consensus meeting agreed that adequate assessment in perinatal care is an urgent priority worldwide. A special section of the recommendations was devoted to technology assessment, advocating, for example, the evaluation of technology before widespread use (A detailed description of technology assessment is found in chapter 6). In addition, the participants recommended periodic evaluation of technology that is already part of accepted practice, not only because technology changes over time but also because most technology in accepted practice has never been adequately evaluated. How should such technology assessment be encouraged, if not enforced? It is clearly inadequate and will not improve significantly unless stern measures are taken. The comprehensive assessment required cannot be left to the industry that develops the machines or the physicians who use them.

Further, after assessment, technology should be used only in situations in which it has been demonstrated to be effective. Such limitations on use mean some type of technology control, another task that cannot be delegated to industry or physicians. The participants thus strongly recommended the making of government controls similar to those found in most countries for the assessment and regulation of drugs. Each country must evaluate each type of prenatal technology in the light of its particular social, economic and health system conditions. Such an evaluation must be used to develop means to control the importation, manufacture, diffusion and use of technology on pregnant women.

The risk approach to prenatal care

The concept of a risk approach to care of pregnant women was the subject of considerable debate at the consensus meeting. The definition of risk groups forms the basis of current obstetrical practice. The idea is simple. Through screening procedures, and the use of a risk scoring system that gives points for each risk factor present, pregnant women are divided into two groups: those with low risk for trouble and those with high risk. Women in the low-risk group receive routine prenatal care, with the possibility that screening at subsequent visits may shift them to the high-risk group. Women in the high-risk group receive special attention and further tests and are often referred to large central hospitals for further care. This approach is intended to prevent problems before they arise, or at least catch them early enough to reduce or eliminate them. It is also designed to ensure that the women most likely to have complications during birth will have them in a setting that provides the expertise and technology to deal with them. The risk approach also provides a rationale for resource allocation. Low-risk pregnant women can receive prenatal care locally without specialised personnel or equipment. These are reserved for the large centres to which women at high risk are sent. In theory, this should reduce the overall cost of and the needs for health personnel for perinatal care.

The risk approach has been enthusiastically incorporated into the perinatal care systems in the industrialised countries of Europe, and is promoted as an important remedy for the struggling systems in developing countries. More recently, concern has been voiced in Europe and North America, particularly by proponents of the social model, about certain limitations and disadvantages of this approach. First, it is based on the medical model notion that pregnancy and birth are risky and dangerous. Seeing birth as life threatening leads to surveillance and quick interference at the first sign of deviation from normal. When the pregnant woman is screened for risk, she incorporates the idea into her perception of her pregnancy, even if she is at low risk. Further, being labelled high risk certainly increases stress, which is not good for pregnant women (Chalmers 1982).

The risk approach defines the birth as the most important issue in maternal health and perinatal care, at the expense of many other decisive phases and events from the beginning of the pregnancy to the postpartum period (that following birth). This view tends to strengthen the role of the obstetrician at the birth (usually limited to the second stage of labour and the moment of birth) and weakens interest in the contribution of the other professionals involved, who may include a midwife, general practitioner, social worker, psychologist, or a physical therapist.

The risk approach makes the pregnant woman a patient. As such, there is a tendency for her to become a passive object on which screening tests are performed. The risk approach focuses more on the risk to the fetus than the risk to the woman, and this intense focus carries the danger that the pregnant woman may come to be seen simply as a container for the baby. Thus, obstetricians have gradually come to consider themselves the advocates for the unborn baby. This has resulted in an extreme situation in North America:

> "The current discourse pits birthing women against their babies and puts obstetricians in the role of adjudicating disputes over whose 'interest' should come first (Gallagher 1987). . . The concept of 'fetus as patient' has led to demands by some doctors and lawyers that pregnant and labouring women be subjected to physical regulation, forced surgery, detention, and to criminal and civil punishment for behaviour deemed dangerous to the fetus. Some judges have ordered caesarean sections performed despite women's refusal and other women have been taken to court for refusing surgical procedures to prevent miscarriage and for taking non prescription drugs" (Ruzek 1991, p. 66).

The woman has not only become passive, but is sometimes viewed as selfish and irresponsible.

As the risk approach creates uneasiness about pregnancy and birth, it is tempting to want every birth to take place in a hospital with all the equipment and specialists available. In hospitals, physicians and machines work to push back the limits on the lives that can be saved. In doing so, they stress the risks involved. Accordingly, they increase their demands for more technology. According to the risk approach, the central high-technology hospital is the pinnacle of the service pyramid. In this self-perpetuating spiral of more risks, more physicians and machines, and more lives saved survival has come to be synonymous with ideal care. Some believe that the risk approach, by focusing on the negative — i.e. what can go wrong, can interfere seriously with attempts to take a positive approach to prenatal care.

Members of the consensus meeting who supported the medical model also expressed concerns about the risk approach. It has two scientific weaknesses. First, the risk approach is built on a scientific inconsistency. Logically, the abnormal cannot be identified without a clear scientific definition of the variations of the normal. Obstetrics lacks this because the risk concept implies that all pregnancy and birth is risky and therefore no pregnancy or birth can be considered normal until it is over. In other words, one cannot claim both the ability to separate normal from abnormal during pregnancy and the inability to determine normality until after birth.

The second scientific weakness lies in the way that risk factors are generated for use in risk scoring systems. Data are taken from large groups of pregnant women to determine relationships between pregnancy and problems at birth. This information is then applied to each pregnant woman to determine her risk score. Every epidemiologist knows that applying population data to individuals is a dangerous scientific game, fraught with weaknesses. It is probably at least partly for this reason that, although risk scales have been developed in a number of countries, their efficacy in the prevention of morbidity and mortality has not been clearly shown. In fact, people are not yet very good at predicting who is really at risk. This means that many women labelled as low risk will have problems. In one country, for example, half the women having complications at birth were from the low-risk group. It also means that many women thought to be at high risk — and thus subjected to all the accompanying extra tests and anxieties — will turn out to have no problems.

The poor experience with the risk approach in Latin America was highlighted at the consensus meeting. In one background paper, Caldeyro-Barcia reviewed the overall Latin American experience and pointed out that risk ratings based on multiple factors have proven to be a non-appropriate technology, especially when transplanted from one region to another with different demographic, socioeconomic, and cultural factors (Caldeyro-Barcia 1985). In another background paper an analysis was made of the new risk system for pregnant women in Cuba. The paper concluded: "This new (risk) system . . . resulted in too many pregnant being put into the high-risk category and many protective measures being taken for pregnant women who possibly did not need them. Validation tests such as sensitivity, specificity, and predictive power were used in this system, and it was found that it suffered from problems in discriminating the risk groups" (Farnot 1985, p. 830).

The value of the risk approach was discussed intensely by the members of the consensus meeting. They agreed that the risk approach is no panacea, although it may be useful in identifying *groups* of high-risk pregnant women and using this information to target such groups for special attention. Information on levels of risk in a population of pregnant women may be useful in planning services and resource allocation. Attempts to apply this risk approach to individual pregnant women, however, must be very slow and cautious, taking account of the limitations and disadvantages and the ways in which to reduce or overcome them. It was also agreed that if the risk approach to pregnancy care is to be used it should always be combined with a more social approach that emphasises prevention and health promotion.

Scientific basis for pregnancy care

Concern was repeatedly expressed about the lack of scientifically based policy for pregnancy care systems and practices in almost every country. An outstanding example of this unfortunate state of affairs is the variations between countries in the systems for routine prenatal visits (WHO 1985, p. 21). They are based on national guidelines that were developed on the basis not of scientific study but of existing practice in each country at the time the guidelines were promulgated.

National perinatal surveillance systems

Most countries do not have systems for collecting data on perinatal events. The importance of having such a national perinatal surveillance system was underlined for the consensus meeting by a description of the system in Czechoslovakia (Stembera 1985). It includes the systematic collection at the national level of data on every pregnant woman in the country, as well as on surveys and experimental intervention in pilot areas. This provides a scientific rationale for the modification of the system of care. While perinatal surveillance systems are feasible in industrialised countries with highly developed health care systems, the participants from Latin America stressed the difficulty of obtaining adequate data in their countries. The use of periodic surveys is a possible solution for such countries; the outstanding perinatal survey conducted in Greece is a model case in point (Tzoumaka-Bakoula 1987).

Another solution for developing countries could be to recruit the assistance of local lay people in collecting data on pregnancy and birth. Such people already know who is pregnant, who gave birth, and where and when. It has been shown that local people can be motivated and trained to collect and record reliably such data. In Turkey, even in areas with high illiteracy rates, studies have demonstrated that birth registration by village people is more accurate than official statistics (personal communication, Ministry of Health, Ankara 1990). The members of the consensus meeting encouraged such innovative methods of collecting information from community and family sources.

In developing national perinatal surveillance systems, it is important to have a group of people in one place, whose sole responsibility is perinatal surveillance and research. Detailed descriptions were presented to the consensus meeting of two national perinatal epidemiology centres, in Mexico and the United Kingdom. Such centres need a multidisciplinary staff, including obstetricians, paediatricians, nurses, midwives, epidemiologists, social scientists and consumers. It is important that the centres be as free as possible from any influence or pressure from clinicians or policy-makers. The functions of the centres should include: the analysis of national statistics, the development of national norms of standards of care, epidemiological research and consultation, and technology assessment

101

and perinatal research, using the tools of anthropology and sociology.

International exchange of information

The exchange of information between countries on pregnancy care and research was felt to be inadequate. There are a number of ways to improve this. The members of the consensus meeting were told of several international collaborative efforts that had been effective. The Latin American Centre for Perinatology and Human Development, located in Montevideo, Uruguay, has played an important role in Latin America and elsewhere (Schwarcz 1985). Unfortunately, this Centre and others like it are little known, because important research from Latin America is rarely published in English, for reasons unrelated to its quality and few North American and European scientists are literate in Spanish. Further, the important collaborative work of perinatal specialists from the Nordic countries provided a different model for international communication. And, in addition to the work of the WHO European Perinatal Study Group (Wagner 1985), WHO is establishing a global network of perinatal collaborating centres to facilitate a better flow of information among countries.

Research

Closely related to the issue of surveillance is the issue of research on pregnancy and pregnancy care. In general, research is not conducted according to established priorities, but determined by the interests of individual researchers. Most is clinical research, performed on relatively small numbers of pregnant women and is observational rather than experimental. In the past, obstetrics had a very poor record for good experimental research. Archie Cochrane, a renowned epidemiologist, in discussing which medical specialties have made the best and worse use of randomised trials, commented:

> "While I had little difficulty in deciding which specialty (at that time — i.e. 1979) had made the best use of trials, I had some difficulty in deciding which one was worst. Surgery, cardiology, and psychiatry were close runners up, but I finally chose obstetrics as the specialty most deserving of the

'wooden spoon' (i.e. worse use). I think I made a reasonable defence of my choice" (Cochrane 1991).

Although the vast majority of studies reported in the obstetrical literature still remain observation rather than experimental, Cochrane goes on to point out that there has been improvement in this situation: "There has been a marked increase in the use of randomised trials in the world of obstetrics" (Cochrane 1991). This is important progress and a recent new textbook in obstetrics, based on information provided by randomised trials, has quickly become an important standard for obstetric practice (Chalmers et al. 1991). Two remaining research issues, however, are clear from this book. There is an enormous gap between, on the one hand, the recommendations made in the book based on a thorough review of the experimental data and, on the other hand, what in reality is everyday practice. The second issue is that some subjects in the book have received adequate experimental study while other subjects are neglected.

The members of the consensus meeting concluded that, as with technology assessment, the nature and quality of research into pregnancy and pregnancy care were far too important to leave to the unsystematic efforts of industry and physicians. Governments must develop means of ensuring that the research done is based on local and national priorities. Such priorities, at all levels, should be established jointly by the users and all types of providers of perinatal care. In setting research priorities, more emphasis should be given to epidemiological research (as opposed to investigations of purely clinical problems), to social research and to research on the content of prenatal care. Research on pregnancy and prenatal care often involves ethical issues such as: is it fair to withhold treatment from a control group; what should be included in 'informed consent' to potential research subjects. Participants recommended that governments ensure that proposed research be reviewed by standing multidisciplinary committees that include the users of pregnancy care, as well as lay people involved in promoting the health of the woman and her fetus.

Role of health professionals

A final issue was the appropriate role of various health professionals (obstetricians, general practitioners, midwives and nurses) in pregnancy care. In Europe, as well as North and South America, the roles of these groups have changed profoundly. In Latin America and some European countries the surfeit of physicians is driving midwives out or leaving them with a minor role as physicians' assistants.

Moving pregnancy and birth care to the hospital has also helped to change the role of the care providers by increasing the role of the obstetrician at the expense of both the midwife and the general practitioner. The members of the consensus meeting noted that these changes carried a risk of further medicalising pregnancy.

Two solutions were proposed to the problem of appropriate roles for providers of pregnancy care. Policy-makers and governments are urged to re-evaluate their human resources for reproductive health services. This would involve studies of midwifery practices and the optimal use of midwives in care for pregnant women. Studies of the appropriate role of obstetricians also would be required, addressing such issues as whether it is appropriate for these specialists to provide routine prenatal care for normal pregnant women, as is the practice in some countries. As an example a Finnish study found that when obstetricians working in a hospital outpatient clinic are caring for pregnant women rather than midwives working in a community maternity centre, the care is more 'provider oriented' and involves more use of technology (Hemminki et al. 1990). All studies should include the social, psychological, economic and institutional factors that influence the training of health personnel, the quality of care provided and service utilisation.

The second solution involved significantly changing the initial training and continuing education of the providers of pregnancy care. Both should include information on the application to pregnancy care of psychological and social support skills, health promotion and health education, epidemiology and anthropology, and technology assessment. The importance of sensitising medical, nursing and midwifery students to all of these was emphasised.

Follow-up

The members of the consensus meeting made several recommendations to facilitate translating its ideas into policy on perinatal care in countries. Most important was the suggestion that follow up birth conferences be organised at national and local level in countries, to take the last step in the consensus process: presenting the recommendations to all interested parties for an open discussion of their relevance to the local situation (see chapter 8). Although convinced of the soundness of its recommendations, the members of the consensus meeting recognised a serious gap between many of the recommendations and current conditions in countries. This necessitates the formulation at national and local level of new policies for the care of pregnant women. The work of the WHO consensus meetings such as the one just held could provide a rational foundation for beginning the reformulation of such policies.

This first meeting in Washington DC on pregnancy care was to be followed by a second meeting on birth care just five months later in Fortaleza, Brazil. Based on the first meeting, we wanted to make some adjustments in the organisation of the following one so that final recommendations would be more specific and there would be more emphasis on how to implement change. The following chapter describes the results of this second consensus meeting.

References

Altman D. & Hytten F. 1989, 'Assessment of fetal size and fetal growth', in *Effective Care in Pregnancy and Childbirth*, eds I. Chalmers, M. Enkin & M. Keirse, Oxford University Press, Oxford.

American College of Obstetricians and Gynecologists 1965, *Standards for Obstetric-Gynecologic Services*, Washington, DC.

—— 1982, *Standards for Obstetric–Gynecologic Services*, Washington, DC.

Banta H. D. 1985, 'Prenatal care — an introduction' *International Journal of Technology Assessment in Health Care*, vol. 1, no. 4, pp. 783–788.

Beech B. & Robinson J. 1993, 'Ultrasound? unsound', *Association for the Improvement in Maternity Services Journal*, vol. 5, no. 1, pp. 3–26.

British Medical Journal 1988, editorial: Radiation and Mental Retardation, vol. 297, pp. 153.

Brown S. (ed.) 1988, *Prenatal Care. Reaching Mothers, Reaching Infants*, Committee to Study Outreach for Prenatal Care, Institute of Medicine, Washington DC, National Academy Press.

Burton B., Schulz C. J. & Burd L. I. 1992, 'Limb anomalies associated with chorionic villus sampling', *Obstetrics and Gynecology*, vol. 79, pp. 726–730.

Caldeyro-Barcia R. 1984, 'Purposes of prenatal care', presented at the Consensus Conference on Appropriate Technology for Prenatal Care, World Health Organisation, Washington DC.

Campbell S. & Little D. 1980, 'Clinical potential of real-time ultrasound', in *Real-time Ultrasound in Obstetrics*, eds M. Bennett & S. Campbell, Blackwell Scientific Publications, Oxford.

Chalmers B. 1982, 'Stressful life events and pregnancy complications: a summary of research findings', *Humanitas*, vol. 8, no. 1, pp. 49–57.

Chalmers I., personal communication.

Chalmers I., Enkin M. & Keirse M. (eds) 1989, *Effective Care in Pregnancy and Childbirth*, Oxford University Press, Oxford.

Chassar Moir J. 1960, 'The uses and value of radiology in obstetrics', in *Antenatal and Postnatal Care*, eds F. Browne & McClure-Brown, 9th edition, J & A Churchill, London.

Cnattingius J. 1984, *Screening for intrauterine growth retardation, doctoral dissertation*, Uppsala University, Sweden.

Cochrane A. 1989, forward in *Effective Care in Pregnancy and Childbirth*, eds I. Chalmers, M. Enkin & M. Keirse, Oxford University Press, Oxford.

Collaborative Group on Drug Use in Pregnancy 1991, 'An international survey on drug utilisation during pregnancy', *International Journal of Risk and Safety in Medicine*, vol. 1, p. 1.

—— 1992, 'Medication during pregnancy: an intercontinental cooperative study', *International Journal of Gynecol and Obstet.*

Crane J. P., Beaver H. A. & Cheung S. W. 1988, 'First trimester chorionic villus sampling versus mid-trimester genetic amniocentesis-preliminary results of a controlled prospective trial', *Prenatal Diagnosis*, vol. 8, no. 355–366.

Creasy R. 1991, 'Preventing preterm birth', *New England Journal of Medicine*, vol. 325, no. 10, p. 727.

Crowther C. & Chalmers I. 1989, 'Bed rest and hospitalisation during pregnancy' in *Effective Care in Pregnancy and Childbirth*, eds I. Chalmers, M. Enkin & M. Keirse, Oxford University Press, Oxford.

Elbourne D., Richardson M., Chalmers I., Waterhouse I. & Holt E. 1987, 'The Newbury maternity care study: a randomised controlled trial to evaluate a policy of women holding their own obstetric records', *British Journal of Obstet Gynecol*, vol. 94, pp. 612–619.

Ershoff D., Quinn V., Mullen P. & Lairson D. 1990, 'Pregnancy and medical cost outcomes of a self-help prenatal smoking cessation program in a HMO', *Public Health Reports*, vol. 105, no. 4, pp. 340–7.

EUROCAT Newsletter 1992, 'Chorionic villus sampling and limb reduction', vol. 6, no. 2.

Ewigman B. G., Crane J. P., Fredric D., Frigoletto F. D., LeFevre M. L., Bain R. P, McNellis D. & the RADIUS study group 1993, 'Effect of prenatal ultrasound screening on perinatal outocme', *New England Journal of Medicine*, vol. 329, no. 12, pp. 821–827.

Farnot U. 1985, 'Use of different systems for classifying populations at risk', *International Journal of Technology Assessment in Health Care*, vol. 1, no. 4, pp. 821–832.

Firth H., Boyd P. A., Chamberlain P., MacKenzie I. Z., Lindenbaum R. H. & Huson S. M. 1991, 'Severe limb abnormalities after chorionic villus sampling at 56–66 day's gestation', *Lancet*, vol. 337, pp. 127–135.

Fraser C. 1983, 'Selected perinatal procedures', *Acta Obstetricia et Gynecologica Scandinavica*, supplement 117.

Froster-Tskenius U. & Baird P. 1989, 'Limb reduction defects in over one million consecutive live births', *Teratology*, vol. 39, pp. 127–135.

Gallagher J. 1987, 'Prenatal invasions and interventions: what's wrong with fetal rights', *Harvard Women's Law Journal*, vol. 10, pp. 9–58.

Goldstein P., Sacks H. & Chalmers T. 1989, 'Hormone administration for the maintenance of pregnancy', in *Effective Care in Pregnancy and Childbirth*, eds I. Chalmers I, M. Enkin & M. Keirse, Oxford University Press, Oxford.

Hassani S. 1978, *Ultrasound in Gynecology and Obstetrics*, Springer Verlag, New York.

Hemminki E., Malin M. & Kojo-Austin H. 1990, 'Prenatal care in Finland: from primary to tertiary health care?', *International Journal of Health Services*, vol. 20, no. 2, pp. 221–232.

Hsieh F. 1991, 'Limb-reduction defects and chorionic villus sampling', *Lancet*, vol. 337, pp. 1091–1092.

Hunter D. & Keirse M. 1989, 'Gestational diabetes', in *Effective Care in Pregnancy and Childbirth*, eds I. Chalmers, M. Enkin & M. Keirse, Oxford University Press, Oxford.

Inch S. 1986, foreword, *Birth*, vol. 13, pp. 3, special supplement 'Forum on Maternity and the Newborn: Ultrasonography in Obstetrics'.

Jackson L. 1991, 'Limb abnormalities and chorionic villus sampling', *Lancet*, vol. 337, p. 1423.

Kotelchuck M., Schwartz J. B., Anderka M. T. & Finison K. S. 1984, 'WIC participation and pregnancy outcomes: Massachusetts Statewide Evaluation Project', *American Journal of Public Health*, vol. 74, pp. 1146–1148.

Kleinman J., Pierre M. B., Adans J. H., Land G. H. & Schramm W. F. 1988, 'The effects of maternal smoking on fetal and infant mortality', *American Journal of Epidemiology*, vol. 127, no. 2, pp. 274–282.

Lancet 1981, 'Bed rest in obstetrics', editorial, May 23, pp. 1137–38.

—— 1884, 'Diagnostic ultrasound in pregnancy', editorial, July 28, pp. 201–202.

Lippman A., Tomkins D. J., Shime J. & Hamerton J. L. 1992, 'Canadian multicenter randomised clinical trial of chorion villus sampling and amniocentesis. Final report', *Prenatal Diagnosis*, vol. 12, pp. 385–476.

Lovell A., Zander L. I., James C. E., Foot S., Swan A. V. & Reynolds A. 1987, 'The St. Thomas's maternity case notes study:a randomised controlled trial to assess the effects of giving expectant mothers their own maternity case notes', *Paediatric and Perinatal Epidemiology*, vol. 1, pp. 57–66.

Macintyre S. 1981, 'Expectations and experiences of first pregnancy', occasional paper no. 5, MRC Medical Sociology Unit, Aberdeen.

Mahoney M. 1991, 'Limb abnormalities and chorionic villus sampling', *Lancet*, vol. 337, pp. 1422–1423.

Mastroiacovo P. & Cavalcanti D. 1991, 'Limb abnormalities and chorionic villus sampling', *Lancet*, vol. 337, p. 1423.

McKinlay J. 1981, 'from "promising report" to "standard procedure": seven stages in the career of a medical innovation', *Milbank Memorial Fund Quarterly*, vol. 59, pp. 374–411.

Meire H. 1987, 'The safety of diagnostic ultrasound', *British Journal of Obstetrics and Gynecology*, vol. 94, pp. 1121–1122.

Miller M. 1989, 'Psychosocial factors related to smoking behaviour during pregnancy', doctoral dissertation, Dept. of Health Education, Temple University, Philadelphia.

Ministry of Health of Turkey 1990, personal communication.

Miny P. 1991, 'Limb abnormalities and chorionic villus sampling', *Lancet*, vol. 337, pp. 1423–1424.

Monni G. 1991, 'Limb-reduction defects and chorionic villus sampling', *Lancet*, vol. 337, p. 1091.

MRC Working Party 1991, 'Medical Research Council European trial of chorionic villus sampling', *Lancet*, vol. 337, pp. 1491–1499.

National Institutes of Health 1984, 'Diagnostic ultrasound imaging in pregnancy', *Consensus Development Conference Consensus Statement*, vol. 5, no. 1, Washington DC.

Neilson J. 1984, 'Screening for small-for-dates fetus: a prospective randomised controlled trial', *British Medical Journal*, vol. 289, p. 1179.

Neilson J. & Grant A. 1989, 'Ultrasound in pregnancy', in *Effective Care in Pregnancy and Childbirth*, eds I. Chalmers, M. Enkin & M. Keirse, Oxford University Press, Oxford.

Newnham J. 1992, personal communication.

Newnham J., Evans S. F., Michael C. A., Stanley F. J. & Landau L. I. 1993, 'Effects of frequent ultrasound during pregnancy: a randomised controlled trial', *Lancet*, vol. 342, pp. 887–891.

Oakley A. 1979, *Becoming a Mother*, Martin Robertson, Oxford.

—— 1984, *The Captured Womb*, Blackwell Publishing, Oxford.

—— 1985, 'A social support and perinatal outcome', *International Journal of Technology Assessment in Health Care*, vol. 1, no. 4, pp. 843–854.

—— 1985b, 'Social support in pregnancy: the "soft" way to increase birthweight?', *Soc Sci Med*, vol. 21, no. 11, pp. 1259–1268.

—— 1986, 'The history of ultrasonography in obstetrics birth', special supplement: Forum on Maternity and the Newborn, *Ultrasonography in Obstetrics*, December 1986.

Pagel M., Smilkstein G., Regen H. & Montano D. 1990, 'Psychosocial influences on new born outcomes: a controlled prospective study', *Soc Sci Med*, vol. 30, no. 5, pp. 597–604.

Reece L. 1935, 'The estimation of fetal maturity by a new method of x-ray cephalometry: its bearing on clinical midwifery', *Proc Royal Soc Med*, vol. 18, p. 489.

Reid M. & Garcia J. 1989, 'Women's views of care during pregnancy and childbirth' in *Effective Care in Pregnancy and Childbirth*, eds I. Chalmers, M. Enkin & M. Keirse, Oxford University Press, Oxford.

Rhoads G., Jackson L. G., Schlesselman S. E., de-la-Cruz F. F., Desnick R. J., Golbus M. S., Ledbetter D. H., Lubs H.A., Mahoney M. J., Pergament E., et al. 1989, 'The safety and efficacy of chorionic villus sampling for early prenatal diagnosis of cytogenetic abnormalities', *New England Journal of Medicine*, vol. 320, pp. 609–617.

Rush D. 1989, 'Effects of changes in protein and calorie intake during pregnancy on the growth of the human fetus', in *Effective Care in Pregnancy and Childbirth*, eds I. Chalmers, M. Enkin & M. Keirse, Oxford University Press, Oxford.

Ruzek S. 1990, 'Defining risk: the assessment of new birth technologies', presented at NICHD–SSRC Conference West Virginia, USA, May 1, 1990.

Ruzek S. 1991, 'Women's reproductive rights: the impact of technology' in *Women and New Reproductive Technologies: Medical, Psychological, Legal, and Ethical Dilemmas*, eds J. Rodin & A. Collins, Lawrence Erlbaum Assoc., Publishers, Hillsdale, New Jersey.

Salmond R. 1937, 'The uses and value of radiology in obstetrics', in *Antenatal and Postnatal Care*, ed. F. Browne, Second Edition, J & A Churchill, London.

Salvesen K., Vatten L., Eiknes S., Hughdahl K. & Bakketeig L. 1993, 'Routine ultrasonograpy in utero and subsequent handedness and neurological development', *British Medical Journal*, vol. 307, pp. 159–64.

Schmidt-Jensen 1992, personal communication.

Schwarcz R. 1985, 'Perinatal health and regional activities of the Latin–American centre for perinatology and human development', *International Journal of Technology Assessment in Health Care*, vol. 1, no. 4.

Sexton M. & Hebel J. 1984, 'A clinical trial of change in maternal smoking and its effect on birth weight', *Journal of the American Medical Association*, vol. 251, pp. 911–915.

Shepard T. 1991, 'Limb-reduction defects and chorionic villus sampling', *Lancet*, vol. 337, p. 1092.

Shiono P., Klebanoff M. A. & Rhoads G. G. 1986, 'Smoking and drinking during pregnancy: their effects on preterm birth', *Journal of the American Medical Association*, vol. 255, no. 82–84.

Stembera Z. 1985, personal communication.

Stewart A., Webb J., Giles D. & Hewitt D. 1956, 'Malignant disease in childhood and diagnostic irradiation in utero', *Lancet*, vol. 2, p. 447.

Tzoumaka-Bakoula C. 1987, 'The Greek National Perinatal Survey: design, methodology, case ascertainment', *Paediatric & Perinatal Epidemiology*, vol. 1, pp. 43–51.

Tzoumaka-Bakoula C., Lekea-Karanika V., Matsaniotis N. S., McCarthy B. & Golding J. 1990, 'Birthweight specific perinatal mortality in Greece', *Acta Pediatrica Scandanavia*, vol. 79, pp. 47–51.

UNICEF 1992, 'Drug use in pregnancy', *The Prescriber*, January 1992.

USA Today/International edition 1993, editorial Sept. 18, pp. 7A.

Villar J. & Belizan J. 1986, 'The evaluation of methods used in the diagnosis of intrauterine growth retardation', *Obstet Gynecol Survey*, vol. 41, pp. 187–199.

Wagner M. 1985, 'Health services for pregnancy in Europe', *International Journal of Technology Assessment in Health Care*, vol. 1, no. 4, pp. 789–798.

Wallace H. 1988, 'Infant mortality', in *Maternal and Child Health Practices*, ed. H. M. Wallace, 3rd edition, pp. 411–426, California Third Party Publishers, Oakland.

World Health Organisation 1984a, 'Diagnostic ultrasound in pregnancy: WHO view on routine screening', *Lancet*, vol. 2, p. 361.

—— 1984b, 'Working group on fetal diagnosis of hereditary diseases', *Bulletin of the World Health Organisation*, vol. 62, pp. 345–355, Geneva.

—— 1985, *Having a Baby in Europe*, Public Health in Europe Series no. 26, European Regional Office, Copenhagen.

—— 1992, *Working Group on Risk Evaluation of Chorionic villus sampling*, report, Regional Office for Europe Maternal and Child Health Unit, Copenhagen.

Yankauer A. 1984, 'Science and social policy', *American Journal of Public Health*, vol. 74, no. 10, p. 1148.

Chapter 6

Technology for Birth: A Consensus Meeting in Fortaleza, Brazil

Imagine that you are a midwife: you are assisting at someone
else's birth. Do good without show or fuss. Facilitate what is
happening rather than what you think ought to be happening.
When the baby is born, the mother will rightly say:
"We did it ourselves".

Lao Tzu, The tao of leadership (5th century B.C.)

Introduction

The consensus meeting on Appropriate Technology for Birth began
with an overview of current services for birth in Europe and the
Americas (Wagner 1985; Schwarcz 1985). In Europe, except for The
Netherlands, the trend was towards all births taking place in hospitals equipped with all the technology available. While the midwife
remained the primary birth attendant for normal birth in almost all
countries, her role had been gradually eroded. In general, the use of
technology in birth is gradually increasing across Europe. Although
variations within and between countries are great, levels of use have
not yet reached the extremes generally found in North America and
some private hospitals in Latin America.

Large parts of the population in Latin America receive no official
health care. In many countries, women have low status, and often a
high rate of illiteracy. There is a surplus of physicians in the cities.
Midwives in Latin America have very low status although they exist
in all countries. There is an extensive system of unofficial healers,
but its size is unknown. Traditional healers and empirical midwives
(midwives trained through an informal apprenticeship — also

called lay midwives, traditional midwives or traditional birth attendants) are recognised officially in very few places.

In urban areas of Latin America, most births take place in big hospitals, handling 20,000–50,000 births a year. To accommodate these births, in many large hospitals there are high rates of induction of labour, episiotomy, forceps deliveries and caesarean sections. This leaves no time, space or possibility for proper attention to be paid to the emotional and social aspects of birth. The small affluent urban population can purchase high-technology birth services from the private health care sector. In rural areas, most births take place at home, often under quite primitive conditions and with an empirical midwife in attendance. Because empirical midwives are not recognised by the official health system in most places, they cannot refer complicated births to a hospital.

These facts showed that birth care in the countries of Europe and North and South America has at least two characteristics: inappropriate use of birth technology and of human resources for birth care. The participants started with the feeling of facing an immense task. How could consensus be reached on what birth care should be (as opposed to what it is)? How could changes in policy be promoted?

The consensus meeting was presented with descriptions of innovative programs for birth services that combined the medical and social perspectives. In The Netherlands, for example, over one third of all births are planned home births, attended solely by a midwife (Phaff 1986). Further, several review papers documented Dr Araújo's project in Fortaleza, in which the empirical midwives in rural areas have been brought into the official system of care (Araújo 1985; Janowitz 1985). Other obstetrical care services were described which had critical attitudes towards technology and respect for the emotional, psychological and social aspects of birth. The participants found these unusual programs important aids in its task. One of the recommendations took note of innovative services and encourages them as models to influence obstetrical views (see appendix for all recommendations from this meeting).

Birth as a normal process

As an effective and dramatic way to document the divergence in views of birth, the organisers of the meeting asked one representative of each interested party to present a paper on birth as a normal process. Anyone listening to the seven resulting papers found it hard to believe they were all talking about the same thing.

The obstetrician said that birth is normal when there are no pathological deviations and no need to intervene. According to the epidemiologist, birth is normal when it is an entirely physiological process, although he added that the tendency to intervene has limited knowledge about normal physiology. The midwife asked (rhetorically) if the not-abnormal were normal. Answering this question in the negative, she proposed that having a baby is a normal process in life, regardless of outcome, even when complications arise. She concluded that birth is normal if it is seen as normal by the woman involved, if it mirrors her way of living. The psychologist defined birth as a normal developmental crisis that is decisive in personal emotional development towards womanhood and motherhood. The anthropologist stated that the modern world is involved in a process of 'abnormalising' birth. Anthropology has described the diversity of human societies, each with an extremely rich and varied repertory of techniques and forms of childbirth. People in each of these societies value their kind of birth as effective. The sociologist indicated that sociology does not see birth as a normal process but as a social process, which is not quite the same thing. Sociological research adds up to the statement that nothing is intrinsically normal or natural about birth: what happens depends on the woman's personality and circumstances. Whether birth is seen and treated as normal is a function of who has the power to define normality, and who lacks the power to make and maintain an alternative definition. The user of birth services concluded that birth is normal when the woman controls it.

In the panel on birth as a normal process and the general discussion that followed, several overarching issues arose. The first was the domination of birth by health professionals and its consequences. The fact that different professional groups were asked to write papers on this issue tells, in part, why birth must be seen as a normal process. Today, birth is often considered an abnormal event. It is an episode in the lives of women and families that is not part of everyday life but an occasion for medical surveillance and treatment. Thus, to think about the possible normality of birth requires a deliberate shift of focus. This was not necessary before birth became the province of experts. Obstetricians and paediatricians are not the only experts who have helped to make birth abnormal. Other professional groups have also participated and benefited, including psychologists, sociologists, anthropologists, epidemiologists, technicians and other members of the commercial world surrounding birth. Despite their different perspectives, all these groups actually collaborated in transforming birth into a professional subject.

Intense discussion ensued over the midwife's assertion of the normalcy of birth regardless of the outcome. Indeed, it seemed possible to differentiate between holders of the medical and social perspectives simply by their response to the question of whether birth is a normal process when it ends with a dead baby. No consensus was reached on the answer, but the participants agreed the issue of the normalcy of birth is worth a lot of thought by everyone involved.

Further, the participants agreed that no one really knows what a normal birth is. The WHO European Perinatal Study Group had raised this important issue in its review of current birth care: by 'medicalising' birth, i.e., separating a woman from her own environment and surrounding her with strange people using strange machines to do strange things to her in an effort to assist her (and much or all of this may sometimes be necessary), the woman's state of mind and body is so altered that her way of carrying through this intimate act must also be altered and the state of the baby born must equally be altered. The result is that it is no longer possible to know what births would have been like before these manipulations. Most health care providers no longer know what 'non-medicalised' birth is. This is an overwhelmingly important issue. Almost all women in most developed countries give birth in hospital, leaving the providers of the birth services with no genuine yardstick against which to measure their care. What is the range for length of safe labour? What is the true (i.e., absolute minimum) incidence of respiratory distress syndrome of newborn babies? What is the incidence of tears of the tissues surrounding the vaginal opening if the tissues are not first cut? What is the incidence of depression in women after 'non-medicalised' birth? The answer to all these and many more questions is the same: no one knows. The entire modern obstetric and neonatological literature is essentially based on observations of 'medicalised' birth (WHO 1985a).

Social factors in birth

One of the major issues discussed at the consensus meeting was the role of social factors in birth and birth services. Building on the discussions of social factors in the earlier meeting on pregnancy care as well as a number of papers presented at Fortaleza, consensus evolved on three general principles which are reflected in a number of final recommendations: centrality of women; respect for the psychological and social aspects; different professions providing different care.

Centrality of women

The centrality of women was felt to be as important in birth care and formulating policy on birth care as in pregnancy care and policy. Again, the key to action on this belief was informed choice. Unfortunately there is lack of informed choice in many countries as shown by the results of a WHO survey (table 1).

One of the recommendations, for example, emphasised the value of women's mutual aid groups in giving social support to the woman when she gives birth and in providing her with the information necessary for making proper, informed choices at this time. Women more experienced with birth can work with the pregnant woman in drafting a written plan for her hospital birth that includes her wishes about the use of various procedures and types of technology. The plan can be presented to the hospital staff, ideally before the birth, so the woman and the staff can discuss and perhaps negotiate the best way to achieve her goals.

Another recommendation proposed that the woman choose someone to be with her during the birth and that this person have easy access for visits during the postnatal period. Much scientific literature shows the value of a companion (often called a doula) in supporting the woman and acting as her advocate, to ensure she has the

Procedure	No. of countries offering	
	choice	no choice
Shaving	5	18
Birth method	0	23
Birth position	3	20
Anaesthesia/analgesia	10	13
People present	10	13
Choice of doctor	8	15
Holding dead newborn	11	12
Electronic fetal monitoring	5	18
Episiotomy	1	22

(WHO 1985a, p. 25)

Table 1: *Women's choice in selecting routine procedures in uncomplicated births in official services in 23 survey countries.*

type of birth appropriate for her. Scientific research has shown that this shortens labour and significantly reduces complications and the necessity for obstetrical intervention (Hemminki et al. 1990; Klaus et al. 1986; Sosa et al. 1980; Kennell et al. 1988; Hofmeyer et al. 1991). After reviewing the scientific literature, Keirse, Enkin and Lumley conclude: "It is inappropriate for hospitals to take it upon themselves to exclude any category of support person from labour and birth. Where women have strong preferences for who should be with them at this time, these should be respected" (Keirse et al. 1991, p. 813). It is important to remember that in 126 of 127 non-industrialised societies from which data is available it is an established practice that a women is present with the labouring women during her entire labour (Murdock & White 1969).

A recent analysis of the randomised clinical trials on the effect of social support during labour on perinatal outcome concluded: "It would appear that continuous support during labour is an essential ingredient of the labour that has unfortunately been left out when maternity care moved from home to hospital in the early 1930s. Randomised trials of continuous emotional and physical support during labour have resulted in multiple benefits, which include a shorter labour, significanlty less medication and fewer medical interventions, including caesarean section, forceps, and epidural anasthaesia" (Klaus et al. 1992). The authors point out other benefits: "They [doulas] have also been associated with positive social outcomes such as decreased maternal anxiety and depression, increased breastfeeding and increased satisfaction with interpersonal relations with partners".

Using a doula is another example of simple, appropriate technology which can save money. It has been estimated that if every woman in the United States had a supportive woman with her conitinously throughout labour, the reduction in interventions such as caesarean sections and epidurals would reduce maternity care costs by more than two billion dollars a year (Klaus et al. 1992). For all these reasons, the particpants unanimously agreed to the recommendation for the labouring woman to have the choice of a companion throughout birth.

Two other recommendations were made in an effort to guarantee all women the right to informed choice about the policy on and nature of the birth care in their communities. The first stated that the whole community should be informed about the various birth care procedures available. Each hospital should make freely available to the public it serves, information on its rates of anaesthesia, episiotomy, forceps or vacuum extraction, caesarean section and perinatal mortality. Hospitals that do so recognise their responsibility to the people in their communities. In the United States two States, Massachusetts and New York, have already passed a law to guarantee access to such data and the idea is spreading. A book *The New Good Birth Guide* (Kitzinger 1983) based on a survey of all the institutions in which to give birth in the United Kingdom, provides this type of information and has been a best seller in that country. The Director of the National Perinatal Epidemiology Unit in the United Kingdom said that this book has probably done more than any other single publication, scientific or popular, to improve maternity care in Britain (Chalmers 1989, personal communication). The participants agreed that information on birth care procedures would allow each woman to make better choices for the birth of her baby, and provide women in the community with a good data base from which to make policy recommendations.

The second recommendation also addressed the public disclosure of information. The consensus was that the results of assessment of birth care technology should be disseminated to health professionals, the users of birth services and the general public. Here the principle is similar: usually research on birth technology is used on and ultimately paid for by the public, and thus researchers are responsible to the public. Information on technology assessment would allow each woman to make a better choice about the technology to be used on her and provide a data base for policy recommendations. One way to facilitate public access to research data is to involve the people on whom technology is to be used in conducting the assessment.

Respect for the psychological and social aspects

The second general principle arising from the discussion of social factors in birth was the need for obstetrical care services to adopt an attitude of respect for the psychological and social aspects of birth care. This requires that training in birth care should aim to improve students' knowledge of the social, cultural and ethical aspects of birth. Two recommendations were directed to this principle. The problem, of course, is how to implement them, given current conditions in birth and birth care.

A consideration of the social factors in birth must include the nature of the social interaction between the mother, the infant and the family during and after birth. The importance of a companion during labour and birth has already been mentioned. Equally important, persons of the woman's choice should have free access to her for visits during the remainder of her hospital stay. If implemented, this would guarantee opportunities for family and friends to have adequate contact with the mother and new baby. While most hospitals in Canada, the United States and Western Europe already have policies in accord with this recommendation, many hospitals in Latin America and almost all in Eastern Europe permit no non-professionals except the woman to enter the labour and birth rooms (WHO 1985a). In these countries, the father of the child and other family members, including other children, have little or no access to the mother and the new baby in the hospital.

The reason often given for these restrictive visiting policies is the danger of bringing infectious agents into the hospital. Considerable research has shown, however, that this is not a problem; such visiting is not associated with increased infection or illness in mother or baby. The importance of this subject justifies quoting the scientists who thoroughly reviewed the literature on maternity hospital practices and infections of mother and baby.

"The various restrictive and interventionist policies that have been introduced in the care of hospitalized mothers and babies in an attempt to control nosocomial infection were conceptualized through induction based on theoretical considerations, rather than through deduction from empirical evidence, derived from controlled trials — that is, they were based on what *should* work rather than what *does* work. Gradually the various elements of this wholesale and poorly controlled experiment on women and their babies have been challenged with evidence from randomised controlled trials, and studies using other designs. Williams and Oliver (1969), for example, described how in one nursery some of the long standing procedures were removed sequentially while monitoring colonization rates in newborn infants. The removal, one after the other, of rules for wearing caps, masks, and hairnets; for delivery room baby bathing; for restricting access of mothers and students to the nursery; and for initial scrub brushing of hands and gowning while doing incubator care, was not associated with any significant rise in colonization rates.

"Yet, many restrictive and costly practices remain in force today. For example, recent survey data from 712 American doctors and institutions revealed that the gowning rule persists in 73% of newborn nursery settings, despite the lack of evidence that this ritual has any beneficial effect (Cloney & Donowitz 1986). As mentioned earlier, many hospitals invoke concern about infection as a reason for restricting or forbidding siblings to visit, although studies using concurrent and historical control groups have been unable to detect any adverse effect of sibling visiting on infant colonisation rates (Umphenour 1980; Wranesh 1982; Maloney et al. 1983; Kowba & Schwirian 1985). This segregation is particularly ironic in the light of the evidence already presented suggesting that earlier and longer contact between babies and their mothers after birth may well have contributed to the welcome decline in staphylococcal infection in newborn infants. Observational data continue to give support to the notion that early and increased contact between mothers and their newborn infants reduces the risk of bacterial colonisation. In a recent study (Rush et al. 1987), colonisation rates were more than twice as high among babies who had spent less than 50% of their hospital stay with their mothers than among those who spent more than 50% of the time rooming-in" (Rush et al. 1991, p. 1339).

There was agreement during the discussion that a more important implicit reason for restricted visiting was the convenience of the hospital staff. The more recent scientific literature clearly shows the importance of adequate contact with family and friends around the time of birth for the psychological and social wellbeing of all family members (Rush et al. 1991); this consideration must override any inconvenience to hospital staff. The presence of relatives and friends after a birth is a recognition of the importance of the event in the life of the family and community.

The scientific research on the attachment (or bonding) between the mother and infant at the time of birth and in the first few days afterwards was reviewed. This is a subject which has received considerable attention in the literature including a number of controlled trials. An excellent review of this work is given by Thomson and Westreich (1991). While not all research on this subject meets the highest standards, in general the data overwhelmingly support both recommendations made at the conference: allowing healthy newborn infants to remain with their mothers (rooming-in) and promoting the immediate beginning of breastfeeding, even before the mother leaves the birth room. Research has shown that separating the mother and infant after birth may lead to postpartum depression in the mother and developmental problems in the infant. A woman who puts her newborn infant to her breast within the first 20 minutes after birth breastfeeds longer and more successfully. A geographical pattern similar to that for family contact is found. Most hospitals in Canada, the United States and Western Europe allow rooming-in and promote immediate breastfeeding. In Latin America such practices are found in only a few hospitals; in Eastern Europe they are almost unheard of and are just beginning as experiments in a few places.

Different professions, different care

The way in which the various health professions participate in birth care is a third key issue. As pointed out in earlier chapters, through historical accident three health professions are vying for some degree of control of birth care. In general, each group has a different view of birth. Obstetrics has a medical perspective, midwifery, a social one, and general practitioners, a view somewhere between the two. As a result, the current situation is somewhat confusing and, in some places, chaotic or confrontational.

Obstetrics

Obstetrics is a specialty with a long history of turmoil. The specialty is a joining together of two strange bedfellows, surgeons and midwives. The surgical heritage leads to an interest in intervention and technology while the midwifery heritage encourages less intervention and a humanistic approach. Within the profession one finds conflict between conservative and progressive obstetricians. Regardless of how many women practice obstetrics the specialty is male dominated. Recently in many countries this male hegemony has experienced frequent criticism from the women's movement, who express concern for men's attempt to control women's reproductive lives.

In Europe, obstetricians are mainly hospital-based specialists who concentrate on complicated births. In a few countries, they may also practise outside the public hospital, in a private hospital or clinic, but even here the tendency is to focus on problem births. With the coming of the risk system, the obstetrician often attends the births of women labelled as high risk even when they have not experienced complications, expanding the role of this profession in Europe. The public and policy-makers perceive obstetrics as the highest level of expertise on birth, so it is the most important — if not the only — health profession to contribute to policy-making on birth care, including care for normal births. In some European countries, general practitioners attend some normal births or provide first-level back-up to midwives attending normal births. Nevertheless, most complicated births are referred to the obstetrician. In general, as the role of obstetrics in birth has expanded in Europe, the role of general practice has declined.

In the United States and Canada, obstetricians attend great numbers of normal births, in addition to high-risk or complicated births. This extraordinary situation is found in only a few places elsewhere in the world, and health professionals (including obstetricians) from other countries cannot understand its rationale. While general practitioners and family practitioners also attended normal and sometimes even complicated births in the past, they rarely do so any more, partly because of its drain on their lifestyle and partly because of reimbursement and malpractice issues.

In Latin America, most obstetricians are hospital-based specialists managing difficult or high-risk births, although they may also attend normal births among the few affluent women in the cities. As in Europe, obstetricians have growing influence on policy on birth services and practices. General practitioners attend many normal births in the cities and more developed rural areas of Latin America. As more and more physicians are trained, they attend an increasing number of births.

Midwifery

Midwifery has been a legitimate and well established health profession in Europe for hundreds of years. The midwife is still the birth attendant at the majority of normal births in nearly every European country. Most women not only expect the presence of a midwife but feel it is their right. Studies show that women prefer midwives to care for them (Flint 1991). In the majority of European countries, midwives go to midwifery school without previous professional training; this is called direct entry training. In a small number of countries, some or all train first as nurses. Whatever the type of training, every European country has only one type of midwife — formally trained and officially certified — and she is called simply a midwife.

Recent decades have seen a significant change in midwifery in most of Europe. In general, the midwife's importance has been attacked, her status as an independent health professional eroded, and her practice shrunk. The geographical distribution of this trend is interesting; the role of midwives decreases as one goes further east and further south in Europe. Midwifery has been diminished in a variety of ways. First, in many countries the directors of midwifery schools are obstetricians, and physicians give much of the instruction. Second, the legislation or regulations determining what midwives may do at a birth have changed. For example, in some countries midwives may no longer perform an episiotomy; in one country, they may perform the episiotomy but not sew it up. Nevertheless, in a few countries, such as Denmark and The Netherlands, midwifery (not without a struggle) has managed to remain a strong, independent health profession, with sole responsibility for attending the majority of normal births.

> "The Dutch midwife, who does not have a prior qualification in nursing, is trained and recognised as an autonomous practitioner, a specialist in normal childbirth, legally permitted to perform a few intranatal interventions, including episiotomy and perineal suturing, but barred from using instruments. The pregnant woman can refer herself directly to a midwife and so long as she remains within certain defined risk criteria, the midwife will undertake complete maternity care with a free choice of conducting the delivery in the woman's home or in hospital, retaining her own control and using only her own permitted methods" (Tew & Damstra-Wijmenga 1991).

In other countries there is a clear resurgence of midwifery. Hard data is beginning to substantiate the widespread observation that women cared for by midwives have less interventions than women under obstetric care (Runnerstrom 1969; Flint 1991). Furthermore at least one study suggests that, at least for women at low risk, the midwife is the *safest* birth attendant. "Analysis of national perinatal statistics from Holland, 1986, demonstrates that for all births after 32 week's gestation mortality is much lower under the non-interventionist care of midwives than under the interventionist management of obstetricians at all levels of predicted risk." (Tew & Damstra-Wijmenga 1991) These findings are consistent with the observation that in the Nordic countries (Denmark, Sweden, Norway, Finland), which have lower perinatal mortality rates than any other country in Europe or North America, over 70% of births have a midwife as the only birth attendant and there is never a doctor in the room. These are some of the reasons behind a recent report from the British House of Parliament recommending a strong, central role of midwives in maternity care (House of Commons 1992).

The situation of midwifery in Canada and the United States can only be described as chaotic. Midwifery has been illegal in Canada, although a handful of midwives practise in every province. Ontario Province passed new legislation in 1990 to bring midwifery into the official health care system for the first time. In 1993 two further provinces acted: British Columbia recognised midwifery as a legitimate health profession; Quebec began official programs to start midwifery practice on an experimental basis. Because of a number of court cases on birth care and a consequent rise in the cost of malpractice insurance, many obstetricians and general practitioners no longer attend births. Without a cadre of midwives in place, birth care in Canada is becoming more and more uncertain. While Ontario is presently certifying the approximately 100 already practising midwives, retraining them when necessary, and will start Canada's first ever midwifery school in the mid 1990s, it will be a long time before there are adequate numbers of midwives in Canada.

The United States has three types of midwife, and every state has its own legislation on whether midwives (or certain types) can practise and what they are allowed to do. Nurse-midwives, a title and concept not found outside North America, train first as nurses and then train as midwives. They are permitted to practice in nearly all States but there may be restrictions on where and how they practice. Direct entry midwives do not train first as nurses but go directly to midwifery training. There are various educational models for direct entry training, most using a mix of conventional (classroom) and apprenticeship training. The legality of practice of direct entry midwives varies widely among States, from fully certified and registered to no legal status. Empirical midwives (also called lay or traditional) are trained only through an apprenticeship system. In some States they can take examinations, be certified and registered for practice while in other States they have no legal status and in some areas even may be arrested on criminal charges if they assist at birth (see chapter 1). Controversy still rages over the appropriate role for midwifery in the United States.

Some midwives in the United States work independently in free-standing birth centres, an alternative which has been shown by a nationwide collaborative study to be safe and effective (Rook et al. 1990). But many doctors and hospitals see such centres as competition and as a result many doctors who have provided medical backup to birth centres have been sanctioned through loss of hospital privileges and other means. In 1991, while in Des Moines Iowa, a leading practising obstetrician told me that the only birth centre in his city was stealing his patients and he wanted it stopped. A few months later the only physician in that city willing to provide medical backup to the birth centre retired and the centre was forced to close.

In the United States the issue of who is to give maternity care to poor women is acute. In many of the largest cities, the majority of practising obstetricians refuse to give care if the women's bill is to be paid by public funds. These same doctors frequently block attempts to use midwives as a solution. For example, in 1991 the California Medical Association successfully stopped a bill to expand midwifery services from passing the State legislature (personal communication, State Senator Killea, 1992). Meanwhile a private hospital in Los Angeles hired security guards to patrol the hospital parking lot to stop poor women in active labour from gaining access to the emergency room where the hospital is obliged to provide assistance (*Cable News Network* 1989). And in 1992 the County of Los Angeles, desperate to increase the number of poor women receiving prenatal care, tried to expand their prenatal service but could find no obstetricians to staff prenatal clinics and the county did not consider using midwives instead.

The evidence suggests that the United States government is perhaps doing less than it might to promote midwifery. In 1991, the State of Alaska was considering an important bill to expand midwifery in that State. I, representing the European Regional Office of WHO, wrote to the Governor of Alaska explaining why WHO strongly advocates midwifery. The top civil servant in health services in the United States Federal Government, rather than appreciating that WHO was trying to promote midwifery in his country, wrote to the

Director General of WHO complaining that WHO should not mix in internal affairs.

In Latin America, while the excess of physicians is becoming apparent in most countries, the number of nurses has grown very little and the number of formally trained midwives has decreased markedly. Midwifery survives as an officially recognised health profession only in a very few countries such as Chile and Argentina. This changing mixture of birth attendants has resulted in an official maternity care system characterised by spiralling costs, the overuse of technology, and the increasing medicalisation of birth, with decreasing attention to social factors. Although the disappearance of midwives as birth attendants early in this century is now being reversed in North America, the exclusion of midwives continues in the parts of Latin America reached by official health systems.

In many countries of Latin America, however, some areas are still not served by official health care and there are sizeable groups of people who choose to use alternative services, even when the official ones are available. As a result large numbers of births in Latin America are still attended by empirical midwives. With a few exceptions, they are not recognised as professionals by the government. Their exclusion from the official health system eliminates the possibility for the referral of women with problems, thus reducing the accessibility of official care and the options available to the woman who develops complications in birth. In addition, empirical midwives neither benefit from the knowledge in obstetrics and formal midwifery nor contribute their own knowledge of the local culture of birth and traditional birth practices to other health professionals. The field trip made by the Fortaleza meeting demonstrated clearly the many advantages of integrating empirical midwives into the official health care system (Araújo 1985; Janowitz et al. 1985).

WHO studies have shown that attempts in many countries to eliminate traditional health practitioners (such as lay or empirical midwives in the Americas) through legislative and other means have only driven these practitioners underground. An English barrister, after carrying out a study for WHO, wrote:

"Legislation prohibiting the untrained TBA (empirical midwife) from practising is rarely enforceable. In the few countries where such prohibitions have been enacted, (empirical midwives) continue to work, accepted by the community and preferred to the modern health system; the real effect of such legislation has been to force (empirical midwives) to work in secret or to prevent them from being trained. Yet they are tolerated and sometimes found indispensable by health centres. Legislation should facilitate training of (empirical midwives) and authorize them to perform tasks within their competence, rather than set down unenforceable and unrealistic prohibitions" (Owens 1983, p. 447).

It appears that some people will always want the services of such practitioners, who will always perpetuate their tradition. A WHO meeting report has made some important statements with regard to promoting empirical midwives:

"It is now almost universally acknowledged that unless the traditional health practitioners (including empirical midwives) are properly recognised, and articulated with the national health system to implement strategies to achieve health for all by the year 2000, countries will never be able to achieve adequate health coverage for all their populations . . . Almost everywhere, attempts to upgrade the skills and knowledge of empirical midwives and to mobilize them to play an effective role in the health system have met with resistance from organized groups of health professionals with vested interests in maintaining the status quo . . . The development of a policy favourable to empirical midwifery depends upon an enlightened understanding of the nature of such care, and the role and resources of its practitioners, many of whom possess a fund of wisdom, knowledge, and experience that can only serve to improve the quality of care that countries provide for their populations . . . Empirical midwives constitute a major and valuable reserve of human resources that must be better utilized within every country's national health service, if the health status of populations is to be improved . . . Governments should formally recognise and legitimize the practice of empirical midwives . . . In countries where existing legislation is not supportive of empirical midwives, supportive policies should be adopted as a temporary measure until the more time-consuming process of legal reform can be carried out . . . Where existing legislation presents a barrier to the promotion of empirical midwifery, it should be repealed, or amended, and ultimately replaced by supportive legislation. The experience of countries shows that legislation prohibiting the practice of empirical midwives does not succeed" (WHO Report 1985b).

The participants in the consensus meeting tried to determine the national policies in North and South America that produced this chaotic situation or permitted it to evolve. As it must be expected that shortages of formally trained midwives will exist for some time in the United States and Canada as well as Latin America, the promotion of empirical midwives in all the Americas is important.

Policy on personnel for birth care

Policy on personnel for perinatal care is part of larger policies on health personnel and health care in general. In other words, the people who decide what health care should include also decide who should provide it, including who should attend birth. This causes at least two problems. First, in many countries these policies are not determined mainly through a careful, rational assessment of what is needed and what resources are available. Other, less rational factors predominate, such as the influence of the most powerful groups in the health sector, special interest groups (including commercial interests) and particular people.

Second, even if policies on health care and personnel are based on rational assessment, it is inappropriate to apply the principles used for assessing general health care needs to maternity care needs. The birth process creates needs different from any other that the health care system must meet. Effective hospital staffing patterns on a surgical ward, for example, are likely to be inappropriate for a maternity ward. To preserve the social qualities of birth, the maternity ward will need a different mixture of personnel, working hours, hospital and community responsibilities. The forces that determine policies for modern health services obscure the view of birth as a normal process, and thus contribute to its medicalisation. The tendency for birth services to move from the primary care level in the community to the secondary and tertiary levels in the hospital has had a detrimental effect on policy on perinatal care personnel. Birth is considered just another hospital service to be provided. The availability of many types of practitioner to assist at birth, however, provides the opportunity to formulate new policy that makes adjustments in the numbers, responsibilities and combinations of personnel. This would provide a pattern of personnel use appropriate to primary health care.

The meeting reached agreement on policy on the providers of birth care. First, every country needs to work towards a rational policy that respects the unique nature of birth, its place in the family and culture, and local conditions. Very little research has been reported on the personnel needed for birth care, including the optimal mixture of workers assisting at birth. Appropriate health personnel development requires information on health problems and this, in turn, requires epidemiological studies of population needs. Countries need to study their patterns of birth and birth care. Then, with the assistance of all interested parties, they should draw up new policies for the providers of this care. It is hoped that these new policies will be based on the following ideas concerning the balance of obstetrics and midwifery on which there was consensus at the meeting. Midwives are the best experts on normal birth; obstetricians are hospital specialists who devote all their time and expertise to assisting at difficult births. This division of responsibility and labour, between two strong and respected professions seems to create the best conditions for optimal birth care.

When this balance is achieved, there are not only fewer deaths but also a tendency towards lower obstetrical intervention rates and more possibilities for a truly normal birth. The mutual respect and give-and-take can balance the medical and social perspectives and bring forward the best each has to offer. The efforts of midwives to preserve the normalcy of birth can counterbalance the tendency of obstetricians to intervene quickly when signs of trouble appear. The result can be obstetrical intervention rates adequate to meet the needs of complicated births but not so excessive as those in some countries. For these reasons, the final recommendations (see appendix) included that the training of professional midwives or birth attendants be promoted; care during normal pregnancy and birth, and following birth, should be the duty of this profession.

Another recommendation also related to new policies for health workers attending birth: empirical midwives. As a result of the visit to Dr Araújo's project, as well as the review papers and discussion at the meeting, the whole group agreed on the benefits of integrating empirical midwives into the perinatal care system. Everyone involved would profit: empirical midwives, other health care workers and, most importantly, the women giving birth. Both formally trained and empirical midwives emphasise the social perspective, which stresses normality and social and cultural sensitivity. Recognition of this view creates a better balance in the maternity care system. As Dr Araújo wrote in his review paper for the first consensus conference,

> "The success achieved [by the project in Fortaleza] was due, most of all, to the degree to which we were able to win the confidence of these [traditional] birth attendants during their training. Since all they had previously received from the medical profession was harsh criticism or, at times, even promises of help that were never kept, their unreserved cooperation was only obtained by showing them that we fully recognised the inestimable value of the services they were providing by attending to births in their communities" (Araújo 1985).

Accordingly, the participants enthusiastically agreed that the informal perinatal care system (including empirical midwives) must coexist with the official birth care system, and collaboration between them must be maintained for the benefit of the mother. Such relations, when neither is held to be superior, can be highly effective.

Determining appropriateness

The issue of the appropriateness of certain types of technology used during birth was a central theme. The current situation and general principles for appropriate birth technology and its assessment were discussed. Further, specific types of technology (the artificial induction of labour, amniotomy, the positioning of the woman's body, the drugs given, electronic fetal monitoring and caesarean section) were reviewed, to illustrate the issues and because of their importance to birth care and controversial nature.

130

The healthy opposition between enthusiasm for and scepticism about birth technology has a long and respectable history. For example, the introduction of forceps in the eighteenth century sparked much controversy. A sceptical midwife said in 1760 that:

"A few of the midwives, dazzled with the vogue into which the instruments brought the men, attempted to employ them but soon discovered that they were at once insignificant and dangerous substitutes for their own hands, with which they were sure of conducting their operations both more safely, more effectively and with less pain to the patient" (Oakley 1987).

The healthy opposition within the meeting in Fortaleza helped the participants find the right balance in their search for consensus.

One issue was the definition of appropriateness. This clearly depends on the group that makes the definition, which is, as the social scientists in the group pointed out, composed of the people who own and use the technology in question. In general, these people have been physicians, but many in the group favoured the extension of the power of definition to all interested parties.

Again, the use of birth technology in the industrialised countries of Europe and North America is characterised by not only excess but great variation, even among the most prestigious university hospitals. Such variations raise doubt among epidemiologists and other scientists, policy-makers and the public about what really constitutes appropriate use.

The situation in the developing countries of Latin America is even more critical because of the lower level of resources and the greater distance between Latin culture and high technology:

"Whatever the intrinsic value of Western obstetrics, it is quite evident that the Euro–American way of birth has emerged as a seductive standard for most developing nations which aspire to modernisation. Many countries have designed local and national versions of the Western technology for birth that are unmanageable, counter-productive and unacceptable for large segments of the population. In their urge to modernise the national obstetric care delivery system, many health planners in Latin American countries tend to promote certain Western technical practices for which there exists no universal scientific evidence and which contradicts local behaviours grounded in the traditional birthing systems. Apparent technological progress is therefore pure facade, detrimental to large groups of people" (Bibeau 1985, p. 6).

What, then, is the reason for the continuing expansion of the birth machine in Latin America? A review paper by two prominent Latin American obstetricians stated that:

"For many years, programs in obstetrics [in Latin America] have been synonymous with new discoveries and applications of new technologies. In spite of clear proof that some techniques that were universally accepted, used and appraised were far from beneficial and caused maternal and fetal damage, obstetricians still have an almost mystical faith in each new technology offered to obstetrical practice. There is a certain mystic attraction for what is complex, electronic, and somewhat mysterious. Perhaps that is why demanding better proof of efficiency before a new technology is accepted meets with such resistance" (Pinotti & Faundes 1985, p. 1).

The primary need

If much of the use of birth technology is inappropriate, the primary necessity is a system of assessment, so that new policies on birth technology and its use can be based on reason. Although the main reason for assessment is to guide decisions on a particular type of technology, at the policy level the results of assessment can be used to decide how a drug, piece of equipment or procedure should be used in a particular country. Should it be imported? Should its use be regulated, or limited to certain health professions?

From the policy-maker's point of view, the key problem is often the limited financial resources for the health sector. As a result, choices must be made, by policy-makers and the public, in which technology assessment can be helpful. In addition, clinicians (such as physicians and midwives) and pregnant women can use assessments directly, in deciding on the types of technology to offer and to accept.

There was strong consensus on every country's need for a national system for technology assessment. This was the subject of two recommendations:

"Countries should develop the potential to carry out cooperative surveys to evaluate birth care technology; Governments should identify, within the structures of their health ministries, units or departments to take charge of promoting and coordinating the assessment of appropriate technology".

Three countries presently have units involved in assessing birth technologies: the Office of Technology Assessment in the United States (United States Congress, Washington DC 20510–8025), the National Perinatal Epidemiology Unit in the United Kingdom (Radcliffe Infirmary, Oxford) and the Institute for Mother and Child in Czechoslovakia (Nabr. K. Marx 157, 14710 Prague-Podoli). Countries could benefit from looking carefully at these pioneering efforts.

Although experience with technology assessment is limited, it is already clear that useful assessments must include all interested parties. Thus the recommendation:

"Technology assessment should be multidisciplinary and involve all types of providers who use the technology, epidemiologists, social scientists and health authorities. The women on whom the technology is used should be involved in planning the assessment as well as evaluating and disseminating the results. The results of the assessment should be fed back to all those involved in the research as well as to the communities where the research was conducted".

The units in the United States and the United Kingdom are evolving methodology for this purpose.

Elements of comprehensive assessment

At least five kinds of effects should be assessed: benefits and risks; financial costs; social effects; effects on the health care system; effects on the skills of health professionals. These aspects are listed in decreasing frequency of inclusion, although comprehensive assessments cover all five.

The first and most basic measurement is of the efficacy and risks of technology. While efficacy always tends to be assessed, studies that show a desired efficacy tend to be more frequently published, read and quoted than those that show no efficacy. This is understandable in the face of clinicians' wish to help the people who come to them with a specific need. There is an inherent positive bias in the medical literature. At a recent meeting of a European Perinatal Society, a leading German Professor of Obstetrics presented a paper on the History of Obstetrics. The paper listed a series of only positive advances in the field in the past 150 years. During the discussion, my suggestion that such a list was incomplete without including the negative side, for example the thalidomide disaster and the diethyl-stilboestrol tragedy, precipitated an angry rejection.

Clinicians are less interested in negative technology assessment. The other side of the efficacy coin — risk — is less frequently assessed in any systematic or experimental way, in part because lay people are more likely to be concerned about risks than clinicians. This should not be surprising since it is the patients who take the risk and experience the undesired side effects.

Efficacy (the probability of a desired effect) can be measured empirically in statistical terms. But the importance of that desired effect to the individual and/or society is a social value judgement. Risk (the probability of an undesired effect) can be measured empirically and stated statistically. But the importance of that undesired effect to the individual and/or society is a social value judgement. (Note that since nothing is completely free from risk, nothing is 'safe' — there are only degrees of safety.) Therefore the first principle is the necessity for all interested parties to keep the difference between fact and value judgement clearly in mind.

The importance of a desired effect can only be judged by the person or persons needing that effect. The importance of an undesired effect can only be judged by the person or persons who would suffer that undesired effect. Thus, the second principle is that only those on whom the technology is to be used can possibly make the value judgements on the importance of desired and undesired effects and the balance between the two. The role of the provider of the service is to measure and report on the scientifically proven efficacy and risk so that the individual consumer of the service can make a truly informed judgement and choice on whether he or she wishes that technology, and so that society can make a truly informed judgement and choice on whether they wish that technology to be offered.

At the present time there is confusion of terms concerning these terms. Words like 'benefit' and 'safety' are used frequently without careful definition. Whatever words are used, it is most important for everyone to insist on clear definitions of terms and a clear understanding of meaning when discussing desired and undesired effects of technology. It is also important for all interested parties to keep the two principles mentioned above firmly in mind and to be aware that all too often the providers of services unfortunately do not limit themselves to facts but also make value judgements whether to offer a particular technology, and its importance.

Next is the assessment of financial costs. Cost is rarely assessed by clinicians, but the rising cost of health care and shrinking resources is promoting many more cost analyses, particularly by epidemiologists, health economists and government agencies.

Third, the examination of the social elements of technology includes the legal, ethical, social and cultural implications. Until recently these were rarely addressed; consumer groups in a few countries brought their importance to the forefront. As all interested parties take part in technology assessment, social elements will undoubtedly receive much more attention.

Fourth, the effects of technology on the health care system encompass both any changes in the system's infrastructure necessary to use the technology, and the influence of technology on subsequent diagnostic and therapeutic practices. These were given little thought before the introduction of electronic fetal monitoring during labour. The way in which the introduction of ultrasound scanning during pregnancy has tended to move prenatal care from clinics to hospitals is an example of this (see page 75).

Like ultrasound scanning, fetal monitoring significantly affected the health care system. For example, it further justified, in some people's minds, the need to hospitalise all women giving birth. It also affected the organisation of labour wards, how often the labouring women were visited personally by staff and where the staff spent their time. If the monitoring screens were gathered at a central location, for instance, staff could sit in front of a bank of screens and not go to the women. As the use of the electronic monitor increased during the 1970s, the caesarean section rates began to rise precipitously. It was several years, however, before a connection was recognised

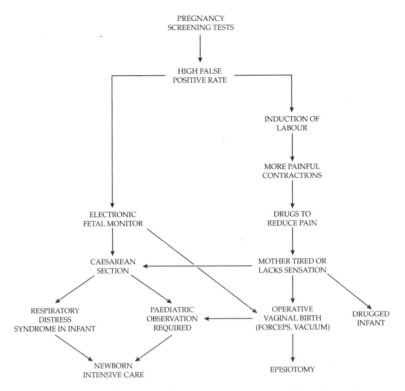

Figure 2: *Postulated chain of diagnostic and therapeutic interventions in perinatal services. Arrows do not represent cause and effect but rather an increased chance that the subsequent event will take place. (WHO 1985a, p. 98).*

between the use of the monitor and subsequent diagnostic and therapeutic action (including operative birth by forceps, vacuum extraction and caesarean section). Although technological intervention in obstetrics may create chain reactions of further diagnostic and therapeutic intervention (figure 2), the effects on the health care system are seldom assessed.

As the fifth aspect of assessment, the impact of the use of technology on the skills of practitioners should be measured. As labour is increasingly monitored electronically, for example, the human ear is used less for the task; midwives and physicians thus lose the skill of auscultation of the fetal heart. Worse, newly trained professionals may never learn this skill and be totally dependent on the machine. The assessment of this aspect of technology use is still very rare.

Organising assessment

Technology assessment in a country needs to be systematic. Because resources for this task are limited, priority must be assigned to particular types of technology. In the United States, assessment activities have proliferated in both the public and private sectors, but there is little co-ordination. As a result, several assessments may be made of some drugs, procedures and machines, while others are ignored. Although no country yet has a system that solves this problem, the Office of Technology Assessment has developed a model organisational system. It has four simple steps.

The first is the identification of the technology to be assessed. A list can be drawn up of all intervention used in a field such as birth. With an idea of the total deserving testing, decisions can be made about which types to choose. Clearly, these decisions must be made by a group including all interested parties. The criteria for deciding what to test are complicated but can include: widespread use, the presence of safety problems, a significant potential for benefit, public concern, high costs.

The second step is collecting data, often using experimental methods such as controlled clinical trials. It should be truly comprehensive, covering all five aspects of assessment. The testing phase, especially if experimental, can be expensive. For this reason, one approach is that developing countries not collect much original data on efficacy and safety. A better strategy for these countries may be to obtain such information from industrialised countries and then make local assessments of the costs, social effects and impact on their health care systems.

Another approach argues the opposite: do the research first in developing countries where research costs are lower, there are more births and higher rates of negative outcomes and thus smaller sample size is needed. Many developing countries, for example in Latin America, have well trained obstetricians and epidemiologists capable of high quality research. Then such research can be replicated in developed countries. There are outstanding examples of such an approach — the kangaroo method of managing small newborns discussed in chapter 7 was first developed and studied in Colombia and is now being replicated in developed countries.

The third step involves synthesis: pulling together all the information, evaluating it and reaching conclusions on the use of the technology. A synthesis must be made for the use of people who need its result but lack the time or sometimes the expertise to make one themselves. The consensus approach used by the three WHO meetings on perinatal technology is an example of this process. Far too little is known about how best to promote consensus statements so as to change practice (see chapter 8).

The fourth step is giving the information to the people who will make decisions about technology (including policy-makers), use it (health care workers) or be subjected to it (women, in the case of birth technology). This step is probably the most seldom taken, especially to inform the third group. Hence the recommendation: *"The results of the assessment of technology used in birth care should be widely disseminated, to change the behaviour of professionals and give a basis to the decisions of users and the general public"*. Current procedures for giving out such information are flawed. For example, it is well known that simply providing health care workers with a written report or a list of journal articles does not change their practices. In addition, policy-makers and the public may well have questions about the use of technology that the information collected does not answer; there may be too much, too little or irrelevant information. The involvement of all interested parties in assessment is one way to help solve this problem.

After the dissemination phase, policy-makers, practitioners and the public should return to the identification phase, that is, to report their reactions to the people who made the original decision to test the technology. These responses can determine whether the assessment was helpful and pertinent. Adopting this formal system for assessing birth technology can help to ensure that under emphasised areas are covered and assessments are done properly, and can serve as a brake on the tendency of the birth machine towards unchecked expansion.

Measures to control birth technology

The first step in improving the use of birth technology is creating a system of assessment. Unless some form of control measure follows, however, no great advance can be expected. The use of pharmaceuticals in medical practice sets an important precedent. In most countries, regulations permitting the prescription of a drug by a physician or over-the-counter use by the public have been tied to prior, officially approved assessment, to bring drug use under reasonable control. Today, new drugs cannot be used until after careful assessment and approval by a government agency. In contrast, except in the United States, a new machine that may be useful in health care can be used the day after its invention. For this reason, the consensus meeting recommended measures to promote control of birth technology. These recommendations covered two possible control mechanisms: government policies and the influence of the public.

Two recommendations directly addressed government control. *"Health ministries should establish specific policies about the incorporation of technology into commercial markets and health services"*. Few health ministries have taken over the control of health technology from commercial interests. In concert with clinicians, industry has been responsible for the discovery and refinement of much important technology. But the need to promote rapid, widespread use, to profit from the investment in research and development has too often resulted in inadequate assessment and unjustified claims of efficacy and safety.

The consensus meeting agreed that the responsibility of ministries of health — to protect the health of the people, mainly through the services of their health care system — included controlling the incorporation of technology into these services. This is easier said than done, particularly when the decision involves an expensive machine. Ministry staff have sometimes described to WHO staff the frequent pressure to approve and purchase a particular type of technology for a particular hospital. The mass media may add to the pressure with dramatic stories about how the machine saved a life or some patient died because of its absence. The first line of defence against such pressure for a ministry of health is to have clear, specific policies to control the incorporation of technology.

"Governments should consider developing regulations to permit the use of birth technology only after adequate evaluation." This recommendation ties assessment to control, giving teeth to the assessment process. Almost every country has made this link in drug control, but to date only the Food and Drug Administration in the United States has tried to control technology. The considerable problems experienced in the United States in their attempt to control medical technology have been described earlier. The participants felt that this control step was so important that national health care services should refrain from purchasing new equipment until the results of assessment were known.

The control of birth technology can also be promoted by public influence. To exert this influence, the public must first be fully informed about the results of assessments of birth technology and the procedures and practices in birth care used in the hospitals and elsewhere in the community. Armed with this information, the community can state its opinion and participate in the formulation of policy on the use of birth technology. This can be accomplished through means such as:

- the organisation of consumer groups;
- letters or telephone calls to or personal contact with the mass media, organisations of health professionals and appropriate government bodies;
- the organisation of public meetings; and
- participation as consumers in research and in consensus conferences.

At an individual level, women can tell their birth attendants opinions on birth technology and their wishes about its use on them.

Review of specific practices by the consensus meeting

The meeting evaluated and made recommendations on a number of specific practices: shaving the pubic area, giving an enema, amniotomy, induction of labour, the positioning of the woman during labour and birth, the use of drugs for pain relief, electronic fetal monitoring, episiotomy and caesarean section. The scientific data available on each were reviewed in papers and each was discussed, and sometimes debated, before a recommendation was drafted. With some effort, the Group reached consensus on the appropriate use of all these types of technology.

Shaving and enema

The participants agreed rather quickly that there was no indication for pubic shaving or giving an enema before delivery. Both procedures are routinely used in the hospital before abdominal surgery; their widespread use at the time of admission of the woman in labour reflects the transformation of birth into a medical (or, perhaps more accurately, a surgical) event. That these practices are still found in many hospitals in industrialised countries is illustrated by data from Australia showing that of private patients 26.9% are shaved and 32.0% given an enema while among publicly funded patients 19.7% are shaved and 23% given an enema (Lumley 1988).

In the early part of this century, the preparation of women admitted to a maternity hospital in New York included: "They were given an enema followed by a vaginal douche with bichloride of mercury. Their heads were cleansed with kerosene, ether, or ammonia and their nipples and navels doused with ether. Charity (poor) patients, who were assumed to harbour an abundance of germs, had their pubic hair shaved, whereas that of private patients was merely clipped" (Mahan & McKay 1983).

There are no benefits to either shaving or enema. The claim that the enema reduces faecal contamination and possible consequent infection of the woman or baby has proved to be unfounded (Romney & Gordon 1981; Drayton & Rees 1984). Likewise the idea that shaving reduces infection has been scientifically disproven (Kantor et al. 1965).

In addition, both procedures have drawbacks, important to women although minor to many clinicians, and illustrating the contrast between the medical and social view of technology. Shaving disfigures the woman, and makes her feel less like she is having an experience that is part of normal life and more like a dependent hospital patient awaiting surgery. The enema is painful and humiliating, and has similar effects in increasing the woman's feeling of loss of control of her body and of the situation.

Medical anthropologists have described how both these procedures are highly symbolic in converting the labouring woman into a hospital patient and in defining who is now to control her body. This symbolic value may explain the persistence of both procedures as routines in many maternity wards, even when scientific evidence of their uselessness has been presented to the staff.

Amniotomy

Amniotomy, intentionally breaking the bag of waters (also called the fetal membranes) in an effort to start or accelerate labour, seems to be a simple and benign procedure, and is routinely used in some hospitals. Many people believe that, since the bag of waters ruptures spontaneously during labour, an artificial rupture is not really much of an intervention. In fact, one clinical trial showed that, when the fetal membranes were still intact at the beginning of labour and the labour proceeds without complication, they remained intact in two thirds of the women until the second stage of labour (Schwarcz et al. 1975). This trial revealed amniotomy to be an artificial manoeuvre that disturbs the physiological timing of the spontaneous rupture of the fetal membranes during labour.

Several randomised controlled trials show that amniotomy early in the first stage of labour (the period of cervical dilation) shortens labour (Schwarcz et al. 1975; Laros et al. 1972; Guerresi et al. 1981). These trials found that the length of the first stage of labour was shortened by around 30 to 60 minutes but that it was rare for the second stage to be shortened.

BENEFIT

The benefit of amniotomy, then, is the shortening of the first stage of labour by about an hour. Because the effects of several types of birth technology may include shorter labour, the participants discussed the benefits that might result. The consensus was that shortening the duration of normal labour may not necessarily benefit the fetus and newborn baby.

The issue of the length of labour is contentious. In recent years, some obstetricians have tried to quantify the progress of labour using a special chart that indicates the elapsed time and compares it with the timing of an 'optimal' labour. This practice emphasises the clock and implies that deviation from the optimal time curve is dangerous. Since extremely long labours can lead to trouble, the tendency has been to assume that short labours are better. Except for extreme cases, however, the duration of labour is not correlated with increased harmful consequences for woman or fetus. The participants (including the obstetricians) agreed that the recent focus on optimal duration of labour is not constructive in general, is not based on sound scientific principles that respect the normal physiological variability of labour, and often results in premature and unnecessary intervention. A review of the literature on monitoring the progress of labour concluded: "Slow progress should alert one to the possibility of abnormal labour, but should not automatically result in intervention. In view of the importance of labour progress and the amount of discomfort that slow progress can provoke in the woman, the fetus, and the caregivers, it is rather surprising that so few of the many guidelines to care that have been suggested have been substantiated by solid research evidence" (Crowther et al. 1991).

The length of the first stage varies widely and depends on many factors, which certainly includes the mental state of the woman. Thus, shortening the length of the first stage by one hour may be considered a minor, not a major, benefit. Although the length of the second stage is less variable and more important, amniotomy has less influence on it. A review on the augmentation of labour states: "None of the studies discussed thus far specifically addressed the question of whether or not amniotomy is effective in augmenting slow or prolonged labour. As far as I am aware, this issue has never been addressed in a published report of a randomised controlled trial" (Keirse 1991, p. 955).

RISKS

What are the risks of amniotomy? Although it is generally believed that the risk of infection increases six hours after the rupture of the membranes, this may be the result of vaginal examinations as well as the passage of time. Ironically, then, amniotomy may increase the importance of the length of labour. A potentially serious risk lies in the fact that the intact bag of waters provides a cushion that protects the fetal head as it is forced through the birth canal and, at the same time, serves as a wedge helping to dilate the cervix during the earlier stages of dilatation. The minor benefit of early amniotomy may be gained at the expense of increased trauma to the fetal head; one study found a higher incidence of caput succedaneum (a swelling of the skin on the top of the head) and misalignment of the cranial bones (Caldeyro-Barcia et al. 1974). Although no harmful effects can be directly attributed to these results, they may indicate similar disturbances in the brain. A prospective trial has shown an association between the rupture of the membranes and increases in signs of possible fetal distress during labour on an electronic fetal monitor (Schwarcz et al. 1973).

Another potential risk of amniotomy arises because, with the water gone, every contraction of the uterus may compress some portion of the umbilical cord, which the waters had cushioned. The compression of the cord can lead to umbilical occlusion; no blood can flow through the umbilical cord from woman to baby. If this lasts 60 seconds or more, the fetus will receive too little oxygen (have hypoxia), and the chemical balance of the blood will be upset. Research has shown that amniotomy produces a reduction of maternal uterine blood flow of sufficient length to lead to metabolic and respiratory acidosis (Martell et al. 1976).

The question is whether these potential risks to the fetal head and oxygen supply brought on by early amniotomy leads to harm. The research on the risks, while highly suggestive, is not yet conclusive because of inadequate numbers and some methodological problems. More research is necessary to confirm or refute such possible long-term effects.

Given the questionable benefit of amniotomy and the potential serious risks involved, it was agreed that the procedure should not be done routinely as, for example, is done in the so-called 'active management of labour' promoted by O'Driscoll (O'Driscoll et al. 1984). While O'Driscoll states that this active management scheme reduces caesarean section rates, this claim is "made on the basis of poorly controlled observational data" (Keirse 1991, p. 958) and 4 controlled trials do not substantiate the claim. The consensus at the meeting was that amniotomy should rather be restricted to a few complicated and serious situations once labour has started:

> *"Normally rupture of the membranes is not required until a fairly late stage in the delivery. Artificial early rupture of the membranes, as a routine process, is not scientifically justified."*

Induction of labour

The induction of labour is one method of elective delivery. Here, the word elective means chosen — by the physician rather than the child-bearing woman. The procedure has an interesting history providing some valuable lessons. Technology for inducing labour is historically linked to that of induced abortion by the common intention to prod the uterus into action. A wealth of effort has taken two main directions: mechanical and hormonal.

HISTORY

Labour was induced, without the benefit (or hazard) of modern technology by empirical midwives. They gave women natural agents to promote childbirth, such as ergot, and advocated the use of nipple stimulation, orgasm and sexual intercourse to start or speed up labour. With the emergence of obstetrics as a profession, a range of compounds for inducing labour was eagerly tried throughout the nineteenth and early twentieth centuries: hot water, creosote and tar, quinine, castor oil and iodine, to name but a few. In addition, under the mechanical heading, many different objects were inserted into the uterus or vagina — stomach tube, tampon, seaweed, toy balloon, piece of wax, animal bladder.

The modern era of induction begins in the mid-1950s when oxytocin was separated out from other components of pituitary extract, and a synthetic form was developed and could be produced on an industrial scale. Opinion varied, however, as to how and where pregnant women should be given the new compound. Some obstetricians tried putting it in women's mouths or noses; some suggested the rectum or direct injection into the amniotic sac. Eventually the intravenous method emerged as the most popular, when mechanical devices to control the delivery of the drug appeared in the late 1960s.

The ease and efficiency of this new technique assisted a change characteristic of the introduction of all birth technology. Early on, the use of oxytocin was limited to a few specific conditions for which it had been clearly shown to have benefit, such as a prolonged pregnancy of 44 weeks' gestation or more. Gradually these carefully proven indications expanded. If induction of labour was beneficial for a pregnancy of 44 weeks, how about 43 weeks or 42? This common problem in the use of technology has serious consequences. As the indications expand, the benefit weakens but the hazards remain constant. As a result, the hazards outweigh the benefits. In the case of induction of labour, another reason for use began to emerge: the choice to have labour and birth at an optimal time. The optimal time was, of course, when physicians were normally in the hospital — during the day on weekdays. It was hard to separate the intended benefit of such 'daylight obstetrics' to the woman and child (ensuring that the best quality of care would be on hand) from the convenience of the physician. In any case, all these factors resulted in a steep rise in induced labour in many countries. In England and Wales, 13% of labours was induced in 1966, and 39% in 1974 (Chalmers & Richards 1977).

By the beginning of the 1980s, several factors produced a reconsideration of the indications for induction of labour. Studies began to document some of its hazards (Chalmers et al. 1978). Some of these hazards can be serious such as an increased likelihood of neonatal hyperbilirubinemia. Some of the leading obstetricians who had helped to introduce and promote induction became alarmed at its excessive use. Dr. Turnbull, late Professor of Obstetrics at Oxford University, whose early work on oxytocin intravenous drips stimulated its rapid spread, told a group of visitors in 1985 that the extreme overuse of induction made him wonder if he should ever have helped to develop this particular technology. The overuse of induction for 'daylight obstetrics' was reflected in studies made in Canada, England and Wales, Scotland, the United States and other countries. By the simple means of analysing all births in a given country or region by day of the week and time of day, a number of researchers have shown that the proportion of births taking place during daylight on weekdays is far greater than would result from random distribution (Macfarlane 1978, 1884; Phillips et al. 1982; Paccaud et al. 1984; Evans et al. 1984).

That excessive induction continues and is related to social rather than medical factors is shown by data from Australia. The use of oxytocin for induction or augmentation in the State of Victoria in 1988 varied between 29.1% and 31.9% in tertiary level teaching hospitals and between 36.5% and 42.8% in primary level metropolitan suburban hospitals. While all these rates are quite excessive, the hospitals with the lowest risk women (and the most private patients) all had higher rates when, medically speaking, they should have had the lowest rates (Lumley 1988).

Consumer groups and the mass media became alarmed and started talking about birth for physicians' convenience, while some women began to demand that labour be induced when it was convenient for them and their families. As a result, the initial enthusiasm for induction wavered and induction rates in at least a few countries such as the United Kingdom and Australia began to fall (Lumley 1988).

But induction continues as a widespread practice in a number of countries. The WHO study (WHO 1992) found the following rates of oxytocin use (as a percent of all births): Greece 80%, Finland 41%, the State of Victoria (Australia) 37%, United Kingdom 20%, United States 12%. The WHO Report comments on these rates as follows:

> "A disturbing finding of this study was the tendency in some countries to 'hurry labour along' with oxytocin. It is most unlikely that 20–80% of women in the participating countries needed oxytocin induction or augmentation, or benefited by it. There are situations when induction of labour is clearly beneficial: to avoid maternal mortality or morbidity from fulminating pre-eclampsia; or to avoid prolonging the psychological distress of carrying a dead foetus (Chalmers and Kierse 1991)."

> "Post-term pregnancy, another indication for induction of labour, is a rare occurrence; its true incidence is only 4–6% of pregnancies of 28 weeks or more (Crowley 1991).

> "Augmentation of labour for slow progress is an intervention that has a place in obstetrical care only after other more simple measures have been tried. Allowing women the freedom to walk around and to eat and drink as tolerated are at least as effective as oxytocin augmentation (Keirse 1991).

"A number of investigators have shown that oxytocin induction, and perhaps augmentation, has been used for the convenience of physicians, women or both (Macfarlane & Mugford 1986; Oakley & Richards 1990; Cartwright 1979). This practice, as well as a widely held (but scientifically unfounded) belief that slow progress is the most frequent complication of labour, must account for the excessively high rates of oxytocin use in several countries. Oxytocin use for these reasons should be discouraged.

"Oxytocin use is not without risks. The findings of this study are consistent with others which have documented a positive association between oxytocin use and operative vaginal delivery (Crowley 1991). Induction of labour with oxytocin increases the incidence of neonatal hyperbilirubinemia (Keirse 1991). Uterine hyperstimulation can also occur with oxytocin use and may lead to inadequate placental blood flow oxygenation and fetal compromise (Keirse 1991). Rarely, uterine rupture or iatrogenic preterm delivery occur as a result of oxytocin use (Keirse & Chalmers 1991). However, Chalmers and Keirse report that in at least one population, the gestational age and birth weight distributions were shifted downwards as elective delivery became more widely used (Chalmers & Keirse 1991; Newcombe & Chalmers 1977).

"This pattern — initial enthusiasm and later disenchantment — is frequently found in the use of birth technology. It is clearly not related to the rational use of technology (which is based on scientifically proven indications)" (WHO 1992).

FINDINGS

In spite of the wide swings in the use of induction of labour, benefits remain when this technique is applied for certain specific indications. Since hazards are now known to be associated with induction it important to limit its use. Initial assessments of birth technology, done by clinicians with a medical perspective, usually emphasise benefit, while concern for hazards is much higher among people with a social perspective, particularly those on whom the technology is used. For example, a survey showed that procedures such as induction of labour are much more popular with obstetricians than with midwives or women (Cartwright 1979). A more recent study reveals the significant increase in pain experienced by the woman receiving oxytocin (Hemminki et al. 1985). This pain may lead to the increased use of pain medication, which can lead to a drugged infant and an exhausted labouring woman, the latter, in turn, can lead to slowed labour which increases the chance for forceps or caesarean birth. This chain of events (figure 2) illustrates a most important characteristic of birth technology, namely the tendency for one intervention to lead to another, resulting in a geometric escalation of technology use. Further, the hazards of induction of labour are of sufficiently significance and well enough documented that its use is a legitimate indication for electronic fetal monitoring to quickly detect any of the possible complications brought on by this procedure.

The participants had little difficulty in agreeing to recommend that

> *"Birth should not be induced for convenience, and the induction of labour should be reserved for specific medical indications. No geographic region should have rates of induced labour over 10%."*

Although not included in this recommendation, the feeling of the group was that some of the more traditional, non-invasive techniques such as walking around and nipple stimulation should be more widely tried to induce or speed up labour, before resorting to more hazardous modern technology. Scientific research substantiates this feeling. For example, one clinical trial found that ambulation during labour reduced the need for pharmacological augmentation by half and reduced the need for analgesics by two-thirds (Flynn et al. 1978). Another trial reported ambulation to be more effective than oxytocin in restoring normal progress in labour when dystocia has occurred (Read et al. 1981). Two trials found breast stimulation (nipple stimulation) to be effective in inducing labour (Salmon et al. 1986, Elliot and Flaherty 1983). Another trial compared the efficacy in inducing women with prolonged pregnancies through pharmacological methods and a physiological method (breast massage). The breast massage was as effective as the drugs, and of course caused fewer medical complications (Rokiki and Krasnodebski 1988).

Positioning during labour and birth

Until about 200 years ago, the preferred birth positions worldwide were more vertical than horizontal. The birth chair, for example, dates back to at least the Babylonian culture of 2000 B.C. Ancient Egyptian art depicts Cleopatra giving birth in a kneeling position. Surveys of present traditional cultures find that nearly all use more vertical birthing positions (Dundes 1987). The evidence suggests that the adoption of horizontal positions (both the dorsal position — lying flat on the back, and the lithotomy position — lying flat on the back with legs up in stirrups) came into western obstetrics as a result of two factors: the first obstetricians were surgeons (who were used to having their patients in the lithotomy position) and inter-professional struggles between surgeons (favouring horizontal positions) and midwives (favouring vertical positions) in the sixteenth and seventeenth centuries.

CRITERIA FOR CHOICE

There are seven criteria which may or may not be included in deciding on the most desirable positions for women during labour and birth (Caldeyro-Barcia 1985). The first is the woman's preference. Choosing her own position reduces the woman's pain and discomfort, and as the woman is the principal, active participant in birth, her wishes should be respected whenever possible. Research shows that given the choice, women in the first stage of labour prefer to be seated, standing or walking about and to have freedom to change positions and move at will (Caldeyro-Barcia 1980; Chamberlain & Stewart 1987). During the second stage of labour, squatting is the preferred position during uterine contractions and pushing, while a seated, slightly reclining position is the preferred position between contractions (Sabatino 1984; Caldeyro-Barcia 1984). In one very large series of births, with freedom of choice of position, no women chose the lithotomy position, although it was offered, because they felt it to be uncomfortable and to restrain freedom of movement (Caldeyro-Barcia 1980).

The second criterion is the cultural factor: respecting the preferred position of the cultural group of the birthing woman.

The third criterion for deciding on the woman's position during labour and birth is facilitation of the progress. Randomised trials have shown that duration of the first stage of labour was 25% shorter in the group using vertical positions compared with the group using horizontal positions. This difference in duration increased to 35% with women having their first baby (Diaz et al. 1980; Flynn et al. 1978). Another randomised controlled study found that for woman having their first birth, the duration of the expulsion period was significantly shorter in the group using the birth chair than in the group using the lithotomy position (Nagai 1982). Several other trials comparing upright with supine labour found shorter labours in the upright group (Caldeyro-Barcia 1978, 1979; Liu 1974; Mitre 1974).

The fourth criterion is fetal and neonatal health. In the randomised trials comparing the use of the birth chair with the lithotomy position in the second stage of labour, babies whose mothers had used a birth chair had statistically better blood chemistry values indicating less fetal hypoxia (Nagai 1982; Caldeyro-Barcia 1984). None of the studies, however, found differences between the two groups in Apgar scores, which measure the condition of the baby at birth.

The fifth criterion which might be used is physiological changes in the labouring woman including blood flow and the ability of the uterus to contract effectively. Several studies show that the supine position causes the uterus to compress both the main blood vessel carrying blood to the baby from the mother's heart (aorta) and the main blood vessel carrying blood to the mothers's heart from the baby (inferior vena cava), thus compromising the flow of blood to and from the baby (Ueland & Hansen 1969; Eckstein & Marx 1974; Abitol 1985). Other studies show that the intensity of the uterine contractions is less when the labouring woman is on her back (Miller et al. 1982; Roberts et al. 1983). During the first stage of labour, research has demonstrated that the uterine contractions are more intense in a standing position than in a seated one and that they are more efficient in dilating the cervix when the woman is in a vertical position (Mendez-Bauer et al. 1975). During the second stage of labour pushing is strongest when squatting, less strong when sitting and weakest when lying down (Caldeyro-Barcia 1980; Sabatino 1984; Caldeyro-Barcia 1984; Mengert & Murphy 1933). In summary "The results of these studies suggest that the supine position can adversely affect both the condition of the fetus and the progression of labour by interference with uterine haemodynamics and compromising the efficiency of uterine contractions" (Roberts 1991, p. 884).

The sixth criterion is the functional anatomy of the birth canal. Research has shown that the vertical positions, particularly squatting, provide for more effective expulsion (Notelovitz 1978), a wider canal for the fetus to go through (Borrel & Fernstrom 1957) and a downhill rather than uphill birth (Notelovitz 1978).

The seventh criterion is the preference of the obstetrician. During the first stage of labour most obstetricians prefer the woman to be in bed because it is easier to examine her, palpate the abdomen and listen to the fetal heart. While many claim that it facilitates electronic fetal monitoring, the recent addition of telemetry to the machine allows the monitor to proceed regardless of position and even when the woman is ambulatory. During the second stage of labour most obstetricians prefer the woman in the lithotomy position because of their training they are used to assisting births in this position. In addition, the lithotomy position makes it easier to intervene. In contrast, where midwifery has maintained some independence, labouring women have retained the option to choose their own positions.

CHANGES IN PRACTICE

In summary, the first six criteria strongly favour the vertical positions during the first and second stages of labour and birth. Only the convenience of some birth attendants favours the horizontal positions. Nevertheless, the vast majority of hospital maternity units in Latin America and virtually all in Eastern Europe place all women in the horizontal positions. In western Europe, Canada and the United States, however, the labouring woman in the hospital is gradually being allowed to choose her own positions during the first stage of labour, and sometimes in the second stage. This change is the result of both increasing appreciation of the scientific findings and women's active participation in choosing the circumstances in which they give birth.

The birth chair is one reason for the increase in the use of vertical positioning in hospitals in Europe and North America. The woman can sit in the chair, and adjust it to achieve positions similar to squatting. The chair also makes care by the birth attendants easier than, say, when the birthing woman is squatting on the floor. To a certain extent, the chair accommodates the needs of the birth attendant and thus represents something of a compromise. Most birth chairs are elegant, mechanical and very expensive; these fit nicely with the rest of the birth machinery in the hospital and are more acceptable to physicians. "Special beds or chairs . . . can tap a great commercial market of increasingly elaborate birth chairs" (*Lancet* editorial 1990). In contrast, the rural birth centres visited by the participants in the consensus meeting had home-made wooden birth chairs that functioned well and cost little. Some western hospitals have discovered that fabric sacks filled with beans can make an excellent cheap chair for labour and birth. Using a cheap cushion which allows the woman to sit comfortably on the normal hospital bed, a clinical trial found significantly shorter second stages and significantly fewer forceps deliveries with the cushion (Gardosi et al. 1989).

After the field trip and a discussion of the review papers, it was readily agreed that *"Pregnant women should not be put in a lithotomy position during labour or delivery. They should be encouraged to walk about during labour and each woman must freely decide which position to adopt during delivery"*. Women in labour tend to be overly compliant and do what they are told to do or what they perceive the health care providers want them to do. Over a century ago a report stated that women in labour ". . . will, in great measure be guided by the arrangements which are made for her confinement and will assume the posture for which they are specially adapted" (Rigby 1857). Thus in this recommendation, the word 'encouraged' is crucial.

Use of drugs for pain relief

The use of drugs for pain relief during birth was also considered. The participants began by agreeing on a few general principles for medication and birth. As birth is a physiological process, there is no justification for the routine administration of medication during labour or birth. Medication should be used only for the treatment of complications, and only when its efficacy for such complications has been scientifically demonstrated. Because all drugs have side effects, careful account must be taken of those that may be undesirable for both the woman and the fetus or newborn baby. In addition, consideration should be given to trying other kinds of intervention before resorting to medication.

In Europe and North and South America, an excess of medication is routinely administered during birth. The results of this widespread practice are:

- the use of medication that is frequently without indication or benefit;
- frequent undesirable side effects that interfere with the normal progress of labour and endanger the health of the woman and fetus or newborn;
- unnecessary high costs.

This situation results from both the medical model's view of birth and the tendency in modern society to turn to pharmaceuticals to solve any problem.

Medication for pain relief in birth is of three types: analgesics (pain relievers), anxiety suppressants (tranquillisers) and anaesthesia, most commonly epidural block (anaesthesia placed in the sac around the lower spinal cord). All three relieve the pain associated with childbirth to a greater or lesser extent. This benefit must be balanced carefully against the hazards.

The analgesics and anxiety suppressants share a dangerous side effect: they act as depressants of the central nervous system (including the respiratory centre) in the woman and the fetus or newborn baby. The depression of the woman's breathing lowers the amount of oxygen, increasing the amount of carbon dioxide in her blood and that of her fetus. It also interferes with her active participation in the birth and with her psychological interaction with her partner and family. This diminishes the quality and significance of the birth experience.

The depression of the brain of the fetus reduces its ability to resist hypoxia. This depressant effect may be seen on the electronic fetal monitor as an increasing variability of the heart rate. The depression of the central nervous system in the newborn infant reduces the Apgar score by causing flaccid muscles (muscular hypotonia), poor reflexes and inadequate or no breathing.This requires the birth attendants to revive the baby through resuscitation and other invasive procedures. After birth, the pharmacological depression of the woman, her baby or both interferes with bonding and the initiation of breastfeeding.

Another possible risk of using drugs for pain relief during labour is that the infant, so exposed, has an increased chance to become a drug addict in later life. A series of studies at the Karolinska Institute in Sweden found that if the mother used inhalation of nitrous oxide during labour, the infant had a statistically significant increased chance of developing amphetamine addiction in later life (Jacobson et al. 1988).

Further studies by the same group showed that infants born following the use of opiates or barbiturates or nitrous oxide during the birth had an increased risk for adult opiate addiction (Jacobson et al. 1990).

In hospitals in industrialised countries the great majority of women receive medication for pain during labour. In a survey in Australia in 1988, 71% received some form of pain relief. The most widely used method was nitrous oxide (74.4%), followed by pethidine (66.4%), epidural (17.0%), and general anaesthesia (3.2%) (Lumley 1988).

The last decade has seen an extraordinary proliferation of epidural anaesthesia. While travelling for WHO, I have conducted an informal survey of hospitals in greater Europe, the United States, New Zealand and Australia between 1989 and 1992. I found the percentage of birthing women at each hospital receiving epidural anaesthesia ranged from 10% to 70% with the majority of hospitals reporting between 20% and 50%. Confirmation of this proliferation is the statement that epidural anaesthesia is "now used in as many as 24% of labours in larger units in the United Kingdom" (*Lancet* editorial 1990). Data collected in Australia in 1992 showed the use of epidural in one large hospital as approximately 30% for publicly funded women and "somewhat higher in the private section". In another large hospital 48.5% of all women giving birth had an epidural (Wagner 1992).

In my same informal survey nearly every obstetrician queried insisted that epidural anaesthesia is 'safe' and they confirmed that women are routinely offered epidural as a 'perfectly safe option'. When asked about risks, the nearly uniform response was that problems arise only in inexperienced hands. As a result, epidural is largely responsible for the blossoming of the specialty of obstetric anaesthesia.

In reality, what is known about epidural anaesthesia? An important review of the scientific literature states:

"Although millions of women have been offered epidural block for pain relief in labour over the past 20 years or so, fewer than 600 women have participated in reasonably well controlled comparisons with other forms of pain relief. Inevitably, therefore, many important questions about the effects of epidural block during labour remain inadequately answered" (Howell & Chalmers 1992, p. 99).

Is epidural block effective? Only two clinical trials asked the woman about pain control (Robinson et al. 1980; Philipsen & Jensen 1990). Both studies found epidural block more effective but both studies also found there were women for whom it didn't work: in one of these studies 8% of women failed to get pain relief from epidural block (Philipsen & Jensen 1990).

What are the risks of epidural anaesthesia? Because so little experimental research has been done, only a few risks are scientifically proven but they cannot be considered minor. On the basis of several clinical trials, there is "solid evidence that epidural block prolongs the second state and can increase the use of instrumental delivery" (Howell & Chalmers 1992, p. 101). Since instrumental delivery (forceps or vacuum) carries proven increased risk for both woman and baby, it is hard to justify describing this technology simply as 'safe'. Although the evidence is not as solid, data strongly suggests the likelihood that epidural can also increase the use of caesarean section, another not innocuous intervention (Thorp et al. 1989; Philipsen & Jensen 1989). Some authors suggest that, if using epidural block, it can be combined with oxytocin in an attempt to avoid instrumental delivery (Frasier 1991). This suggestion is a classic example of one intervention leading to a second intervention in order to prevent a third intervention.

The list of possible but as yet not conclusively proven risks of epidural block during labour is long. Possible short term risks to the woman during labour and just after birth include fever, drop in blood pressure — a serious side effect if not immediately corrected, predisposition to malrotation of the descending baby, severe headache (Fusi et al. 1989, Philipsen & Jensen 1989; Howell & Chalmers 1992). Regarding long term adverse effects to the woman, there is considerable data now suggesting chronic backache (MacArthur et al. 1990). In addition, chronic headache, bladder problems, tingling and numbness and sensory confusion have been observed (Kitzinger 1987; Newburn 1990).

Far too little research has been done on the possible risks of epidural anaesthesia to the baby (Scanlon 1981; Avard & Nimrod 1985). The few studies done indicate possible risks: rapid breathing during the first few hours after birth (Bratteby et al. 1979), neonatal hypoglycaemia (Swanstrom & Bratteby 1981a), problems with lipid metabolism (Swanstrom & Bratteby 1981b). The research on whether the baby is alert enough at birth (Apgar) is still inconclusive.

Another adverse effect of epidural anaesthesia is that the procedure makes it impossible for the woman to stand, walk or assume any of the vertical positions. The importance of this temporary disability to the progress of labour and birth has just been discussed.

In view of the serious lack of data on epidural block during birth and the importance of the proven and suspected risks, why is it called safe and why is this technology so strongly promoted by the medical profession? One study showed that 63% of obstetricians viewed epidural as improving their own job satisfaction (Cartwright 1979). Furthermore, 1992 saw a new publication — The International Journal of Obstetric Anaesthesia — further legitimation of the rapidly expanding specialty of obstetrical anaesthesia which is built on an epidural foundation (Chalmers 1992).

Other forms of pain relief during labour have become popular in some places. A survey of birthing in Greece showed that in 50% of all births in that country, the birthing woman is put sound asleep with a general anaesthesia during birth (Tzoumaka-Bakula 1987). Such a widespread practice, fraught with risks and completely without scientific justification, is not found, to our knowledge, anywhere else in the world.

The number of undesirable side effects associated with medication to reduce pain during childbirth encourages greater emphasis on the use of alternatives (Simkin 1991). A number of factors may reduce or eliminate the need for drugs. The preparation for childbirth during pregnancy, if it emphasises birth as a normal part of family life and encourages the woman to believe that she (and her body) can handle this event, has been shown to reduce the need for pain relief (Kitzinger 1978). It has also been demonstrated that the pain can be reduced through close personal support from a sympathetic birth attendant or a family member or close friend who is with or near the woman throughout her labour (Keirse et al. 1991). Further, pain can also be alleviated through a variety of non-pharmaceutical techniques, including massage, the application of heat and cold, hypnosis, reflexology, transcutaneous electrical nerve stimulation, acupuncture and acupressure, music, immersion in warm water (Simkin 1991). In Europe and North America, immersion during labour is an increasingly popular alternative: more and more maternity hospitals in Western Europe now have large bathtubs for labouring women who wish to use them. Allowing the woman to choose and change her position at will, and to move and walk freely also reduces pain (Caldeyro-Barcia 1979).

If the woman in labour is not heavily medicated and is able, through alternative means, to cope with the pain, eventually her body comes to her rescue with the release by her hormonal system of a substance called beta-endorphin. This endogenous 'drug' has effects similar to morphine, relieving pain and producing a sensation of wellbeing, but lacks the dangerous side effects and may well benefit the fetus as well.

On the basis of these facts, it was unanimously agreed by the participants that: *"During delivery, the routine administration of analgesics or anaesthetic drugs that are not specifically required to correct or prevent a complication in delivery, should be avoided"*.

The electronic fetal monitor (EFM)

At the meeting, a great deal of attention was given to the use of the electronic fetal monitor during labour. With the possible exception of ultrasound scanning, no other type of perinatal technology has seen such a rapid acceptance by physicians and widespread use. Neither phenomenon, however, was based on scientifically proven efficacy. Like other kinds of birth technology, the electronic fetal monitor first proved to be valuable for specific complications during labour. Then the indications for use gradually broadened beyond the scientific justification. By the early 1970s, it was used routinely on every labouring woman in a number of hospitals in

Europe and the Americas. A few researchers then took up the challenge of determining the value of this routine use.

Randomised controlled trials were mounted. By the early 1980s, five were completed, studying a total of about 4000 labouring women. All five showed the same result: no improvement in the health of the mother or baby resulted from routine use of EFM. In 1984, the final results of a randomised controlled trial on about 13,000 women in Dublin, Ireland were reported. Nevertheless, the practice continued to spread as if the results of the trials did not exist. By 1991 it was estimated that approximately 75% of all births in the United States use EFM (Ruzek 1991).

EFFICACY

Although it is quite unusual to get consistent results in medical research, it can be said unequivocally that no differences in perinatal death rates were shown in any of the presently completed 8 randomised clinical trials comparing the use and non-use of EFM: there is no scientific evidence that fewer babies die if EFM is used on all women during labour (Grant 1991; Ruzek 1990).

Probably the most commonly given excuse for the routine use of EFM during labour continuing even to the present time is to prevent brain damage to the fetus. And yet, the randomised controlled trials showed no differences in the following measures: Apgar score at birth, cord blood gases at birth, need for newborn intensive care and long-term neurological status. The large Dublin trial showed fewer seizures in newborn infants with routine monitoring. Further analysis, however, found that these seizures occurred mostly in babies whose mothers had received oxytocin to start or accelerate labour. If these cases are removed, the rates of seizures in babies were identical. Further, a follow-up study done when the babies were 1 year old showed no difference in the number of neurological handicaps (MacDonald et al. 1985). In summary, the Dublin trial results point to the use of oxytocin during labour as a serious intervention that is an indication for electronic fetal monitoring.

The issue of whether EFM reduces brain damage to the offspring received its biggest surprise with the publication of a randomised clinical trial which assessed the neurological development at 18 months of age of 2 samples of children, one group born prematurely whose heart rates were monitored electronically during birth and compared with the other group of children born prematurely whose heart rates during birth were monitored by auscultation. The incidence of cerebral palsy was 20% in the EFM group and 8% in the group that was monitored by auscultation ($p < 0.03$) (Shy et al. 1990). That the use of EFM should possibly increase the incidence of cerebral palsy may be the result of birth attendants focusing on the monitor rather than the overall condition of the woman and baby. The authors admitted to being unprepared for such a negative finding and a flurry of letters in subsequent issues of the same journal indicated that many others resist data which is against their beliefs. Nevertheless, an editorial in the same issue stated: "Clearly, the hoped-for benefit from intrapartum electronic fetal monitoring has not been realised. It is unfortunate that randomised controlled trials were not carried out before this form of technology became universally applied" (Freeman 1990, p. 625). The fact that the cerebral palsy rates have remained the same for the past 30 years in spite of widespread EFM is further evidence of the lack of efficacy of EFM to reduce neurological sequelae (Paneth & Kiely 1984). These results echo those of the other randomised controlled trials: there is no scientific evidence that routine EFM during labour improves the condition of the baby at birth or reduces the possibility of brain damage.

> "The act of throwing into stark relief the unreliability of intrapartum EFM as a predictor of long-term neurological outcome threatens two other much more important beliefs: that the use of EFM can prevent cerebral palsy and that intrapartum asphyxia is the cause of cerebral palsy. It is no wonder that there is resistance to collecting relevant evidence and giving it credence. 'I had not properly realised, until this time, the power of wish to distort and deny — and its prevalence in this complex situation, where enthusiasm of doctors and the distress of patients, might lie in an unconscious collusion, equally concerned to wish away an unpalatable truth' (Sachs 1982)" (Lumley 1988a, p. 306).

Two factors closely associated with the efficacy of the electronic fetal monitor are the way in which it is used, and the skill of the person who interprets the tracing. If there were one scientifically proven, right way to employ the monitor, in general clinicians would be assumed to adopt that method. In reality, all hospitals and physicians have different policies on how and when to use the electronic fetal monitor. Some clinicians use it only for special indications, which vary. Others prefer routine intermittent monitoring of all women, using an external device, reserving internal devices for special indications. Some prefer continuous external or internal monitoring. The systematic use of scalp blood sampling is not very common, even though research makes it clear that this increases reliability.

The skill of the person interpreting the tracing is a sensitive issue, central to the usefulness of the machine. Some physicians disregard findings of the randomised trials on the grounds that clinicians now have greater skill in reading the tracings. Such a statement is an admission that the science of interpreting the tracings is still in its infancy.

If the efficacy of routine EFM is nil, what about its efficacy for high risk or complicated cases? An obstetrician, well known for his expertise with the monitor, wrote:

> "The fetal monitor cannot always distinguish the difference between stress and distress of the foetus. Only 30–40% of the time, with ominous fetal heart rate patterns, are the infants actually acidotic [i.e. truly distressed]. There is a tendency to overcall fetal distress, based on a fetal heart rate pattern which on review, is not ominous at all" (Haverkamp 1985, p. 13).

Problems with the interpretation of fetal heart rate strips also were shown by a collaborative study carried out in a number of European countries (Derom 1987). Two outstanding experts were selected from several countries and all were sent the same set of clinical records which included monitor tracings. There was no agreement among the physicians on the interpretation of the tracings or how to manage the cases. In a similar study, 12 experts, selected for their scientific and clinical contribution to EFM, had considerable disagreement over the interpretation of EFM tracings (Cohen et al. 1982). A well known scientist concluded: "There are no universally agreed definitions of an abnormal EFM pattern" (Lumley 1988, p. 303). Furthermore, another study found 37% of tracings to be difficult or impossible to interpret (Keegan et al. 1985). In summary, the variation in the way the electronic fetal monitor is used and the difficulties in interpreting the tracings contribute to the doubts about the value of using this machine on all women and gives rise to concern about its efficacy for some of the complications of labour and birth.

RISKS OF ROUTINE USE

At first glance, the electronic fetal monitor appeared relatively innocuous; then, researchers took a second glance. In the early 1970s, when the use of the monitor was spreading, the caesarean section rate in many countries began to rise precipitously. These simultaneous increases could, of course, be a coincidence. But when the randomised controlled trials of EFM were reported, they showed more operative births in the groups of women who had received EFM. After a careful review of all these EFM clinical trials, Grant concludes:

> "The randomised comparisons of different methods of intra-partum fetal monitoring (with policies of operative delivery for 'fetal distress') are very consistent in the suggested effect of EFM on operative delivery rates. As might be expected, rates are higher in all the intensively monitored groups, with a typical increase of about one-third, regardless of whether fetal blood pH estimate was available. However, the use of pH assessment has an important modifying effect on the *types* of operative delivery, tending to limit the increased use of caesarean delivery and promote the use of operative vaginal delivery" (Grant 1991, p. 862).

In other words, the use of EFM increases the likelihood that forceps, vacuum extractor or caesarean section will follow. As some operative births result in harm to the woman or baby, such births must be considered a risk of routine electronic monitoring. This is another link in the chain of diagnostic and therapeutic intervention (see figure 2).

In addition, it is unfortunately a great temptation for a busy birth attendant in a hospital to focus on the monitor screens or strips rather than on the labouring woman. This decrease in human attention may be responsible for slowing or stopping the labour; the obstetrical diagnosis of this condition (called dystocia) is more common in electronically monitored women. Some evidence suggests that a further hazard may be an increase in infections in both baby and woman when electronic monitoring has been used.

FACTORS IN THE POPULARITY OF THE MONITOR

As routine monitoring of all women during labour has been scientifically shown to have no benefit and to carry the risk of increasing the frequency of subsequent invasive intervention, the popularity of the practice may seem a mystery. Perhaps the first explanation is the fascination that technology holds for health workers. An obstetrician has written:

> "We are so busy keeping up with this new technology, buying it, learning how to use it, admiring it — that we are not stopping to ask ourselves what problem does it solve? Visualisation and imaging, while of enormous interest to us, may not be the place to spend our money" (Haverkamp 1985, p. 14).

Midwives and nurses, for example, may take great pride in their new skill to read and interpret monitor tracings.

Another reason for the popularity of the electronic monitor during labour is the advantages to the staff in the hospital. The ideal of one-to-one attention by a birth attendant is impossible to achieve in many hospitals because of budget restrictions and variations in the number of women in labour at any given moment. Electronic fetal monitoring is perceived as better than ignoring labouring women for long periods. The monitor also gives the birth attendant more control; it is easier to leave the labouring woman and do other things. Even at the National Maternity Hospital in Dublin — the scene of the largest of the trials of the monitor — which has a long-standing policy of continuous personal bedside support for all labouring women, women were left alone more often when the monitor was used.

The economic interests of the manufacturers of the monitor also play a role. The extensive promotional and educational efforts they direct towards health personnel have an unmeasured but likely significant impact on increasing reliance on the machine (see earlier discussion of monitor manufacturers paying the expenses of doctors coming to a meeting to evaluate the monitor).

In addition, the industry has been slow to improve the inaccurate, cumbersome, uncomfortable and restrictive nature of the machines. An obstetrician suggested that:

"It is high time that we had a new generation of smaller and more intelligent fetal heart rate monitors which, together with telemetry, might make fetal monitoring in labour more effective and less intrusive" (Sawers 1983).

Another factor in the popularity of the monitor is a faith that abnormal electronic monitor tracings reflect abnormal conditions, and the concomitant belief that the reason behind the results of the randomised trials lies not in the technology but in the expertise of the user. This belief also includes the conviction that the monitor can predict brain damage before it occurs. Thus, the higher caesarean section rates associated with the monitor in the research is believed to be justified, despite the results of the trials. Rather than interpreting the caesarean section births as unnecessary, grateful parents and relieved doctors believed that the operations prevented brain damage. The extremely high rate of false positive diagnoses of fetal distress is explained away; a high caesarean section rate is seen as a small price to pay to save large numbers of babies from impairment. These beliefs are based on incorrect thinking and are not scientific (Simkin 1986).

In countries where more and more physicians are being sued for negligence, the electronic fetal monitor is a popular form of insurance. It is difficult to defend the non-use of this machine to juries who are facing grieving parents and brain-damaged children. Juries are easily convinced that the use of the monitor prevents death or disability. In these countries, therefore, physicians tend to allow the standards of practice for birth care to be determined in the court room (Simkin 1986).

In view of all the issues involved in using the electronic fetal monitor, as well as the high cost of buying and maintaining the equipment, great concern was expressed at Fortaleza about the spread of this machine to developing countries. An obstetrician from the United States who has done considerable research on EFM wrote:

"When the principal problem in one country appears to be malnutrition, or sepsis in another, or no access to prenatal care in a third, it seems frivolous to focus on the technology seemingly appropriate at the hour of delivery, rather than on the overall state of maternal and child health. In our opinion, electronic fetal monitoring is not going to have any dramatic effect on perinatal mortality or morbidity if extended universally to Latin America. In the United States, the technology is in place, yet the prenatal care and nutritional support for poor mothers is diminishing. And thus it appears that low birth-weight is on the rise and as we might expect, fetal and neonatal death rates are turning upward after many years of steady decline" (Haverkamp 1985, p. 15).

Such concerns led the participants strongly to recommend that governments in all countries be urged to control the spread of this particular piece of the birth machine. In summary, they stated that:

"There is no evidence that routine intrapartum electronic fetal monitoring has a positive effect on the outcome of pregnancy. Electronic fetal monitoring should be carried out only in carefully selected medical cases (related to high perinatal mortality rates) and in induced labour. Countries where electronic fetal monitors and qualified staff are available should carry out investigations to select specific groups of pregnant women who might benefit from electronic fetal monitoring. Until such time as results are known, national health care services should abstain from purchasing new monitoring equipment."

An interesting post-script to this recommendation came in 1988 with an official joint statement from the American Academy of Pediatrics and the American College of Obstetricians and Gynecologists:

"It has been shown that intermittent auscultation at intervals of 15 minutes is equivalent to continuous electronic fetal heart rate monitoring . . . For low-risk patients in labour, the fetal heart rate may be monitored by auscultation" (American Academy of Pediatrics and American College of Obstetricians and Gynecologists 1988, p. 67).

Episiotomy

Two of the participants published an article just before the meeting (Thacker & Banta 1983). It reviewed over 350 books and articles on episiotomy published since 1860 and this article was used during the meeting as the basis for discussion.

Except for the cutting and tying of the umbilical cord, episiotomy is the most common surgical procedure in birth care. Although widespread, its use varies greatly between and within countries. The extremes are perhaps represented by the rates of episiotomy for all births in The Netherlands (8%) and Hungary (essentially 100%). While the overall rate in United States hospitals is reported to be 62.5% (Thacker & Banta 1983) the rate is around 20% in birth centres staffed by midwives, and is even lower in home births. Rates in Canadian hospitals are similarly high: one study in Quebec found a rate of 82.5% (Rocheleau-Parent 1980). "Despite the increasing evidence that high North American episiotomy rates cannot be easily defended, rates for primiparous women in excess of 80% are commonplace" (Klein 1993). The rates in Western Europe are considerably lower: 28.4% in Belgium (Buekens et al. 1985), 28.2% in France (Rumeau-Rouquette et al. 1979). On the basis of visits to many hospitals in every Eastern European country, I have observed the rates to approach 100% — episiotomy is a routine procedure done on essentially every birthing woman in every hospital in Eastern Europe.

Debate on the management of the perineum (the area surrounding the vaginal opening) during birth has endured for centuries. The widespread use of episiotomy as a solution, however, came with the advent of the specialty of obstetrics. Even today, the data show that the widespread and frequent use of episiotomy is much more characteristic of physicians than midwives. Indeed, the question about episiotomy in the medical literature has almost always been how, rather than whether, to cut. The relative advantages and disadvantages of cutting straight down (midline) and of cutting diagonally (mediolateral) have long been argued in the literature. This issue is not yet resolved; in North America, obstetricians favour the midline approach and those in Europe and elsewhere prefer the mediolateral incision.

To understand the widespread use of episiotomy at present, the procedure must be seen as part of the medical or surgical approach to birth. Thus, an obstetrical text states that episiotomy:

> "substitutes a straight, clean surgical incision for the ragged laceration that otherwise frequently results. Furthermore, the episiotomy is easier to repair and heals better than a tear" (Pritchard & MacDonald 1980).

The most recent edition of another highly respected obstetrical text-book not only continues to recommend episiotomy but also dismisses recent published careful analyses of the scientific literature questioning the procedure (Cunningham et al. 1989).

Other characteristics of the usual obstetrical approach to birth care increase the need for episiotomy: using forceps, the lithotomy position, speeding up the labour, and the use of pain relief such as epidural analgesia and general anaesthesia. All increase the stress on the perineum and decrease the opportunity of the perineal tissues to stretch naturally, thus increasing the risk of tears. Episiotomy rates, at least in the United States, increased as hospital births increased. Episiotomy can be seen as one of the final links in the long chain of diagnostic and therapeutic intervention during medically-oriented birth care.

BENEFITS

Three benefits are claimed for episiotomy by obstetricians. First, it is said to prevent the severe (third degree) tears in the perineum that extend to the anus and/or rectum. Such tears are related to a number of factors, including low parity (the number of previous births the woman has had), breech presentation, abnormal tissue stiffness, speeding up the second stage of labour, the use of forceps, and inexperience or lack of skill in the birth attendant. As a result, there are great differences in the frequency of third-degree tears in women who have no episiotomy (ranging from 0% to 6.4% in this group) and in those in which the surgical cut is extended by tearing (0–23.9%) (Thacker & Banta 1983). Six studies have adequately analysed the relationship of episiotomy to laceration. One study was a retrospective case control investigation on the relationship of episiotomy to third degree tears in 21,278 singleton births (Buekens et al. 1985). Rather than finding fewer tears with episiotomy, they found more: 1.4% of births with episiotomy had third degree tears compared with 0.9% of the births without episiotomy ($p<0.01$). They conclude:

> "Third degree tears were not more frequent in deliveries without episiotomy. No other benefit of routine use of episiotomy has been demonstrated clearly in the literature and evidence of unwanted effects such as postpartum pain and discomfort are accumulating (Kitzinger & Walters 1981;

Reading et al. 1982; Thacker & Banta 1982). Our data is thus in agreement with the suggestion of Thacker and Banta (1983) that episiotomy is needed in no more than one in every five deliveries" (Buekiens et al. 1985 pp 823).

The other 5 studies are prospective random controlled trials (Sleep et al. 1984; Harrison et al. 1984; Stewart et al. 1983; Flint & Poulengeris 1987; Klein et al. 1992). A careful review of 4 of these trials concludes:

"Liberal use of episiotomy is associated with higher overall rates of perineal trauma. There is no evidence that this policy [liberal use of episiotomy] reduces the risk of serious perineal or vaginal trauma" (Sleep et al. 1991, p. 1137).

The most recent randomised controlled trial found very similar results: "Restricting episiotomy use in primiparous women was associated with similar sutured perineal trauma to the liberal or routine approach. Multiparous women in the restricted episiotomy group more often gave birth with an intact perineum" (Klein et al. 1992). It is important to note that in this trial 47 women suffered third or fourth degree perineal tears and 46 of them were in women who had episiotomy.

The five prospective trials agree with the retrospective study: episiotomy does not protect from serious perineal tears.

Some birth attendants, particularly midwives, use a number of techniques to prevent laceration: massage and stretching of the perineum during pregnancy, massage of the perineum and the application of warm compresses to the perineum during labour, immersion of the woman in water during labour, slowing down of the second stage, and gradual stretching of the perineum through careful control of the descending fetal head. In Kazakhstan (formerly of the USSR) a number of these techniques are routinely used on all women during pregnancy and birth. An episiotomy rate of 3.5% and an overall tear rate of 6% is reported (Houd 1983).

Unfortunately, the relationship of these techniques to the prevention of tears during birth has received little scientific study. Overall, the scientific literature does not indicate that episiotomy reduces the number of tears during birth.

The second benefit claimed for episiotomy is the prevention of long-term damage to the pelvic floor (the muscles and ligaments that hold the reproductive organs in place). There are few studies to support or refute this hypothesis; only one has been found that is not scientifically flawed. In this randomised controlled trial pelvic floor function was measured with electromyographic (EMG) perineometry. "No difference between trial groups was found in postpartum perineal pain, antepartum and 3-month postpartum EMG perineometry, and urinary and pelvic floor symptoms" (Klein et al. 1992). We are left with scientific evidence that this second claimed benefit is not justified.

In addition, the decreases in family size over the past century may have resulted in a decrease in the number of times a woman's pelvic floor is stressed, and reduced the frequency of this complication of childbirth. Again, there are no data to assess this possibility. It is also claimed that damage to the pelvic floor can cause prolapse of the genitals and urinary stress incontinence and that episiotomy prevents such incontinence. Since 5–10% of women have this debilitating symptom after having a baby (Stanton 1980), it is important to know if episiotomy reduces it. A review of the literature on this question states: "Whatever the aetiology of postpartum stress incontinence may be, there is no good evidence that more liberal use of episiotomy is protective against this distressing symptom" (Sleep et al. 1991, p. 1140).

The third presumed benefit of episiotomy is to protect the baby from the adverse consequences of an extended second stage of labour, including lack of oxygen and trauma to the head, which has been said to lead to cerebral palsy and mental retardation. As stated earlier, the importance of the length of the various stages of labour and birth is still debated, raising doubts about the advisability of a policy favouring fast labour. Research that has tried to show that a longer second stage of labour is bad for the baby has failed to find this result or has been poorly designed, with questionable interpretation of results. Conversely, some studies suggest that speeding up the second stage may be bad for the baby but here, too, data are insufficient. In summary:

"There is no evidence to suggest that, when the second stage of labour is progressing and the condition of both mother and fetus is satisfactory, the imposition of any arbitrary

169

upper limit on its duration is justified. Such limits should be discarded" (Sleep et al. 1991, p. 1141).

No follow-up studies have been done to find out if there is a relationship between episiotomy and cerebral palsy or mental retardation. Studies of these two conditions suggest that they originate — for the most part — before labour and birth. Furthermore, and most importantly, neither of the two clinical trials which looked at this issue found any evidence that episiotomy reduces trauma to the fetal head (Sleep et al. 1984; Harrison et al. 1984). In the most recent trial the authors state: "Reports based on adequate sample size for this outcome (Reynolds & Yudkin 1987) have indicated the safety for the fetus when a restricted approach to episiotomy was undertaken" (Klein et al. 1992).

Episiotomy is likely to have repeated the pattern frequently found in technology use. A clear benefit from using the procedure for a specific condition is followed by a tendency gradually to increase the indications until the procedure is routine. In extreme cases, such as severe fetal or maternal distress, or a very prolonged expulsion stage in which the perineum is apparently responsible for lack of progress, episiotomy has a place. This has led in some places to a routine use that has no scientific justification. No surgical procedure, even one that seems rather trivial to the people who perform it, should be widely used without convincing evidence of benefit. People who use a type of technology routinely and claim a benefit have an obligation to prove their claims through adequately designed clinical research. As yet, no published study adequately proves the claimed benefits of episiotomy.

RISKS

Any surgical procedure has risks such as blood loss and infection. Considering the frequency of episiotomy, the lack of research on this procedure is extraordinary. A few studies on how to cut, however, have reported complications; they give some unsystematic information on risks. First, there may be an unsatisfactory anatomical result; the incision (and hence the vagina) may be sewn too tightly, too loosely or crookedly. A study reported these complications in 50% of episiotomy cases, but the scientific literature gives no clear indication as to whether long-term anatomical results are better with or without episiotomy. Increased blood loss occurs in about 10% of women undergoing the procedure (Thacker & Banta 1983).

Pain after an episiotomy is almost certainly the most common complication; it occurs to some degree in every case. It normally receives more serious consideration from the women subjected to episiotomy than the people who perform it. No study has focused on this complication. Nevertheless, studies of pain medication and different episiotomy techniques report moderate to severe pain in up to 60% of women with episiotomy and the need for at least some pain relief in 85%. The significance of this pain is indicated by the extensive literature on testing different types of pain killers for episiotomy (Thacker & Banta 1983). In one randomised clinical trial which followed up on the women found that the group in which 51% of the women received episiotomy experienced the same amount of pain at 10 days and 3 months postpartum as the group in which 10% received episiotomy (Sleep et al. 1984). The other trial that followed the women also found no difference between trial groups in postpartum perineal pain (Klein et al. 1992). Birth produces a painful perineum and it is not yet clear whether episiotomy is more painful than natural tears.

Painful sexual intercourse after episiotomy is seldom mentioned in the obstetrical literature, but a few studies show that it is fairly common. Nearly two thirds of the women with episiotomy in one study reported pain or discomfort on sexual intercourse in the first six weeks after giving birth and nearly one quarter reported persistently painful sex after three months. A different study showed 19% of women who had episiotomy as having painful intercourse for more than three months, compared with 11% of women having a tear (Thacker & Banta 1983). On the other hand, the randomised clinical trial by Sleep et al. found that although the group with 51% episiotomy resumed sexual intercourse somewhat later than the group with 10% episiotomy, at 3 months and 3 years postpartum both groups had nearly identical proportions of women with pain on intercourse (Sleep & Grant 1987). Likewise, the most recent trial reports: ". . . women with intact perineums began sexual intercourse approximately 1 week earlier than those experiencing any other perineal outcomes. Pain on resumption of sexual intercourse, 3-month postpartum sexual satisfaction, and the proportion of women not beginning sexual intercourse by 3 months postpartum were also similar in the 2 groups" (Klein et al. 1992).

Infection is a recognised complication of any surgical procedure, including episiotomy. Infection resulting from episiotomy causes a measurable but poorly quantified amount of illness. Rates of infection directly attributable to the result of episiotomy are not found in the literature, although one study found positive cultures in 76% of episiotomies, despite the use of sterile technique (Thacker & Banta 1983). What is more surprising is that deaths from episiotomy have been reported by three studies in the United States (Golde & Ledger 1977; Shy & Exchenbach 1979; Ewing et al. 1979). These deaths were from complications usually found when the episiotomy extends into a third or fourth degree tear such as excessive blood loss, haematoma formation and infections.

Unfortunately, the emotional sequelae from episiotomy are neglected. Anecdotal evidence suggests women may feel sexually assaulted and traumatised. One several occasions, when addressing women's groups in industrialised countries concerned about the mutilation of female genitalia in Africa as a result of female circumcision, I have suggested that since charity begins at home they might do well to focus on the widespread excessive episiotomy in their own countries which could conceivably also be perceived as unnecessary female genital mutilation.

The risks of episiotomy are more severe than often appreciated. Severe pain, painful sexual intercourse, infections or a deformed vagina can have an important effect on the life of an otherwise healthy woman, particularly when she is responsible for the care of a new baby and, usually, the maintenance of a good relationship with a partner.

FINDINGS

Clearly, a decline in operative, interventionist obstetrics would reduce the need for episiotomy. This was conclusively shown in a careful, brilliant analysis of the data from the most recent randomised control trial on episiotomy (Klein et al. 1993). The physicians involved in the trial were divided according to their belief and perineal management style into: low episiotomy users (0–50%); mid episiotomy users (50–75%); high episiotomy users (76–100%). By analysing the data according to these 3 groups, they found:

"The primiparous women cared for by physicians with the lowest episiotomy rates in both arms of the trial sustained the lowest rate of third/fourth degree tears and had the highest rate of intact perineums. By contrast, the group of physicians with the highest episiotomy rate, including several physicians who used episiotomy in primiparous women 100% of the time, attended almost no primiparae with an intact perineum, and primiparae under their care had a severe perineal tear rate of 22% . . . Caring for primiparous women with similar infant weight distribution in both trial arms, the high episiotomy users also employed more procedures of induction, augmentation, epidural and/or forceps. As well, the high episiotomy users had the highest caesarean section rate for their non-randomised primiparous women . . . In summary: physicians with the highest episiotomy rates not only had a different perineal management and perineal trauma pattern, but they saw the clinical situation differently, and their interventionistic style resulted in more severe perineal trauma for the primiparous women under their care . . . The intensity with which physicians adhere to the belief that episiotomy benefits women, is well illustrated by the behaviour of the high episiotomy users within our trial, who were unwilling or unable to reduce their rate according to the protocol" (Klein et al. 1993).

These findings have implications far beyond the issue of episiotomy by showing that a doctors' obstetrical intervention rates are, to a great extent, a function of their belief system and consequent obstetrical management styles. This is an important field for further study and has broad implications for strategies to modify intervention rates.

What would be a reasonable episiotomy rate if there were a more balanced, conservative attitude towards episiotomy? Where birth care is less aggressive and where midwives are most often the principal birth attendants, episiotomy rates tend to be 5–20%. A more recent review of the scientific literature on episiotomy than the review used in Fortaleza concludes:

"There is no evidence to support . . . claims that liberal use of episiotomy reduces the risk of severe perineal trauma, improves perineal healing, prevents fetal trauma, or reduces the risk of urinary stress incontinence after delivery. Episiotomy should be used only to relieve fetal or maternal distress, or to achieve adequate progress when it is the perineum that is responsible for lack of progress" (Sleep et al. 1991, p. 1141).

This suggests that an overall episiotomy rate of 20% is perhaps the most reasonable goal for today's hospitals. Lower rates could be reasonable in birth centres and home births, from which women likely to have complications are excluded. To achieve such rates, birth attendants — physicians and midwives — need improved training and experience with the methods that may help to increase the natural ability of the perineal tissues to stretch, which reduce the tendency for tearing and thus the need for episiotomy.

Further research on episiotomy, using randomised controlled trials, is urgently needed to examine: the efficacy and safety of the procedure; the relationship between episiotomy and long-term pelvic relaxation, infection and pain; and the efficacy of methods to increase the natural distensibility of the perineum.

Reaching consensus on episiotomy was not easy. There was ready agreement on both the lack of scientific justification for the routine use of episiotomy and the need to try alternative methods to protect the perineum. But a proposal that a 20% rate of episiotomy be recommended as a goal for hospital birth aroused strong debate, and finally had to be dropped. The final recommendation, then, was: *"The systematic use of episiotomy is not justified. The protection of the perineum through alternative methods should be evaluated and adopted".*

Caesarean section

Caesarean section epitomises the present crisis in dealing with the birth machine. Because it is a major surgical procedure, good data exist to monitor its prevalence, revealing an increase in its use that can only be described as epidemic. Caesarean section is the ultimate contribution of the medical approach to birth: the most dramatic obstetrical intervention, unequivocally capable of saving the lives of both women and babies. Today, many if not most obstetricians do not attend births: they perform fetal extractions through the vagina or an abdominal cut. In fact, some obstetricians propose that all fetuses be extracted through caesarean section; women who insist on vaginal births should be required to sign a special consent form (Feldman & Freiman 1985). Some women, too, request or demand that a caesarean section be scheduled.

EPIDEMIC INCREASES IN USE

In most industrialised countries, about 5% of all births were by caesarean section in 1970. The figure for 1980 was more than twice as high. By 1985 the figure was three to four times as high in a number of industrialised countries. More recent figures suggest that this increase is continuing in most countries, although there is considerable variation.

Since 1980 several studies have looked at international variations in caesarean section rates in industrialised countries. The WHO European Perinatal Study Group was the first, reporting a four fold variation among the Western European countries having data available (Bergjo et al. 1983). By 1986 the caesarean section rate in the United States had risen to a shocking 24% with Canada not far behind (Notzon et al. 1987). The addition of North America produced a sixfold variation among industrialised countries since countries such as Czechoslovakia and The Netherlands maintained national rates of 5–10% (Notzon 1990).

The most recent study of caesarean section rates among countries was another investigation by the WHO European office (Stephenson 1992). The study was conducted to compare patterns of obstetrical practice in 12 countries: Australia (State of Victoria); Canada (Quebec Province); the Czech and Slovak Federal Republic (Czech Republic); Denmark; Finland; Greece; Hungary; Israel; The Netherlands; Slovenia; the United Kingdom (Scotland); and the United States (Washington State). The study period was 1983–1988. The WHO report summarises the findings:

> "Caesarean section rates varied three fold among the participating countries. Caesarean section rates increased in all countries over the observation period. Those countries with the highest rates had smaller net increases in rates of caesarean section in the latter years of the observation period. The countries with the lowest rates had more modest and gradual, but relentless increases. There was a decrease in the caesarean section rate during the last year of observation in Australia, Denmark and Finland" (Stephenson 1992, p. 1).

Caesarean section rates vary as much within a country as between countries. A Birth Guide giving details from all hospitals in Denmark in 1991 found a caesarean section rate of 23.9% in one Jutland hospital and 9.9% in another (Houd 1992). In Scotland a study found the caesarean section rate varied between 4.9% and 19.6% in smaller hospitals and between 8.7% and 17.4% in larger hospitals (McIlwaine 1985). Some of this within country variation might be the result of referring high risk pregnant women to secondary and tertiary level care hospitals for birth. The recent WHO study looked at this possibility with interesting results (Stephenson 1992). Indicators that a hospital was a referral centre (size of maternity service, availability of neonatal intensive care, being a teaching hospital) correlated with higher caesarean section rates in some countries and not others. Looking, for example, at some data (table below) from this report one sees that while Australia, Czechoslovakia and the United Kingdom appear to have an effective referral system that results in much more caesarean section done at tertiary level hospitals, in countries such as Canada and the United States, so much caesarean section is done everywhere that the referral system does not result in significantly more caesarean section done in referral hospitals.

On the other hand, caesarean section rates do appear to be greatly influenced by who is the birth attendant. Even in the United States, where about one in four births is by caesarean section, two studies have found greatly reduced caesarean section rates when midwives are the primary caregivers at birth. Of 11,814 women admitted to 84 freestanding birth centres in the United States (staffed by midwives with physician backup for complications), 4.4% had caesarean section (Rooks et al. 1989). The second study was a more in depth comparison of one birth centre (midwives in charge) with a hospital in the same city (physicians in charge) (Baruffi et al. 1990). After taking into account all variables, the caesarean section rate was two and one-half times lower in the birth centre. The researchers concluded that diverging philosophies about managing birth at the two facilities offer the most likely explanation for the contrast in caesarean section rates. Two scientists in the United Kingdom, after looking at wide variations in obstetrical interventions including caesarean section in that country conclude: "The treatment women received depended most of all on where they lived, which hospital they went

Country	Procedure	Neonatal Intensive Care Unit Level						p
		I		II		III		
		x	SD	x	SD	x	SD	
Australia 1987	caesarean	9.1	9.1	16.3	5.3	13.3	9.0	++
	inst. vag.	10.4	8.1	13.2	4.5	13.7	9.3	NS
Canada 1987	caesarean	15.8	7.5	18.5	3.9	22.0	1.5	NS
	inst. vag.	10.9	9.6	13.7	9.3	19.0	9.1	NS
Czech. 1987	caesarean	6.0	2.6	6.6	2.6	9.5	2.9	+++
	inst. vag.	1.6	1.1	1.4	1.2	1.6	0.8	NS
Finland 1988	caesarean	14.6	3.4	—	—	14.4	5.6	NS
	inst. vag.	5.2	1.9	—	—	5.2	1.8	NS
Israel 1987	caesarean	6.6	0.0	11.0	2.7	10.0	1.9	NS
	inst. vag.	3.4	0.0	5.4	2.4	5.3	2.3	NS
Slovenia 1987	caesarean	7.3	2.6	—	—	9.2	0.0	++
	inst. vag.	3.1	1.1	—	—	1.1	0.0	++
U.K. 1987	caesarean	1.1	3.5	—	—	14.1	2.9	+++
	inst. vag.	2.5	3.3	—	—	10.5	3.8	+++
United States (1987)	caesarean	15.9	10.2	17.1	7.5	17.6	3.4	NS
	inst. vag.	6.2	6.8	9.2	7.4	11.5	8.4	NS

Test statistics: Student's t; one-way ANOVA

+	$p < 0.05$
++	$p < 0.01$
+++	$p < 0.001$
NS	not significant

(Stephenson 1992)

Table 2: *Hospital-specific caesarean section and instrumental vaginal delivery rates by hospital neonatal intensive care unit level, according to country, most recent year*

to, and the particular doctor or midwife they saw" (Chalmers & Richards 1987). It is impossible at this point not to make the observation that only in those industrialised countries with the highest caesarean section rates such as the United States and Canada does one find both the widespread practice of obstetricians giving primary care to normal (low risk) pregnant and birthing women combined with very few practising midwives.

In all these industrialised countries, the primary justification for caesarean section birth must be to save the life of the woman or baby. While maternal mortality rates are so low as to make cross national variation not significant, perinatal mortality rates vary considerably. Many physicians feel the increasing caesarean section rates are justified believing they have led to lower perinatal mortality rates. Hence a key issue becomes: do the caesarean section rates in countries correlate with their perinatal mortality rates? Researchers who have looked at cross national variations in caesarean section rates in the last ten years and compared these rates with perinatal mortality rates have failed to find any significant correlation. The first WHO European office study found: "An increase in the number of operative deliveries will, at best, have a very small impact on perinatal mortality rates" (Bergsjo et al. 1986). A review of caesarean section rates in the European Economic Community found that the number of caesarean section births had very little impact on perinatal outcome (Thiery & Derom 1984). A study carried out by the National Centre for Health Statistics in the United States comments: "The comparison of perinatal mortality ratios with caesarean section and with operative vaginal rates finds no consistent correlation across countries" (Notzon 1990). A review of the scientific literature on this issue states: "A number of studies have failed to detect any relation between crude perinatal mortality rates and the level of operative deliveries" (Lomas & Enkin 1991).

Since it is true that caesarean section does save babies lives, why has a correlation between caesarean section rates and perinatal mortality rates not been found? As indications for the procedure broaden and rates go up, lives are being saved in a smaller and smaller proportion of all the caesarean section cases. But the risks of the procedure do not decrease with increasing rates. Eventually it is only logical that a point is reached at which the procedure kills almost as many babies as it saves. This possibility is, for the most part, invisible to obstetricians; they may experience the cases in which babies' lives are saved, but very often may not see the death of a baby, for example, from respiratory distress syndrome in a neonatal intensive care unit, hours or days after caesarean section.

The situation in the developing countries is different but equally alarming. Because of the location of the meeting and the availability of good data, caesarean section in Brazil was reviewed. Although not necessarily representative of the situation in all developing countries, this example was valuable. In 1981, caesarean section accounted for 30.9% of all births in Brazil — a rate higher than that in any industrialised country (Faundes 1985). An in-depth analysis showed the lowest caesarean section rates in the poorest states in Brazil, where the need for such a procedure is greatest, and the highest in the richest states, where malnutrition and chronic disease are lowest and families smallest (table 3). Why is this so?

At a meeting in 1982, a group of the most distinguished professors of obstetrics in Brazil listed what they considered to be the most important influences on the high rate in their country (Faundes 1985):

1. Better follow-up of maternal care during pregnancy with adequate identification and monitoring of those cases where obstetrical risks exist;
2. Indiscriminate use of the procedure where there is no clear medical indication such as for tubal sterilisation.
3. Some women are not psychologically prepared for vaginal delivery;
4. Lack of adequate competence by some doctors to handle a vaginal delivery;
5. Convenience and security of the doctor;
6. Health care inefficiency;
7. Failure of prenatal care to give orientation to the pregnant woman about vaginal delivery.

The Brazilian obstetricians wrote:

"There is no question that the caesarean delivery has become a cultural phenomenon that goes beyond the purely medical factors — the acceptance of the caesarean delivery by Brazilian women is clear" (Faundes 1985).

They explained the women's acceptance in terms of the worship of the body by western culture; the sexual function of women is considered both extremely important and to be connected to the anatomical condition of the genital organs. The obstetricians thought that many women believed that vaginal delivery permanently stretches the vagina and thus damages women's sexual function. Further, this notion did not originate in lay opinion, but was publicly promoted by influential obstetrical professors at national medical conferences.

Monthly family income (equivalent to number of minimum salaries)	Percentage of caesarean deliveries in		
	Sao Paulo	Rio de Janeiro	Brazil
<1	26.6	24.2	16.7
1–2	32.9	29.4	22.2
2–3	33.9	33.0	27.6
3–5	45.3	43.7	36.2
5–10	52.4	49.6	45.9
10+	63.4	67.9	57.6

(Faundes et al. 1985)

Table 3: *Percentage of caesarean deliveries by family income in the States of Sao Paulo and Rio de Janeiro and for all of Brazil.*

While such cultural beliefs may be widely held, only women who can pay for private health care or have adequate health insurance can act on them to get the caesarean section they desire. The most extreme examples of this phenomenon are found in the largest cities in Brazil. Here, about two thirds of the richest women have caesarean section births and some private hospitals have caesarean section rates of over 90% (table 3). As a result, Brazil has the highest ever recorded national caesarean section rate, 32% (Notzon 1990). While Brazil illustrates the extreme of these cultural contributions to rising rates, the same factors exist to a lesser extent in many other countries, developing and developed.

INDICATIONS

Caesarean section has undoubted benefits for certain complications of pregnancy and birth. The use of the procedure for premature separation of the placenta, eclampsia, placenta praevia, or a pathologically small pelvic outlet has saved the lives of many women and babies. For other conditions such as possible fetal distress and prolonged or difficult labour, caesarean section may be beneficial. In these cases, however, the decision to resort to this procedure is difficult and has tended to be made too quickly. Consequently one finds great variation in the frequency of fetal distress and dystocia as reasons given for caesarean section. As seen in the following table, the recent WHO European Office study, for example, found dystocia as the reason for caesarean section in from 9.7% to 33.8% of cases and fetal distress as the reason in from 8.6% to 23.2% of caesarean sections.

Country	Year	Repeat caesarean	Breech	Dystocia	Fetal Distress	Other
Australia	1987	29.9	17.3	23.5	7.3	22.0
Canada	1987	39.0	14.6	31.46	6.4	8.6
Czech	1988	6.4	16.9	20.0	33.5	23.2
Greece	1988	40.8	15.0	17.4	10.8	16.0
Israel	1987	35.4	17.2	9.7	17.4	20.4
Slovenia	1987	23.7	12.5	33.8	10.9	19.1
US (Wash)	1987	36.7	13.0	22.1	2.9	18.0

(Stephenson 1992)

Table 4: *Percent of births delivered by caesarean section by indication and country, most recent year.*

There are also conditions for which caesarean section has become routine, in spite of scientific evidence of a lack of benefit: all cases of breech presentation and all cases in which the woman has had a previous caesarean section. A detailed review of each of the clinical indications for caesarean section is beyond the scope of this book, but it was the task of two consensus conferences, held in Canada and the United States. The conclusions presented here on two of the indications received unanimous agreement at the two conferences and by the participants at the WHO consensus meeting.

The scientific literature and the national consensus conferences recommended that caesarean section not be routinely used for breech presentation; vaginal birth is the best choice in a number of situations. (US Department of Health and Human Services 1981; Canadian Panel 1986) No more than 50% of all breech births should ever require caesarean section. The birth attendant at vaginal breech births needs patience and skill. In many countries, it is the midwives who have maintained these skills. In some medical schools in the United Kingdom, the United States and Scandinavia it is the midwives who teach future obstetricians how to assist at a breech birth (Houd 1991; Gaskin 1991; Flint 1991). But the data from the recent WHO study (table 4) nevertheless suggests routine caesarean section for breech birth in these seven countries (Stephenson 1992).

The obstetrical policy "once a caesarean section, always a caesarean section" has been the most powerful force in the epidemic increase in the use of the procedure. This policy has a multiplier effect on all other indications for caesarean section. "Since over 90% of North American women with previous caesareans have repeat sections and over one-third of all caesareans are repeat operations, professional and public support for vaginal birth after caesarean (VBAC) is crucial if the caesarean section rates are ever to fall" (International Childbirth Education Association 1990, p. 2). This quote was from 1990, ten years after the US Consensus Conference had recommended vaginal birth after caesarean. In 1988 only 12.6% of United States women with a previous caesarean section had a VBAC and the proportion of United States women with a caesarean section scar on their uterus doubled between 1980 and 1988 despite the recommendation of the consensus conference. While the United States struggles to increase its VBAC rate, other countries do it more routinely. Thus table 4 from the recent WHO European study makes it clear that: in the United States, Canada and Greece repeat caesarean section is the norm; VBAC is the norm in Czechoslovakia; while Slovenia, Israel and Australia do some of both.

The scientific data in support of a trial of VBAC is overwhelming (Enkin 1991). Two national consensus conferences, United States (US Department of Health and Human Services 1981) and Canada (Canadian Panel 1986) together with two national obstetrical organisations, United States (American College of Obstetrics and Gynecology 1985) and Canada (Canadian Society of Obstetricians and Gynecologists 1982) have all recommended a trial of labour after caesarean section. And yet one study showed that 80% of practising obstetricians would not try VBAC, even if shown overwhelming evidence of its safety (Sloan 1968).

Because the data are so clear favouring a trial of VBAC and because repeat caesarean section has a multiplier effect, the participants made a separate recommendation against routine repeat caesarean section:

> "There is no evidence that a caesarean section is required after a previous transverse low-segment caesarean section birth. Vaginal deliveries after a caesarean should normally be encouraged wherever emergency surgical capacity is available."

With regard to the indications for caesarean section, then, the situation can be summarised: "Thus the observed differences in operative delivery rates suggest that collectively the obstetrical community is uncertain as to when caesarean section is indicated" (Lomas & Enkin 1991).

RISKS

Yielding to the temptation to do a caesarean section for dubious medical indications or because a woman requests it, to maintain a "honeymoon vagina", could only be justified if such a birth carried no more risk for the woman and baby than a vaginal birth. Starting with risks to the woman, it must first be understood that she has a significantly greater risk of dying from giving birth through a caesarean cut than from giving birth through her vagina. The rate of maternal mortality associated with caesarean section is 4 times that associated with vaginal birth (Petitti 1982). Clearly some of these deaths are related to the condition for which the caesarean section was done. But for women who have an elective repeat caesarean section, any excess death must be that associated with the surgical procedure itself. Since the maternal mortality for elective repeat caesarean section is twice the rate for all vaginal birth (Petitti 1982), there can be no doubt that caesarean section itself carries twice the risk of death for the woman (Enkin 1991). One of the reasons this appalling fact is not sufficiently appreciated is that deaths associated with caesarean section are seriously under-reported. In one United States study, five of the sixteen maternal deaths after caesarean section (nearly a third) had not been reported (Rubin et al. 1981). Nine of these sixteen deaths were found to be due to the caesarean section per se. These nine deaths produced a caesarean-per-se-attributed maternal mortality rate (9 per 15,188 caesarean sections or 59.3 per 100,000 caesarean sections) which was six times higher than the maternal mortality rate for all vaginal births.

The woman having a caesarean section faces dangers other than death including: damage to uterine blood vessels, accidental extension of the uterine incision, damage to the urinary bladder, anaesthesia accidents, wound infections, lower subsequent fertility (Pearson & Rees 1991; Petitti 1985; Sachs et al. 1987; Burt et al. 1988; Kirkinen 1988; McClusker et al. 1988; Hemminki 1987; Eisenkop et al. 1982; Nielsen & Hokegard 1984; Hurry et al. 1984; Hemminki 1985).

Some of these risks are common — for example one in five women have fever after caesarean section (Enkin et al. 1991), most of which is due to various infections.

In addition, there are psychological and social risks. Research shows a connection between the procedure and the development of postpartum depression and other psychological morbidity in the woman (Garel et al. 1987). Other research shows a lower likelihood of successful establishment of breastfeeding. Although the psychological and social consequences of caesarean section have received less extensive study than the medical consequences, they are not less real.

There are also medical risks for the baby. A serious consequence of a high rate of caesarean section is iatrogenic prematurity (the baby is premature because the caesarean section was performed too early, before the end of the pregnancy). As one of the consequences is low birth weight, iatrogenic prematurity can be a grave problem (Benson et al. 1969). Caesarean section also puts the newborn infant at greater risk of respiratory distress syndrome — another major cause of neonatal death.

> "That abdominal delivery (caesarean section) carries an increased risk of respiratory distress has been observed frequently, but there has been more controversy as to whether this is an effect of the mode of delivery itself or of any of several possible confounders. Much documentation now supports the view that the procedure per se is a potent risk factor for infantile respiratory disease syndrome in preterm infants and for other forms of respiratory distress in mature infants" (Hjalmarson 1991, p. 12).

This risk has at least two causes: the absence of an unidentified factor that reduces the risk of this syndrome when there has been a trial of labour, and low birth weight and lung immaturity due to iatrogenic prematurity.

> "Despite the consistent finding that the incidence of respiratory distress syndrome is less among infants whose mothers were allowed to go into labour prior to their section than in those of mothers who were sectioned without the benefit of labour, elective caesarean section without the benefit of a period of spontaneous labour persists as the norm" (Lomas & Enkin 1991, p. 1192).

Such medical problems in babies born by caesarean section lead to an increased number of referrals to neonatal intensive care units. This is one of the final links in the chain of diagnostic and therapeutic intervention (figure 2). Even babies born following subsequent pregnancies after a previous caesarean section have an increased perinatal mortality (Hemminki 1987).

The fact that caesarean section carries serious risks for both woman and baby seems to be one of modern civilisations best kept secrets. Why is it that an article in a leading American obstetrical journal proving that elective repeat caesarean section has a 6 times higher maternal mortality than vaginal birth had no apparent effect on the rapidly rising caesarean section rate in that country? Why can a leading medical journal, in all apparent seriousness, publish an article suggesting that all birth be caesarean section? (Feldman & Freiman 1985). Why is it that when the possibility of caesarean section arises, women are *not* told as part of their informed consent that the procedure increases the chance of their dying and increases the chance that the baby will have a life threatening illness? The reality is rather the opposite. Caesarean section has become such an accepted phenomenon that the redundant phrase 'vaginal birth' has come into common usage, to distinguish it from the euphemistic 'abdominal birth'.

FINANCIAL COST

In view of the increased hospital expenses for this major operation as compared with normal birth, the economic costs to a nation can be staggering. In the United States, for example, the caesarean section rate was 24.1% in 1986; of the 3,731,000 live births, 899,171 were by caesarean section (National Centre for Health Statistics). In this year, the Scandinavian countries, which have some of the lowest perinatal and infant mortality rates in the world, had rates of 10–15% (Stephenson 1992). If the rate in the United States had been 15%, caesarean section births would have numbered 559,650. Since each of the additional 339,521 operations costs US$3000 more than a vaginal birth (Statistical Bulletin 1986), these excess caesarean sections cost more than US$1000 million in one year.

The economic costs of caesarean section go beyond the hospital costs for the woman, to the increased use of expensive neonatal intensive care and to the home. Families may need extra help at home and suffer from loss of earnings. Caesarean section is expensive; the costs are an even more serious matter for countries and people with limited economic resources.

NON-MEDICAL FACTORS INFLUENCING CAESAREAN SECTION RATES

It is clear from the earlier discussion of caesarean section in Brazil that social and cultural factors play a role in caesarean section rates. These factors also play a role in industrialised countries. For example, studies in the United States show that women most likely to receive caesarean section are white and married, have private health insurance and give birth in private hospitals (Stafford 1990; Hayes et al. 1986, Gould et al. 1989; Rock 1988; Carpenter et al. 1987; Kizer et al. 1988; Stephenson 1992). These are the women at lowest risk of any medical complications at birth that might necessitate a caesarean section. One study in California found a caesarean section rate 20–25% higher in women with private medical insurance than in those whose medical care was paid for by government funds or a health maintenance organisation, and more than 35% higher than in women paying for their care themselves (Kizer et al. 1988). The WHO European study (Stephenson 1992), using Washington State in the United States, found 20.3% caesarean section rate in hospitals using government funds and 36.0% in private-for-profit hospitals.

> "In the United States the profit motive explained hospital-specific caesarean section rates that were high even by United States standards. This result was consistent with those reported by other investigators. In the United States many private health insurance packages reimburse physicians and hospitals by the procedure rendered. Therefore, more tests and procedures per patient means more income for the physician and greater revenue for the hospital. For-profit hospitals cater to those in socioeconomic brackets high enough to have private insurance coverage of maternity services. At the population level, women in this income bracket are much lower risk than women who are self-pay or women who are enrolled in public insurance programmes. Further, for-profit hospitals in the state of Washington do not offer high risk obstetrical care or neonatal intensive care. Therefore, it is difficult to imagine how these hospitals could justify medically, their excessive caesarean section rates" (Stephenson 1992).

A second non-medical determinant of caesarean section is part of a larger problem; it is one of the few answers possible to a question that birth attendants ask themselves: "What else is there to do"? Recent birth technology has provided more and more diagnostic information, but the usual obstetrical treatment possibilities during labour and birth are very few. When diagnostic information suggests even a remote possibility of a problem (such as the fetal distress that is sometimes incorrectly diagnosed by the electronic monitor), the temptation to turn to caesarean section is strong. This temptation is increased in countries such as Canada, the United Kingdom and the United States, where physicians are afraid of being sued for malpractice (Rostow et al. 1989; Smith 1990; Cohen &

Estner 1983; Ennis & Vincent 1990). In defensive medical practice, action is safer (for the physician) than inaction. Even when the diagnosis is clear, obstetricians have recently tended routinely to perform caesarean section to respond to conditions for which the evidence does not support its usefulness. To the extent that possible litigation is a determinant of caesarean section, it is a chilling thought to realise that there are physicians willing to pick up a knife and cut open a woman's abdomen because they are afraid they might end up in court.

A third non-medical determinant of caesarean section rates is convenience. A study showed that only 9.6% of the repeat caesarean section in one hospital occurred on weekends (Phillip et al. 1982). But repeat caesarean section is an elective procedure and can be scheduled in advance to fit everyone's convenience. Therefore it is much more surprising that studies of non-elective (i.e. emergency) caesarean section show a distribution skewed to favour both week days and daylight (Hurst & Summey 1984).

> "While it is not possible to give an exact assessment of the extent to which the convenience factor influences the caesarean section rate, the above data leave little doubt that it is important. Of particular concern is the extent to which this factor influences the decision to perform an elective caesarean section for women with a previous section" (Lomas & Enkin 1991).

In other words, it is much more convenient for the doctor to schedule a short surgical procedure in the middle of the day than to worry for hours with a woman in labour in the middle of the night.

Forceps and Vacuum extraction

Although forceps and vacuum extraction were not considered in Fortaleza, a discussion of the birth machine would not be complete without mentioning the important research findings since the conference on this perinatal technology. In the most recent WHO European study on obstetrical interventions (Stephenson 1992), if forceps and vacuum extraction are combined into an instrumental vaginal delivery rate, a ten fold variation in this rate was found among the 12 countries (see table below). Instrumental vaginal birth rates appeared to be decreasing in several countries, remained the same or increased slightly in other countries, and sharply increased in only one country, Greece.

Country	Year	Caesarean	Forceps	Vacuum	Instr. Vaginal	Total Operations
Australia (Vic)	1988	16.1	13.7	0.7	14.4	30.5
Canada (Que)	1988	19.5	10.1	4.3	14.4	33.9
Czech	1988	7.7	1.3	0.2	1.5	9.2
Denmark	1987	12.1	0.3	9.2	9.5	21.6
Finland	1988	14.1	0.3	5.1	5.4	19.8
Greece	1988	16.7	0.5	14.7	15.2	31.9
Hungary	1987	10.2	0.2	2.1	2.3	12.5
Israel	1987	10.2	1.5	3.3	4.8	15.0
Netherlands	1988	7.2	2.4	4.9	7.3	14.5
Slovenia	1987	7.4	0.2	2.4	2.6	10.0
UK (Scotland)	1988	14.4	11.1	0.6	10.8	25.2
US (Wash.)	1988	19.1	6.2	4.8	11.0	30.1

(Stephenson 1992)

Table 5: *Caesarean section, forceps, vacuum extraction, instrumental vaginal delivery, and total operative delivery rates in the most recent year according to country or region.*

In looking at table 5, it is important to note that the four countries with caesarean section rates over 15 and total operative rates over 30 (Australia, Canada, Greece, United States) all have one thing in common: large numbers of obstetricians in private practice caring for normal pregnant and birthing women.

Some argue that as higher rates of caesarean section are reached, they will have a moderating effect on the instrumental vaginal birth rate — in other words caesarean section may tend to replace forceps or vacuum extraction as an intervention (Lomas & Enkin 1991). The WHO data does not substantiate this since, in general, countries with high caesarean section rates also had high instrumental vaginal birth rates. Furthermore in Greece and the United States, both rates rose dramatically in the 1980s (Stephenson 1992). This suggests that in places where there is a rampant interventionist mentality without checks and balances, all interventions increase. On the other hand, in other places such as England and Wales, increasing caesarean section rates have been accompanied by a decrease in forceps and vacuum extraction rates (Welsh Office 1985) suggesting a moderating factor at work (midwives?).

The high instrumental vaginal birth rates in many countries is cause for alarm because these are not procedures without risk. Forceps and vacuum extraction are associated with: pelvic injury to the woman; lowered Apgar scores in the infant; fetal scalp injuries; intracranial injuries to the baby; more use of anaesthesia and analgesia for pain relief; more jaundice in the baby (Vacca & Keirse 1991). The startling variation in use of instruments for vaginal birth is matched by an equally dramatic variation in the use of forceps as opposed to vacuum as seen in the table (Stephenson 1992). In general English speaking countries prefer forceps while the rest of the world has adopted the vacuum extractor as the first choice. Until recently it was believed there was little to choose between the two methods. But a careful review of the scientific work comparing the two revealed that forceps carries significantly higher risk for pain, both during birth and several days after, more trauma to the woman's vagina and perineum, and more need for pain medication for birth (Chalmers & Chalmers 1989). Shortly after this article appeared, in preparation for giving a paper in New Zealand, I asked the midwives of that country to collect data on obstetrical intervention rates from the maternity hospitals. The most alarming finding was an extraordinary rate of operative vaginal birth, essentially all of it being forceps. The operative vaginal rate (essentially all forceps) was 1.4% for home births and in hospitals varied from 5.4% to 23.0% with an average of 14.5%. The following was therefore included in the paper:

"If New Zealand has approximately 58,000 births a year and if the forceps rate is approximately 15%, then approximately

8,700 births a year are with forceps. Extrapolation of data from studies of maternal morbidity of forceps compared to vacuum extraction show that the continued use in New Zealand of forceps as the instrument of first choice results every year in:

- 2,100 unnecessary pudendal blocks and other forms of regional anaesthesia for birth;
- 1,700 women unnecessarily experiencing moderate or severe pain during childbirth;
- 900 more women with severe perineal or vaginal trauma than there need be, and
- 600 women suffering unnecessarily from severe pain for several days after birth" (Wagner 1990).

In visiting a number of the maternity hospitals in New Zealand, my concern for the high forceps rates and the inevitable and unnecessary maternal morbidity that follows was met with general disinterest from the doctors. I have found similar high rates of forceps in Australia (State of Victoria 13.7%, State of South Australia 13.1%) together with similar lack of concern from the doctors (Wagner 1992).

When operative vaginal rates are combined with caesarean section rates the result is the total operative birth rate, i.e. the percent of all babies who are cut out or pulled out rather than being born in the normal way. The result is some rather frightening figures. For example, in Australia, the entire State of South Australia had over a third of all babies born by means of one of these surgical procedures in 1989 (Wagner 1992) and in the largest teaching hospital in Western Australia over half of all babies born to primiparous women in 1987 were surgically removed (Stanley 1992). That over half of new mothers did not have the opportunity to experience normal birth is truly extraordinary and impossible to justify.

FINDINGS

Caesarean section and forceps or vacuum extraction are often performed without medical need, carry serious medical risks to both woman and baby (far beyond those of vaginal birth) and have real social and economic costs to the family and the nation. The participants searched for appropriate responses to this situation. A number of suggestions were made.

The first was the dissemination of information, to health personnel and the general public, on the real risks associated with the procedure. Everyone must come to see caesarean section for what it is — a major surgical procedure with serious risks involved. A second suggestion was to reorient the training of obstetricians, with greater emphasis on assisting at vaginal births. A related proposal urged the strengthening of midwifery to create a more balanced perspective among birth attendants on surgical intervention. It was suggested that each country develop its own standards for the proper indications for caesarean section and use audit systems to monitor and, when necessary, correct practices. Several obstetricians also proposed that a stronger and more active cadre of public health professionals be responsible for ensuring compliance with national standards of practice on caesarean section.

A number of attempts have been made to reduce caesarean section rates. These have been summarised in the recent WHO report:

"How can countries, communities, or hospitals change practice and improve care? Several strategies have been tried with varying degrees of success.

"Consensus conferences are a good first step. These increase awareness about the problem and provide clinical guidelines for appropriate care. They do not, however, seem to have any real impact on the behaviour of physicians and other health providers (Lomas et al. 1989; Domnick-Pierre et al. 1991; Anderson & Lomas 1989; Stafford 1990).

"Clinical review of all births by caesarean section is another strategy (Stafford 1990; Myers & Gleicher 1988). This type of intervention must be initiated at the level of the hospital. Therefore, the success or failure of such an intervention is likely to depend on the motivation of the staff, and the enthusiasm of the chief of obstetrics.

"Community intervention strategies using opinion leaders and educational materials have also met with success (Lomas 1989). One study of this type was a variation of the classic network studies wherein an opinion leader was given an educational intervention designed to produce a change in clinical practice decisions. Others associated with the opinion leaders then gradually modified their practice in accordance with that of the opinion leader.

"The effects of adjunct technologies on obstetrical intervention rates should also be accounted for in future studies. For example, the increase in use of electronic fetal monitoring during labour is blamed, in part, for the substantial rise in the caesarean section rate. Interventions directed towards the reduction of inappropriate use of this technology may also help to stem the tide of unnecessary caesarean sections (Glasser 1988).

"Changes in physician payment, changes in hospital payment, medical malpractice reform and public dissemination of hospital caesarean section rates are among the other strategies that have been suggested as ways to reduce caesarean section rates (Stafford 1990). The type of strategy most appropriate for a given country will depend on the cultural and health systems factors behind the increasing rates. Regardless of the approach taken, the strategy should seek to improve the concordance between actual practice and the scientific basis for practice. It is not so much the rate of obstetrical intervention in a population that is at the heart of the issue, but rather the extent to which interventions are used appropriately to maximise the likelihood of a good outcome" (Stephenson 1992).

Reaching consensus on a final recommendation on caesarean section was not easy. The participants readily agreed on the first sentence: "Countries with some of the lowest perinatal mortality rates in the world have caesarean section rates under 10%". The original draft final recommendation went on to say, "Clearly there is no justification in any specific geographic region to have a caesarean section rate higher than this 10%". On this second sentence there was not consensus. While the majority favoured this, a minority felt strongly that although technically correct, it was an unreasonable standard for many hospitals and countries today. Intense debate, fuelled by everyone's desire for a strong final result, ended with agreement on:

"Countries with some of the lowest perinatal mortality rates in the world have caesarean sections rates under 10%.

Clearly there is no justification in any specific geographic region to have more than 10–15% caesarean section births".

Changing the use of birth technology

The urgency of the need to change the use of birth technology prompted the participants to go beyond the suggestion of solutions usual in most conferences, to finish the meeting with recommendations on implementation strategies.

The first step is for governments to establish formal, clearly visible systems to take charge of promoting and coordinating the assessment of appropriate technology. To be effective, assessment must be tied to control, which can be achieved in several ways. The first recommendation regulates usage in the same way that drug usage is controlled:

"Governments should consider developing regulations to permit the use of new birth technology only after adequate evaluation".

Many of those attending the consensus meeting argued that a second method would be more effective in their countries — insurance companies and/or government agencies can use their purse strings to eliminate any possible financial gain to doctors and/or hospitals from the use of birth technology. In many countries technology use brings hospitals and doctors greater financial rewards. The doctor's fee and the hospital fee for a caesarean section, for example, are higher than that for a vaginal birth. Both government and private insurance companies are beginning to realise that the reversal of this policy makes economic and medical sense. In England a new system requires the local health authority to make contracts for services with local hospitals. WHO European Regional office have held discussions with one local health authority to consider the possibility of not reimbursing a hospital for caesarean sections over 15% of all births in that hospital. For these reasons another final recommendation states *"Funding agencies should use financial regulations to discourage the indiscriminate use of technology"*. A third means of financial control would see national health care services abstaining from purchasing new equipment until it has been adequately assessed and the real need for it determined.

In the long run, perhaps the most important source of change is the dissemination of information. First is the need to disseminate information on examples of good birth care, such as those presented to the meeting. These examples can spread both specific new ideas and a belief in the possibility of progressive change. Research to account for the success of innovative programs would also be valuable. The final consensus recommendation was

>*"Obstetric care services that have critical attitudes towards technology and that have adopted an attitude of respect for the emotional, psychological and social aspects of birth care, should be identified. Such services should be encouraged and the processes that have led them to their position must be studied so they can be used as models to foster similar attitudes in other centres and to influence obstetrical views nationwide."*

Information on the results of research, including technology assessment, is needed for three groups. The providers of birth services should use it to modify their practices. Policy-makers need such information to modify their policies and the general public needs it to influence policy and to choose acceptable kinds of birth technology. The final consensus recommendation on this stated

>*"The results of the assessment of technology used in birth care should be widely disseminated, to change the behaviour of professionals and give a basis to the decisions of users and the general public."*

Although the discussion was not reflected in the recommendations, the participants talked about how to improve the impact of information on birth practices. The commercial world has learned a lot about how to give information to people in a way likely to influence their behaviour. The large gap between what is known about birth technology and how it is actually used attests to the ineffectiveness of methods of information dissemination in the medical world. Some Canadians are trying to use scientific methods to narrow this gap. Since a national consensus conference on caesarean section, they are experimenting with ways of disseminating the final recommendations. Using present caesarean section rates among physicians, hospitals and districts as the baseline, they use various strategies to bring the recommendations to the practitioners in different areas. They then measure changes in the rates to find the most effective strategies.

In one experiment in Canada, (Lomas 1989) different strategies were used to try to implement a particular recommendation of the Canadian Consensus Conference on Caesarean Section: that there be an attempt at vaginal birth after previous caesarean section (VBAC). Simply sending this recommendation to all doctors did not increase the VBAC rate, even though the doctors indicated that they received the recommendation and agreed with it. Holding caesarean section review committee meetings at the hospital every month where each physician had to defend not doing a VBAC also did not increase the VBAC rate. On the other hand, determining the opinion leader in the obstetrical community through questioning all doctors and then providing this leader with an intensive weekend seminar on VBAC did slowly but significantly begin to reduce the VBAC rate. This type of research on how to change practice is urgently needed.

It is also important to disseminate information on birth practices in hospitals. One participant described how birth practices in her country "have come under the consumer microscope" (Beech 1985). Consumer groups play an important role by distributing information to parents on a wide range of subjects related to birth. Mention has been made of the effectiveness of a birth guide, which details the birth practices in all hospitals. Such a guide exists in at least two countries, England (Kitzinger 1983) and Denmark (Houd 1992).

Another important strategy is the national or local birth conference. The first type of birth conference is a general review by all interested parties of current birth care in a country or location. Its purpose is to stimulate public discussion on how to improve birth services. Such conferences have been held in a number of European countries and have proved to be effective (see chapter 8). The second type of birth conference is held to reach consensus on a specific type of birth technology. The conferences on caesarean section in the United States and Canada have been mentioned as examples. Countries can build on the experience of others in developing this new approach and applying what is known about a given type of technology to their own circumstances. The final consensus recommendation at Fortaleza proposed

"National and local birth conferences that include relevant health providers, health authorities, users, women's groups and the mass media should be promoted."

Conclusion

At the end of the meeting in Fortaleza, the participants were exhausted but elated. Some members had been shocked by the extent to which the birth machine was out of control. The elation arose from the real consensus on appropriate birth technology achieved by people who represented all interested parties and came from many parts of the world.

References

Abitol M. 1985, 'Supine position in labour and associated fetal heart rate changes', *Obstet Gynecol*, vol. 65, pp. 481–486.

American Academy of Pediatrics & American College of Obstetricians and Gynecologists 1988, *Guidelines for Perinatal Care*, Second Edition.

American College of Obstetrics and Gynecology 1985, 'Guidelines for vaginal delivery after a previous caesarean birth', *ACOG Newsletter*, February 1985, p. 8.

Anderson G. & Lomas J. 1989, 'Recent trends in caesarean section rates in Ontario', *Canad Med Assoc Journal*, vol. 141, pp. 1049–53.

Araújo J. 1985, 'Obstetrical care by traditional birth attendants in rural areas of the State of Ceara, Brazil', *International Journal of Technology Assessment in Health Care*, vol. 1, no. 4, p. 863.

Avard D. & Nimrod C. 1985, 'Risks and benefits of obstetric epidural anaesthesia: a review', *Birth & Family Journal*, vol. 12, pp. 215–225.

Baruffi G., Strobino D. M. & Paine L. L. 1990, 'Investigation of institutional differences in primary caesarean birth rates', *Journal of Nurse Midwifery*, vol. 35, no. 5, pp. 274–281.

Beech B. 1985, 'The role of consumer advocacy in birth care', presented at the WHO consensus meeting, Forteleza.

Benson R., Bedendes H. & Weiss W. 1969, 'Fetal compromise during elective caesarean section', *Am J Obstet Gynecol*, vol. 105, pp. 579–588.

Bergsjo P., Schmidt E. & Pusch D. 1983, 'Differences in the reported frequencies of some obstetrical interventions in Europe', *British Journal of Obstetrics & Gynecology*, vol. 90, pp. 628–632.

Bibeau G. 1985, 'Health, birth and social change in Latin America: a politico-economic perspective', presented at the WHO meeting on Appropriate Birth Technology, Forteleza.

Borrel V. & Fernstrom I. 1957, 'A pelvimetric method for the assessment of pelvic mouldability', *Acta Radiologica*, vol. 47, pp. 365–370.

Bratteby L. 1979, 'Effect of obstetrical regional analgesia on the change in respiratory frequency in the newborn', *British Journal Anesth*, vol. 51, p. 415.

Buekens P., Logasse R., Dramaix M. & Wollast E. 1985, 'Episiotomy and third degree tears', *British Journal of Obstetrics & Gynecology*, vol. 92, pp. 820–823.

Burt R., Vaughan T. L. & Daling J. R. 1988, 'Evaluating the risks of caesarean section: low apgar score in repeat c-section and vaginal deliveries', *American Journal of Publ Health*, vol. 78, pp. 1312–1314.

Cable Network News 1989, December 14.

Caldeyro-Barcia R. 1974, 'Adverse perinatal effects of early amniotomy during labor', in *Modern Perinatal Medicine*, ed. Gluck, Yearbook publishers, Chicago.

—— 1979, 'The influence of maternal position on time of spontaneous rupture of membranes, progress of labor and fetal head compression', *Birth & Family Journal*, vol. 6, pp. 10–18.

—— 1980, 'Physiological and psychological bases for the modern and humanized management of normal labor', in *Recent Progress in Perinatal Medicine and Prevention of Congenital Anomaly*, Medical Information Service, Inc., Tokyo, Japan.

—— 1984, 'Birth in the sitting position', presented at the Second Symposium on Perinatal Medicine, Campinas, Brazil.

—— 1985, 'Position of the mother during labor and birth', presented at the WHO meeting on appropriate birth technology, Forteleza.

Canadian Panel 1986, 'Indications for caesarean section: final statement of the panel of the National Consensus Conference on Aspects of Caesarean Birth', *Can Med Assoc Journal*, vol. 134, pp. 1348–1352.

Canadian Society of Obstetricians and Gynecologists 1982, 'The increasing caesarean section rate', *SOGC Bulletin*, vol. 3, no. 3.

Carpenter M. W., Soule D., Yates W. T. & Meeker C. I. 1987, 'Practice environment is associated with obstetric decision making regarding abnormal labor', *Obstet Gynecol*, vol. 70, pp. 657–62.

Cartwright A. 1979, *The Dignity of Labor*, Tavistock, London.

Chalmers I. & Richards M. 1977, 'Intervention and causal inference in obstetric practice', in *Benefits and Hazards of the New Obstetrics. Clinics in Developmental Medicine*, eds S. Chard & M. Richards, no. 64, Spastics International Medical Publications & Heinimann Medical Books, London.

Chalmers I., Dauncey M. E., Verrier-Jones E. R., Dodge J. A. & Gray O. P. 1978, 'Respiratory distress syndrome in infants of Cardiff residence during 1965–1975', *British Medical Journal*, vol. 2, pp. 1119–1121.

Chalmers J. & Chalmers I. 1989, 'Forceps or vacuum extractor', *Brit J Obstet Gynecol*, vol. 96, no. 5, pp. 505.

Chalmers I. 1989, personal communication.

—— 1992, Letter to the Editor, *Lancet*, vol. 339, pp. 490.

Chalmers I. & Keirse M. 1989, 'Evaluating elective delivery', in *Effective Care in Pregnancy and Childbirth*, eds I. Chalmers, M. Enkin & M. Keirse, Oxford University Press, Oxford.

Chamberlain G. & Stewart M. 1987, 'Walking through labor', *British Medical Journal*, vol. 295, p. 802.

Cloney D. & Donowitz L. 1986, 'Overgown use for infection control in nurseries and neonatal intensive care units', *American Journal of Diseases of Children*, vol. 140, pp. 680–683.

Cohen A. 1982, 'Electronic fetal monitoring and clinical practice. A survey of obstetric opinion', *Medical Decision Making*, vol. 2, pp. 79–95.

Cohen N. & Estner L. 1983, *The Silent Knife*, Bergin & Garvey Publishers, South Hadley, Mass..

Crowley P. 1989, 'Post-term pregnancy: induction or surveillance?' in *Effective Care in Pregnancy and Childbirth*, eds I. Chalmers, M. Enkin & M. Keirse, Oxford University Press, Oxford.

Crowther C., Enkin M., Keirse M. & Brown I. 1989, 'Monitoring the progress of labor', in *Effective Care in Pregnancy and Childbirth*, eds I. Chalmers, M. Enkin & M. Keirse, Oxford University Press, Oxford.

Cunningham F., Macdonald P. & Grant N. 1989, *Williams Obstetrics*, 18th edition, pp. 323–325, Appelton & Lange, Norwalk, Connecticut.

Derom R. 1987, 'Electronic fetal heart rate monitoring', presented at European Perinatal Society Meeting, Leipzig.

Diaz A., Schwartz R., Fescina R. & Caldeyro-Barcia R. 1980, 'Vertical position during the first stage of the course of labor, and neonatal outcome', *European Journal of Obstet Gynecol Reproductive Biology*, vol. 11, pp. 1–7.

Domnick-Pierre K., Vayda E., Lomas J., Enkin M., Hannah W. J. & Anderson G. M. 1991, 'Obstetrical attitudes and practices before and after the Canadian Consensus Conference statement on caesarean birth', *Soc Sci Med*, vol. 32, pp. 1283–89.

Drayton S. & Rees C. 1984, 'They know what they are doing', *Nursing mirror*, vol. 159, pp. 4–8.

Dundes L. 1987, 'The evolution of maternal birthing position', *American Journal of Public Health*, vol. 77, no. 5, pp. 636–641.

Eckstein K. & Marx G. 1974, 'Aortocaval compression and uterine displacement', *Anesthesiology*, vol. 40, pp. 92–96.

Eisenkop S., Richman R., Platt L. D. & Paul R. H. 1982, 'Urinary tract injury during caesarean section', *Obstet Gynecol*, vol. 60, pp. 591–596.

Elliott J. & Flaherty J. 1983, 'The use of breast stimulation to ripen the cervix in term pregnancies', *American Journal Obstet Gynecol*, vol. 145, pp. 553–556.

Enkin M. 1989, 'Labour and delivery following previous caesarean section', in *Effective Care in Pregnancy and Childbirth*, eds I. Chalmers, M. Enkin & M. Keirse, Oxford University Press, Oxford.

Enkin M., Enkin E., Chalmers I. & Hemminki E. 1989, 'Prophylactic antibiotics in association with caesarean section', in *Effective Care in Pregnancy and Childbirth*, eds I. Chalmers, M. Enkin & M. Keirse, Oxford University Press, Oxford.

Ennis M. & Vincent C. 1990, 'Obstetric accidents: a review of 64 cases', *British Medical Journal*, vol. 300, pp. 1365–1367.

Evans M., Richardson D. A., Sholl J. S. & Johnson B. A. 1984, 'Caesarean section: assessment of the convenience factor', *Journal Reprod Med*, vol. 29, pp. 670–673.

Faundes A. 1985, 'Caesarean Section: when is it appropriate?', presented to WHO Consensus meeting, Forteleza.

Feldman G. & Freiman J. 1985, 'Prophylactic caesarean section at term?', *New England Journal of Med*, vol. 312, no. 19, pp. 1264–1267.

Flint C. & Poulengeris P. 1987, *The 'Know Your Midwife' Report*, Heinemann, London.

Flint C. 1991, 'Continuity of care provided by a team of midwives — the know your midwife scheme', in *Midwives, Research and Childbirth*, eds S. Robinson & A. Thomson, vol. 2, Shapman & Hall, London.

—— 1991, personal communication.

Flynn A., Kelly J., Hollins G. & Lynch P. F. 1978, 'Ambulation in labor', *British Medical Journal*, vol. 2, pp. 591–593.

Fraser W. 1991, 'Oxytocin during the second stage with epidural', in *Oxford Data Base of Perinatal Trials*, ed. I. Chalmers, version 1.2, disk issue 6, record no. 6448, Autumn 1991, Oxford University Press, Oxford.

Freeman R. 1990, 'Intrapartum fetal monitoring—A disappointing story', *New England Journal of Medicine*, vol. 322, no. 9, p. 625.

Fusi L., Steer P. J., Maresh M. J. & Beard R. W. 1989, 'Maternal pyrexia associated with the use of epidural analgesia in labor', *Lancet*, June 3, pp. 1250–1252.

Gardosi J., Hutson N. & Lynch C. 1989, 'Randomised control trial of squatting in the second stage of labor', *Lancet*, July 8, pp. 74–77.

Garel M. 1987, 'Psychological consequences of caesarean childbirth in primiparas', *J Psychosom Obstet Gynecol*, vol. 6, pp. 197–209.

Gaskin I. 1991, personal communication.

Glasser M. 1988, 'Strategies to avoid unnecessary caesarean section', *Journal Family Pract*, vol. 27, pp. 514–518.

Gould J. B., Davey B. & Stafford R. S. 1989, 'Socioeconomic differences in rates of caesarean section', *New England Journal of Med*, vol. 321, pp. 233–9.

Goyert G. L., Bottoms S. F., Treadwell M. C. & Nehra P.C. 1989, 'The physician factor in caesarean birth rates', *New England Journal Med*, vol. 320, pp. 706–9.

Grant A. 1989, 'Monitoring the fetus during labor', in *Effective Care in Pregnancy and Childbirth*, eds I. Chalmers, M. Enkin & M. Keirse, Oxford University Press, Oxford.

Guerrese E., Gori G., Beccari A., Farro M. & Mazzanti C. 1981, 'Influence of spasmolytic treatment and amniotomy on delivery times: a factorial clinical trial', *Clinical Therapy*, vol. 3, pp. 382–388.

Harrison R., Brennan M., North P.M., Reed J. V. & Wickham E. A. 1984, 'Is routine episiotomy necessary?', *British Medical Journal*, vol. 288, pp. 1971–1975.

Haverkamp A. 1985, 'Electronic fetal monitoring: perspectives for industrialised and developing countries', presented at the WHO Conference on Appropriate Birth Technology, Forteleza.

Haynes deRegt R. H., Minkoff H. L., Feldman J. & Schwarz R. H. 1986, 'Relation of private or clinic care to the caesarean birth rate', *New England Journal Med*, vol. 315, pp. 619–24.

Hemminki E., Lenck M., Saarikoski S. & Henriksson L. 1985, 'Ambulation versus oxytocin in protracted labor: a pilot study', *European Journal of Obstet Gynecol Reprod Biology*, vol. 20, pp. 199–208.

Hemminki E., Graubard B. I., Hoffman H. J., Mosher W. D. & Fetterly 1985, 'Caesarean section and subsequent fertility. Results from the 1982 national survey of family growth', *Fertility Sterility*, vol. 43, pp. 520–528.

Hemminki E. 1987, 'Pregnancy and birth after caesarean section: a survey based on the Swedish birth register', *Birth & Family Journal*, vol. 14, pp. 1–17.

—— 1990, 'A trial of continuous human support during labor: feasibility, interventions and mother's satisfaction', *Journal of Psychosomatic Obstetrics and Gynecology*, vol. 11, pp. 239–250.

Hjalmarson O. 1991, 'Epidemiology of neonatal disorders of respiration', *International Journal of Technology Assessment in Health Care*, vol. 7, supplement 1.

Hofmeyer G., Nikodem V. C., Wolman W. L., Chalmers B. E & Kramer T. 1991, 'Companionship to modify the clinical birth environment: effects on progress and perceptions of labor, and breastfeeding', *British Journal of Obstetrics & Gynecology*, vol. 98, pp. 756–764.

Houd S. 1983, personal communication during visit to Khazakstan.

—— 1991, personal communication.

—— 1992, *Fodselsguide* (Danish birth guide), consumer protection organisation, Copenhagen.

House of Commons 1992, *Health Committee second report on maternity services*, Her Majesty's Stationary Office, London.

Howell C. & Chalmers I. 1992, 'A review of prospectively controlled comparisons of epidural with non-epidural forms of pain relief during labor', *International Journal of Obstetric Anaesthesia*, vol. 1, pp. 93–110.

Hurry D., Larsen B. & Charles D. 1984, 'Effects of post caesarean section febrile morbidity on subsequent fertility', *Obstet Gynecol*, vol. 64, pp. 256–260.

Hurst M. & Summey P. 1984, 'Childbirth and social class; the case of caesarean section', *Soc Sci Med*, vol. 18, pp. 621–631.

International Childbirth Education Association 1990, 'Vaginal Birth After Caesarean', *ICEA Review*, vol. 14, no. 3, August.

Jacobson B., Nyberg K., Eklund G., Bygdeman M. & Rydberg U. 1988, 'Obstetric pain medication and eventual adult amphetamine addiction in offspring', *Acta Obstet Gynecol Scand*, vol. 67, pp. 677–682.

Jacobson B., Nyberg K., Gronbladh L., Eklung G., Bygdeman M. & Rydberg U. 1990, 'Opiate addiction in adult offspring through possible imprinting after obstetric treatment', *British Medical Journal*, vol. 301, pp. 1067–1070.

Janowitz B., Wallace S., Araújo G. & Araújo L. 1985, 'Referrals by traditional birth attendants in Northeast Brazil', *American Journal of Public Health*, vol. 75, no. 7, p. 745.

Kantor H., Rember H. I. & Tabio D. 1965, 'Value of shaving the pudendal-perineal area in delivery preparation', *Obstet Gynec*, vol. 25, pp. 509–512.

Keegan K., Waffarn F. & Quilligan E. J. 1985, 'Obstetric characteristics and fetal heart rate patterns of infants who convulse during the newborn period', *American Journal of Obstetrics & Gynecology*, vol. 153, pp. 732–737.

Keirse M. 1989, 'Augmentation of labor', in *Effective Care in Pregnancy and Childbirth*, eds I. Chalmers, M. Enkin & M. Keirse, Oxford University Press, Oxford.

Keirse M., Enkin M. & Lumley J. 1989, 'Social and professional support during childbirth', in *Effective Care in Pregnancy and Childbirth*, eds I. Chalmers, M. Enkin & M. Keirse, Oxford University Press, Oxford.

Keirse M. & Chalmers I. 1989, 'Methods for inducing labour', in *Effective Care in Pregnancy and Childbirth*, eds I. Chalmers, M. Enkin & M. Keirse, Oxford University Press, Oxford.

Kennell J. 1988, 'Medical intervention: the effect of social support during labor', *Pediatric Res*, vol. 23, p. 211A.

Killea, Senator 1992, personal communication.

Kirkinen P. 1988, 'Multiple caesarean sections: outcomes and complications', *British Journal Obstet Gynecol*, vol. 95, pp. 778–782.

Kitzinger S. 1978, 'Pain in Childbirth', *Journal Med Ethics*, vol. 4, pp. 119–121.

—— 1983, *The New Good Birth Guide*, Penguin, London.

—— 1987, *Some women's experiences of epidural*, National Childbirth Trust, London.

Kizer K. & Ellis A. 1988, 'C-section rate related to payment source', *American Journal of Public Health*, vol. 78, no. 1, pp. 96–97.

Klaus M., Kennell J., Berkowitz G. & Klaus P. 1992, 'Maternal assistance and support in labour: father, nurse, midwife or doula?', *Clinical Consultations in Obstet and Gyn*, vol. 4, no. 4, pp. 211–217..

Klaus M., Kennell J. H., Robertson S. & Sosa R. 1986, 'Effects of social support during parturition on maternal and infant morbidity', *British Medical Journal*, vol. 293, pp. 585–587.

Klein M., Gauthier R., Jorgensen S., Robbins J., et al. 1992, 'Does episiotomy prevent perineal trauma and pelvic floor relaxation?', *Current Clinical Trials*, vol. 1, document 10.

Klein M., Gauthier R., Kaaczorowski J., Robbins J., et al. 1993, 'Physicians beliefs about episiotomy and perineal management: Consequences for women under their care. Further results from the McGill University-Univerite de Montreal Episiotomy trial', unpublished manuscript.

Kowba M. & Schwirian P. 1985, 'Direct sibling contact and bacterial colonization in newborns, *J Obstet Gynecol Neonatal Nurs*, vol. 14, pp. 412–417.

Lancet editorial 1990, 'Stand and deliver', vol. 335, pp. 761–762.

Laros R., Work B. A. & Witting W. C. 1972, 'Amniotomy during the active phase of labor', *Obstet Gynecol*, vol. 39, pp. 702–704.

Liu Y. 1974, 'Effects of an upright position during labor', *American Journal of Nursing*, vol. 74, pp. 2202–2205.

Lomas J. 1989, 'Promoting clinical policy change: using the art to promote the science', in *The Challenge of Medical Practice Variations*, eds J. Anderson & S. Mooney, pp. 174–91, McMillan, London.

Lomas J., Anderson G. M., Domnick-Pierre L., Vayda E., Enkin M. & Hannah W. J. 1989, 'Do practice guidelines guide practice? The effect of a consensus statement on the practice of physicians', *N England J Med*, vol. 321, pp. 1306–11.

Lomas J. & Enkin M. 1989, 'Variations in operative delivery rates', in *Effective Care in Pregnancy and Childbirth*, eds I. Chalmers, M. Enkin & M. Keirse, Oxford University Press, Oxford.

Lumley J. 1988, 'Does continuous intrapartum fetal monitoring predict long-term neurological disorders?', *Pediatric & Perinatal Epidemiology*, vol. 2, pp. 299–307.

Lumley J. 1988, *Having a Baby in Victoria*, Victorian Department of Health.

MacArthur C., Lewis M., Knox E. G. & Crawford J. S. 1990, 'Epidural anaesthesia and long term backache after childbirth', *British Medical Journal*, vol. 301, pp. 9–12.

MacDonald D., Grant A., Sheridan-Pereira M., Boylan P. & Chalmers I. 1985, 'The Dublin randomised trial of intrapartum fetal heart rate monitoring', *American Journal of Obstetrics & Gynecology*, vol. 152, pp. 524–539.

Macfarlane A. 1978, 'Variations in numbers of births and perinatal mortality by day of the week in England and Wales', *British Medical Journal*, vol. 2, pp. 1670–1673.

Macfarlane A. 1984, 'Day of Birth', *Lancet*, September 22, p. 695.

Macfarlane A. & Mugford M. 1986, *Birth counts: statistics of pregnancy and childbirth*, Her Majesty's Stationary Office, London.

Mahan C. & McKay S. 1983, 'Preps and enema—keep or discard?', *Contemporary Obstet Gynecol*, Nov., pp. 241–248.

Maloney M. 1983, 'A prospective, controlled study of scheduled sibling visits to a newborn intensive care unit', *Journal American Acad Child Psychiatry*, vol. 22, suppl. 6, pp. 565–570.

Martell M. Belizan J. M., Nieto F. & Schwarcz R. 1976, 'Blood acid-base balance at birth in neonates from labours with early and late rupture of the membranes', *Journal of Pediatrics*, vol. 89, pp. 963–967.

McClusker J., Harris D.R., Hosmer D. W. Jr. 1988, 'Association of electronic fetal monitoring during labor with caesarean section rate and with neonatal morbidity and mortality', *Am J Publ Health*, vol. 78, pp. 1170–74.

McIlwaine G. 1985, 'The rising caesarean section rate — a matter of concern', *Health Bulletin*, vol. 43, no. 6, pp. 301–304.

Mendez-Bauer C., Arroyo, Garcia Ramos C., Menendez A., Lavilla M., Izquierdo F., Villa Elizaga I. & Zamarriego J. 1975, 'Effects of the standing position on spontaneous uterine contractility and other aspects of labor', *Journal of Perinatal Medicine*, vol. 3, pp. 89–100.

Mengert W. & Murphy D. 1933, 'Intra-abdominal pressures created by voluntary muscular effort: relation to posture in labor. *Surg Gynecol Obstet*, vol. 47, pp. 745–751.

Miller F. 1982, 'Effects of position change during labor on intrauterine resting pressure', *Journal California Perinatal Assoc*, vol. 2, pp. 50–52.

Mitre I. 1974, 'The influence of maternal position on duration of the active phase of labor', *International Journal Gynec Obstet*, vol. 12, pp. 181–183.

Murdoch G. & Whiete D. 1969, 'Standard cross-cultural sample', *Ethnology*, vol. 8, pp. 329–369.

Myers S. & Gleicher N. 1988, 'A successful program to lower caesarean section rates', *New England Journal Med*, vol. 319, pp. 1511–1516.

Nagai H. 1982, 'The management of labor with a modern birthing chair and telemetry', in *Tenth World Congress of the Federation Internationale de Gynécologie et d'Obstetrique* (FIGO), Paris.

National Centre for Health Statistics, United States 1986, National Hospital Discharge Data.

Newburn M. 1990, 'Epidural anaesthesia and long term backache after childbirth', *British Medical Journal*, vol. 301, pp. 385–386.

Newcombe R. & Chalmers I. 1977, 'Changes in distribution of gestational age and birthweight among first born infants of Cardiff residents', *British Medical Journal*, vol. 2, pp. 925–926.

Nielson T. & Hokegard 1984, 'Caesarean section and intraoperative surgical complications', *Acta Obstet Gynecol Scand*, vol. 63, pp. 103–108.

Notelovitz M. 1978, 'Commentary on maternal position in labor and birth', *ICEA Review*, vol. 2, pp. 6–7.

Notzon F. C., Placek P. J., Taffel S. M. 1987, 'Comparisons of national caesarean section rates', *New England Journal of Med*, vol. 316, no. 7, pp. 386–389.

Notzon F. 1990, 'International differences in the use of obstetric interventions', *Journal of American Medical Assoc*, vol. 263, no. 24, pp. 3286–3291.

Oakley A. 1987, 'Consequences of Obstetrical Technologies: social, psychological and medical', paper given at International Conference on Childbearing and Perinatal Care, Jerusalem, Israel.

Oakley A. & Richards M. 1990, 'Women's experiences with caesarean delivery', in *The Politics of Maternity Care*, eds Garcia, Kilpatrick & Richards, Oxford University Press, Oxford.

O'Driscoll K., Foley M. & MacDonald D. 1984, 'Active management of labor as an alternative to caesarean section for dystocia', *Obstet Gynecol*, vol. 63, pp. 485–490.

Owens M. 1983, 'Laws and policies on traditional birth attendants', *International Digest of Health Legislation*, vol. 34, no. 3, pp. 441–475.

Paccaud F. 1984, 'Weekend births', *Lancet*, August 25, pp. 470.

Paneth N. & Kiely J. 1984, 'The frequency of cerebral palsy: a review of population studies in industrialised nations since 1950', in *The Epidemiology of the Cerebral Palsies*, eds F. Stanley & E. Alberman, Clinics in Developmental Medicine, no. 87, pp. 46–56.

Pearson J. & Rees G. 1989, 'Technique of caesarean section' in *Effective Care in Pregnancy and Childbirth*, eds I. Chalmers, M. Enkin & M. Keirse, Oxford University Press, Oxford.

Petitti D., Cefalo R. C., Shapiro S. & Whalley P. 1982, 'In-hospital maternal mortality in the United States: Time trends and relation to method of delivery', *Obstet Gynecol*, vol. 59, pp. 6–11.

Petitti D. 1985, 'Maternal mortality and morbidity in caesarean section', *Clin Obstet Gynecol*, vol. 28, pp. 763–768.

Phaff J. 1986, 'The organisation and administration of perinatal services in The Netherlands', in *Perinatal Health Services in Europe*, ed. Phaff J., Croom Helm, London.

Philipsen T. & Jensen N. 1989, 'Epidural block or parental pethidine as analgesic in labor: a randomised study concerning progress in labor and instrumental deliveries', *Eur Journal Obstet Gynecol Reproductive Biology*, vol. 30, pp. 27–33.

Philipsen T. & Jensen N. 1990, 'Maternal opinion about analgesia in labor and delivery. A comparison of epidural blockade and intramuscular pethidine', *Eur Journal Obstet Gynecol Reproductive Biology*, vol. 34, pp. 205–210.

Phillips R., Thornton J. & Gleicher N. 1982, 'Physician bias in caesarean sections', *Journal of the American Med Assoc*, vol. 248, pp. 1082–1084.

Pinotti J. & Faundes A. 1985, 'Appropriate Technology for Childbirth: the Obstetrician's viewpoint', presented at the WHO meeting on appropriate birth technology, Forteleza.

Pritchard J. & MacDonald P. 1980, *Williams Obstetrics*, 16th edition, Appleton-Century-Crofts, New York.

Read J., Miller F. C. & Paul R. H. 1981, 'A Randomised trial of ambulation versus oxytocin for labor enhancement', *American Journal Obstet Gynecol*, vol. 139, pp. 669–672.

Reynolds L. & Yudkin P. 1987, 'Changes in the management of labour: 2 perineal management', *Can Med Assoc J*, vol. 136, no. 10, pp. 1045–9.

Richards M. & Chalmers I. 1987, 'Intervention and causal inference in obstetric practice — how have things changed over the last ten years?', *New Generation*, March.

Rigby E. 1857, 'What is the natural position of a woman during labor?', *Medical Times & Gazette*, vol. 15, pp. 345–346.

Roberts J. 1983, 'The effects of maternal position on uterine contractility and efficiency', *Birth & Family Journal*, vol. 10, pp. 243–249.

—— 1989, 'Maternal position during the first stage of labor', in *Effective Care in Pregnancy and Childbirth*, eds I. Chalmers, M. Enkin & M. Keirse, Oxford University Press, Oxford.

Robinson J., Rosen M., Evans J. M., Revill S. I., David H. & Rees G. A. 1980, 'Maternal opinion about analgesia for labor. A controlled trial between epidural block and intramuscular pethidine combined with inhalation', *Anaesthesia*, vol. 35, pp. 1173–1181.

Rocheleau-Parent L. 1980, 'Accoucher ou se faire accoucher', *Carrefour des Affaires Sociales*, vol. 2, pp. 4–9.

Rock S. 1988, 'Malpractice premiums and primary caesarean section rates in New York and Illinois', *Publ Health Rep*, vol. 103, pp. 459–63.

Rokiki W. & Krasnodebski J. 1988, personal communication, Silesian Medical Academy, Katowice, Poland.

Romney M. & Gordon H. 1981, 'Is your enema really necessary?', *British Medical Journal*, vol. 282, pp. 1269–1271.

Rooks J., Weatherby N. L., Ernst E. K., Stapeton S., Rosen D. & Rosenfield A. 1990, 'Outcomes of care in birth centres: The national birth centre study', *New England Journal of Medicine*, vo.l 321, no. 26, pp. 1804–1811.

Rostow V., Osterweis M. & Bulger R. J. 1989, 'Medical professional liability and the delivery of obstetrical care', *New England Journal of Med*, vol. 321, pp. 1057–60.

Rubin G., Peterson H. B., Rochat R. W., McCarthy B. J. & Terry J. S. 1981, 'Maternal death after caesarean section in Georgia', *American Journal Obstet Gynecol*, vol. 139, pp. 681–685.

Rumeau-Rouquette C. 1979, Naitre en France INSERM, Paris.

Runnerstrom I. 1969, 'The effectiveness of nurse-midwifery in a supervised hospital environment', *Bulletin of the American College of Nurse-Midwives*, vol. 14, pp. 40–52.

Rush J. 1987, 'Rooming in and visiting on the maternity ward: effects on newborn colonization rates', *Infect Control*, vol. 2, suppl. 3, pp. 10–15.

Rush J., Chalmers I. & Enkin M. 1989, 'Care of the new mother and baby', in *Effective Care in Pregnancy and Childbirth*, eds I. Chalmers, M. Enkin & M. Keirse, Oxford University Press, Oxford.

Ruzek S. 1990, 'Defining Risk: The assessment of new birth technologies', NICHD–SSRC Conference on Birth Management, West Virginia.

—— 1991, 'Women's Reproductive Rights: The impact of technology', in *Women and New Reproductive Technologies: Medical, Psychosocial, Legal and Ethical Dilemmas*, eds Rodin & Collins, Lawrence Erlbaum Associates, Hillsdale, New Jersey.

Sabatino J. 1984, 'Birth in the squatting position', presented at the Second Symposium on Perinatal Medicine, Campinas, Brazil.

Sachs O. 1982, 'Awakenings', Picador Press, London (revised edition), pp. 32.

Sachs B., Yeh J., Acker D., Driscoll S., Brown D. A. & Jewett J. F. 1987, 'Caesarean section-related maternal mortality in Massachusetts, 1954–1985', *Obstet Gynecol*, vol. 69, pp. 696–700.

Salmon Y., Kee W. H., Tan S. L. & Jen S. W. 1986, 'Cervical ripening by breast stimulation', *Obstet Gynecol*, vol. 67, pp. 21–24.

Sawers R. 1983, 'Fetal monitoring during labor', *British Medical Journal*, vol. 287, pp. 1649–1650.

Scanlon J. 1981, 'Effects of obstetric anaesthesia and analgesia on the newborn: a select, annotated bibliography for the clinician', *Clin Obstet Gynecol*, vol. 24, pp. 649–670.

Schwarcz R., Althabe O., Belitzky R., Lanchares J. L., Alvarez R., Berdaguer P., Capurro H., Belizan J. M., Sabatino J. H., Abusleme C. & Caldeyro-Barcia R. 1973, 'Fetal heart rate patterns in labours with intact and with ruptured membranes', *Journal of Perinatal Medicine*, vol. 1, pp. 153–165.

Schwarcz R. 1975, 'La Rotura precoz de la membranes ovulares y sus efectos sobre el parto y el neonato Oficina', *Sanitaria Panamericana*, vol. 595, pp. 1–80.

Schwarcz R. 1985, 'Perinatal health and Regional activities of the Latin–American Centre for Perinatology and Human Development', *International Journal of Technology Assessment in Health Care*, vol. 1, no. 4, p. 799.

Shy K., Luthy D. A., Bennett F. C., Whitfield M., Larson E. B., van-Belle G., Hughes J. P., Wilson J. A. & Stenchever M. A. 1990, 'Effects of electronic fetal-heart-rate monitoring, as compared with periodic auscultation, on the neurological development of premature infants', *New England `Journal of Medicine*, vol. 322, no. 9, pp. 588–594.

Simkin P. 1986, 'Is anyone listening? The lack of clinical impact of randomised controlled trials of electronic fetal monitoring', *Birth & Family Journal*, vol. 13, no. 4, pp. 219–220.

Simkin P. 1989, 'Non-Pharmacological methods of pain relief during labor', in *Effective Care in Pregnancy and Childbirth*, eds I. Chalmers, M. Enkin & M. Keirse, Oxford University Press, Oxford.

Sleep J., Grant A., Garcia J., Elbourne D., Spencer J. & Chalmers I. 1984, 'West Berkshire perineal management trial', *British Medical Journal*, vol. 289, pp. 587–590.

Sleep J. & Grant A. 1987, 'West Berkshire perineal management trial: three year follow up', *British Medical Journal*, vol. 295, pp. 749–751.

Sleep J., Roberts J. & Chalmers I. 1989, 'Care during the Second stage of labor', in *Effective Care in Pregnancy and Childbirth*, eds I. Chalmers, M. Enkin & M. Keirse, Oxford University Press, Oxford.

Sloan D. 1968, 'Inconclusive conclusion', *Amer Journal Obstet Gynecol*, vol. 101, pp. 133–136.

Smith R. 1990, 'The epidemiology of malpractice', *British Medical Journal*, vol. 301, pp 621–22.

Sosa R., Kennell J., Klaus M., Robertson S. & Urrutia J. 1980, 'The effect of a supportive companion on perinatal problems, length of labor, and mother-infant interaction', *New England Journal of Medicine*, vol. 303, pp. 597–600.

Stafford R. 1990, 'Alternative strategies for controlling rising caesarean section rates', *JAMA*, vol. 263, pp. 683–687.

Stanley F. 1992, personal communication.

Stanton S., Kerr-Wilson R. & Harris V. G. 1980, 'The incidence of urological symptoms in normal pregnancy', *British Journal Obstet Gynecol*, vol. 87, pp. 897–900.

Statistical Bulletin 1986, National Centre for Health Statistics, United States, vol. 67, no. 3, pp. 2–8.

Stephenson P. 1992, *International differences in the use of obstetrical interventions*, World Health Organisation European Regional Office, Copenhagen.

Stewart P., Hillan E. & Calder A. A. 1983, 'A randomised trial to evaluate the use of a birth chair for delivery', *Lancet*, June 11, pp. 1296–1298.

Swanstrom S. & Bratteby I. 1981a, 'Metabolic effects of obstetric regional anaesthesia and of asphyxia in the newborn infant during the first two hours after birth: arterial blood concentrations', *Acta Pediatr Scand*, vol. 70, pp. 791–800.

—— 1981b, 'Metabolic effects of obstetric regional anaesthesia and of asphyxia in the newborn infant during the first two hours after birth: arterial plasma concentrations of glycerol, free fatty acids and beta-hydroxybutyrate', *Acta Pediatr Scand*, vol. 70, pp. 801–809.

Tew M. & Damstra-Wijmenga S. 1991, 'Safest birth attendants: recent Dutch evidence', *Midwifery*, vol. 7, pp. 55–65.

Thacker S. & Banta H. D. 1983, 'Benefits and risks of episiotomy: an interpretive review of the English language literature, 1860–1980', *Obstetrical & Gynecological Survey*, vol. 38, pp. 322–338.

Thiery M. & Derom R. 1984, 'Review of evaluation studies on caesarean section', Economic Community Workshop, 14 March, Brussels.

Thomson M. & Westreich R. 1989, 'Restriction of mother-infant contact in the immediate postnatal period', in *Effective Care in Pregnancy and Childbirth*, eds I. Chalmers, M. Enkin & M. Keirse, Oxford University Press, Oxford.

Thorp J., Parisi V. M., Boylan P. C. & Johnston D. A. 1989, 'The effect of continuous epidural anaesthesia on caesarean section for dystocia in nulliparous women', *American Journal Obstet Gynecol*, vol. 161, pp. 670–675.

Tzoumaka-Bakoula C. 1987, personal communication.

Tzoumaka-Bakoula C., Lekea-Karanika V., Matsaniotis N. S., McCarthy B. & Golding J. 1990, 'Birthweight specific perinatal mortality in Greece', *Acta Ped Scandin*, vol. 79, pp. 47–51.

Ueland K. & Hansen J. 1969, 'Maternal cardiovascular dynamics. II Posture and uterine contractions', *American Journal Obstet Gynecol*, vol. 103, pp. 1–8.

Umphenour J. 1980, 'Bacterial colonization in neonates with sibling visitation', *Journal Obstetrics Gynecology Neonatal Nurs*, vol 9, pp. 73–75.

United States Department of Health and Human Services 1981, *Caesarean childbirth*, NIH publication no. 82–2067.

Vacca A. & Keirse M. 1989, 'Instrumental vaginal delivery', in *Effective Care in Pregnancy and Childbirth*, eds I. Chalmers, M. Enkin & M. Kierse, Oxford University Press, Oxford.

Wagner M. 1985, 'Health Services for Pregnancy in Europe', *International Journal of Technology Assessment in Health Care*, vol. 1, no. 4, p. 789.

—— 1990, 'Appropriate Technology for Birth', presented at New Zealand Midwife Conference, Dunedin.

—— 1992, 'Appropriate Birth Care in Industrialised Countries', paper given in five Australian cities.

Welsh Office 1985, *Maternity hospital in-patient enquiry*, Cardiff.

Williams C. & Oliver K. 1969, 'Nursery routines and staphyloccal colonization rate of the newborn', *Pediatrics*, vol. 44, pp. 640–646.

World Health Organisation 1985a, *Having a Baby in Europe*, Public Health in Europe no. 26, Regional Office for Europe, Copenhagen.

—— 1985b, *Report of the consultation on approaches for policy development for traditional health practitioners, including traditional birth attendants*, Geneva.

Wranesh E. 1982, 'The effect of sibling visitation on bacterial colonization rate in neonates', *J Obstet Gynecol Neonatal Nurs*, vol. 11, pp. 211–213.

Chapter 7

Care following birth: whose baby is it, anyway?

If you play God you will be blamed for natural disasters

Anonymous

Introduction

There have been extraordinary advances in care in the period following birth (this period includes the first month after birth). Neonatologists and neonatal technology have saved the lives of many newborn infants. Nevertheless, the care of the woman and her new baby varies greatly between and within both industrialised and developing countries.

In Hungary, all births take place in the hospital and the woman and her infant remain there for an average of 10 days. No family member is permitted in the hospital either at the time of birth or during the hospital stay. In The Netherlands, over one third of all births are planned home births and in another one third of all births, the woman and her baby are discharged from the hospital within the first 24 hours after birth. Dutch women can choose any companion in birth, even when they are in hospital.

In Latin America, 40% of all births per year (6 million) take place at home, with an empirical midwife or a family member as birth attendant. The possibility is remote for access to official health services should complications arise for the woman or newborn following birth. Only about 15% of the births in Latin America that take place in hospitals involve any kind of follow-up care once the woman and baby leave the hospital. At the same time, some Latin American neonatal intensive care units have sufficient sophistication and staff to compare favourably with the best units in industrialised countries.

To understand all these differences and the rapid changes in care, the participants at the WHO Consensus Conference on Appropriate Technology Following Birth, by means of several background papers, reviewed the history of the perceptions and management of the first month after birth.

Perceptions and management

The period immediately after birth is a time of rapid physiological and psychological adjustment for the woman and her infant. This is largely controlled by physiological processes and genetic make-up. Anthropological data now suggest that the human species has experienced no significant physiological change for the past one to two million years. Skull and bone structure, the number of chromosomes and probably many behaviour patterns have remained the same. During most of this long period, people lived as hunters and gatherers, a life to which human physiological processes and genetic make-up were adapted. Then, for about 10 thousand years, humans had an agricultural mode of existence, succeeded by 200 years of industrialised society (figure 3).

During this long history of evolutionary adaptation, human beings slowly evolved mechanisms and practices for childbirth and the raising of infants. Meddling with these may result in unforeseen and unintentional harm, since biological adaptation is a very slow process. The seemingly harmless 'modern' practices of moving birth to the hospital, separating the woman from her newborn, placing all healthy newborns in a room together, giving artificial formula during the first day or two, and giving breastfed newborns to their mothers every four hours have all had unpredicted but scientifically proven deleterious consequences for both the woman and her baby.

Respect for the biological mechanisms operating in the woman and baby during the first month after birth needs to be accompanied by an appreciation of the social mechanisms. Social scientists have drawn attention to the ritualistic features of the social component of birth and new motherhood, and pointed out some of the character-

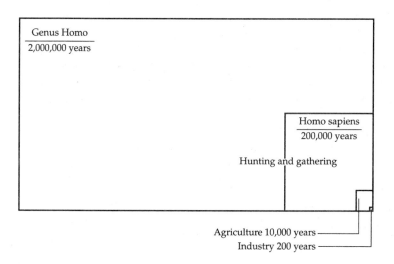

Figure 3: *Schematic diagram illustrating the relative time humans have spent as industrial and agricultural societies compared with their long duration as hunters and gatherers (modified from Lozoff B., Brittenham G. M., Truase M. A., et al.* J Pediatr, *vol. 91, no. 1, 1977.*

istics that these rites of passage share with others, such as those associated with puberty and death. Rituals help to adjust individuals to new positions; the community recognises and makes allowances for the magnitude of what has happened. When modern practices have failed to consider their impact on these social factors, deleterious consequences have also gradually revealed themselves.

In industrialised countries, women began to enter the political arena around 1900. They were encouraged to concentrate on matters befitting their 'special nature'. For this reason and because men had neglected these matters, women were supposed to concentrate on child care, education, facilities for the poor and particularly the 'infant problem': too many babies dying. At the same time, a new concept of public health was developing. Personal hygiene and medical examinations replaced community wide activities, and propaganda encouraging people to wash their hands was pushing aside an environmental approach. A coalition between women and physicians was only one element in a complex social process that resulted in the medical definition of the 'infant problem' and the medicalisation of infant care.

By the 1930s many industrialised countries had developed extensive systems to provide care to newborn infants (called neonatal care), based on the clinical medical model of one-to-one contact between the baby and a health professional. If the baby was born at home, a nurse or physician visited the home, or the baby was brought to a neighbourhood clinic for examination and advice. For babies born in the hospital, services began there. The implications of both situations were the same: infancy is a problem and physicians and nurses are the solution.

This century has also seen the medicalisation of motherhood. Aside from women's obvious biological capacity for reproduction, society sets the status and conditions of motherhood in many senses. An adequate understanding of the first month after birth requires a knowledge of the people who control the mothers' options and physical changes and the kinds of social and medical care provided. A great deal of evidence suggests that the agents controlling and shaping motherhood in industrialised countries are health professionals. This is especially true in the first few days after hospital birth, when these professionals take care of the baby; the mother may feel that her baby is hospital property. The mother's loss of confidence and self-esteem is a dangerously corrosive result of the medicalisation of motherhood.

A medical model for care

In the two decades after the Second World War, the medical model alone was used to develop systems of care following birth. The numbers of women dying as the result of pregnancy and birth had been brought to very low levels in industrialised countries. The number of women dying during pregnancy, birth and shortly after birth had fallen in developed countries to around one death for every 10,000 births (WHO 1991a). With so few women dying there was a gradual and subtle shift in the medical profession's primary concern from the woman to the baby, illustrated by the replacement of the term maternity care with perinatal care. Significant numbers of babies still died around the time of birth. Because of the belief that physicians could cure almost everything, birth and the care that followed it were gradually brought into medical territory — the hospital, despite the lack of evidence to support this move.

By the beginning of the 1970s nearly all births in most industrialised countries took place in the hospital. Newborn infants were then placed in a newborn nursery; newborn care became paediatric and nursing care. Uniformed nursing staff taught women about motherhood; mother care became nursing care. The underlying assumptions were that infancy is dangerous and that women are inadequate mothers without education and assistance from health professionals.

These attitudes spread. Physicians worked to develop infant formula, which was to be superior to breast-milk and could be modified scientifically to fit the needs of any newborn infant. The woman thus felt inadequate as the source of nourishment for her baby. Further, the presence of the newborn infant in the hospital gave the opportunity for frequent examination and observation. This gradually resulted in finding more potential pathology. Natural phenomena such as physiological jaundice came under closer scrutiny and treatment. Staff did not consider that some hospital practices, such as breastfeeding at less frequent intervals, might produce some cases of this jaundice.

Gradually the idea arose of two separate hospital rooms for well and sick babies, and the neonatal intensive care unit was born. A number of factors encouraged the rapid development of these units. Many physicians wished to ally their practice more closely with science and technology. Neonatal care, with the development of an appropriate base in physiological knowledge, appeared to offer an ideal situation in which to build scientific medicine. High technology — including better incubators and machines for artificial ventilation and monitoring respiratory function rapidly evolved. All of this led to the development of a sub-specialty of paediatrics called neonatology. Newborn infant care became more extensive and intensive.

Meanwhile, what happened after the birth to the woman in the hospital? Her baby was taken away from her at the moment of birth and brought to her for occasional visits. Women picked up hospital-acquired infections needing treatment. As the rates of obstetrical intervention increased, more consequences in the woman required care. As more episiotomies were performed, more follow-up treatment was needed (Grant & Sleep 1991). As more drugs and anaesthesia were used during birth, there were more side effects requiring care.

> "For the mother, 'standing orders' were in place for a variety of medications and treatments, including analgesics, laxatives, lactation suppressant, sitz baths, heat lamps, foments, enemas, perineal irrigations and sprays — whether or not the woman had any need for them. Abdominal binders, breast binders, and T-binders were the usual undergarments. Regular physical assessment of fundal height, lochia, stitches, and vital signs were a constant reminder to the new mother that she was a patient in a hospital" (Rush et al. 1991).

The woman's need for care increased with little realisation that much of this resulted from the hospitalisation and medicalisation of the birth.

When the woman and her baby were discharged from the hospital, the feelings of inadequacy generated by the care the woman had received, often combined with feelings of isolation in a nuclear family, led to a need for continued help in the community. Some industrialised countries already had systems to provide such support. Systems of routine check-ups in the home or a neighbourhood clinic for families with newborn babies had been developed in many industrialised countries before the Second World War as a means of combating relatively high infant mortality rates. As these rates fell, the systems continued but shifted their focus to assisting the 'inadequate' woman to care for her infant. Having the baby in the hospital implied that neither the woman nor her home was good enough. Nurses and clinics now had the job of trying to convince the woman that she could manage to raise her baby.

In short, the system of care following birth trains women to use health care providers for any concerns they may have as mothers and thus plants the seed of the medicalisation of childhood and of women's lives.

Introduction of the social model

During the 1960s and 1970s, signs began to emerge of imbalance in the care following birth in industrialised countries. One of the earliest signs was the epidemics of infection in the normal newborn nurseries, which appeared as soon as the infants were collected in the same room. Rather than questioning this practice, professionals reacted by attempting to make the nurseries more sterile. Ironically, this resulted in increased isolation of the newborn infant, which prompted the notion that newborn infants need to be in sterile environments.

The epidemics were iatrogenic; they resulted from bringing birth to the hospital and keeping babies in a nursery. Unfortunately, the treatment of the epidemics caused further iatrogenic effects. Using inappropriate doses of inappropriate antibiotics to combat the infections resulted in epidemics of 'the grey death' (the skin of the newborn infants who died was grey). In addition, as early as the 1940s and early 1950s, the oxygen therapy given to newborn infants was identified as one of the causes of retrolental fibroplasia, a condition leading to blindness (Silverman 1980). In short, the treatment given to the newborn infant created much of the need for further treatment.

The next indication of imbalance in the care of newborn infants was uneven improvement in mortality rates. Although deaths in some categories of newborn infants decreased markedly, the mortality rates for others showed much less improvement. Neonatologists' case-by-case clinical approach clearly showed that neonatal care saved babies' lives. The population-based approach of epidemiology, however, showed that this care might not always do so. Among babies with low birth weight, for example, the mortality rate for the larger infants (weighing 1500–2500 g) definitely improved, while the rate for babies with very low birth weight (less than 1500 g) remained higher. Enormous efforts were made to save those weighing less than 1000 g at birth, with a lower yield for the effort. For example, in one large neonatal intensive care unit in Australia, the percent of very low birth weight babies dying during the 5 years 1977 to 1981 compared with the percent of very low birth weight babies dying during the subsequent 5 years 1982 to 1986, is shown as follows:

Birth weight in grams	Mortality (%)	
	1977–1981	1982–1986
500–799	82	81
800–1199	31	20
1200–1499	2.6	6.8

We see no improvement in the survival of the smallest babies, an improvement in the survival of the slightly larger babies, and a statistically significant worsening of survival of the largest very low birth weight babies (Doyle 1987). The neonatologists at this centre felt that concentrating on the care of the babies under 1200 g may have contributed to the poorer result of babies over 1200 g.

In addition, the issue of the value of newborn care in improving morbidity became less certain. For example, careful studies in Sweden, Australia and England showed that the incidence of the type of cerebral palsy commonly associated with lack of oxygen (anoxia) around the time of birth had not decreased in 20 years and might actually have increased slightly (Hagberg et al. 1984; Jarvis et al. 1985; Stanley & Watson 1988). Figure 4 clearly shows how the fall in perinatal mortality the past 30 years has not been accompanied by a fall in cerebral palsy.

These issues raised questions about the gains resulting from the effort invested in neonatal care.

New scientific data pointed out the next sign of trouble: the suggestion that traditional care is superior to modern care in many cases. For example, a random control trial tested the hypothesis that what industrialised societies consider to be the 'normal' amount of crying in infants is in reality excessive and the result of lack of carrying the baby much of the time during the day such as is done in more 'primitive' societies. The experimental group (i.e. carried) cried and fussed 43% less overall and 51% less during evening hours. The authors conclude: "Supplemental carrying modifies 'normal' crying by reducing the duration and altering the typical pattern of crying

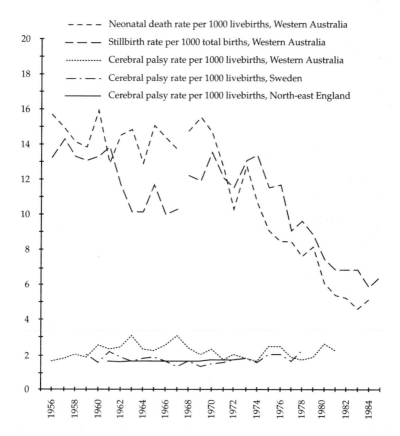

Figure 4: *Trends in perinatal mortality and cerebral palsy, 1956–85 (Stanley & Watson 1988; Hagberg et al. 1984; Jarvis et al. 1985). Gap in neonatal death and stillbirth rates between 1967–68 due to redefinition of 'birth' in Western Australia from one of >28 weeks gestation to one of >20 weeks in 1968. Cerebral palsy data for 1982–85 not yet available due to lag time to accurate diagnosis.*

and fussing in the first 3 months of life. The relative lack of carrying in our society may predispose to crying and colic in normal infants" (Hunziker & Barr 1986).

In another study, stroking the body and passively moving the limbs of very low birth weight babies (700–1500 g) for 15 minutes 3 times a day for 10 days in a neonatal intensive care unit resulted in 47% greater weight gain per day, faster maturation, 6 days shorter hospital stay saving US$3000 per infant (Field et al. 1986). Should we be surprised that science proves that holding and touching infants is good?

Gradually, research conclusively demonstrated that woman-made breast-milk is superior to man-made infant formula. It also began to show that removing the newborn infant from the mother at the time of birth could do serious psychological and social damage to both. Further, research is beginning to suggest that home care following birth may be safer than hospital care, and that mother care may be safer than medical or nursing care, not only for the normal newborn infant but perhaps for larger infants of low birth weight. So the method of care of newborn infants that evolved over millions of years is beginning to be documented scientifically as being in many cases superior to the medical care which has developed over the last 20–30 years.

The worldwide recession of the 1970s brought the necessity of looking at the costs of medical care. This precipitated the beginning of health services research on the neonatal care system. It quickly became evident that, while the entire world was supposedly moving towards more primary health care, birth and newborn care were going the other way, towards the hospital and the specialist. The excessive and inappropriate referrals of newborn infants for special care began to receive notice. The unplanned nature of neonatal care systems became more obvious. In addition, the efficacy of spending an average of approximately US$50,000 on every newborn infant weighing less than 1000 g at birth began to be questioned. Further, questions were raised about establishing more neonatal intensive care units and training more neonatologists where the need was already oversupplied, as in some developed countries, or where basic health care is lacking, as in most developing countries.

The handling of the infant in the hospital during and after birth, and the potential impact on later psychological development, also began to be discussed. For example, research suggested a possible relationship between the early separation of mother and baby and subsequent child abuse and neglect (O'Conner et al. 1980a, 1980b, 1981).

While some groups and authors questioned the management of the infant, the women's movement began to criticise the care of the woman, and the focus of the medical approach on a safe baby, with little concern for the body or feelings of the woman.

By the 1980s, some people suspected that postpartum care for the infant and the mother might to some extent be a house of cards built on a foundation of medicalisation and iatrogenic effects. In industrialised countries, this suspicion and the criticisms that prompted it introduced the social model into care following birth. For example, bonding practices at the moment of birth and the rooming-in of the newborn infant at the mother's bedside were established in many hospitals (WHO 1985). Health care providers acknowledged the superiority of breast-milk and began to encourage breastfeeding. The length of the hospital stay for mother and infant decreased in many industrialised countries; the trend is towards the discharge of healthy mother and infant within 24 hours. In addition, more parents are being allowed into neonatal intensive care units.

Trends in developing countries

Quite a different trend has appeared in developing countries, such as those in Latin America. The need for systems of care following birth was perceived in these countries, but the development of such systems was controlled by the medical profession. Consequently, only the medical model was used. Physicians from developing countries (with high infant and maternal mortality rates and where many women and babies receive little or no perinatal or maternity care) are eager to come to Europe or North America to train as neonatologists. The private sector in health care in many Latin American countries began to replicate the medicalised systems for care following birth developed in industrialised countries. Surveys in Latin America have shown that the interest of hospital personnel is confined to events within the hospital walls. As a result, very expensive neonatal intensive care has started in places that still see many deaths from tetanus of the newborn — an entirely (and cheaply) preventable death. Ironically, these intensive care units are often unable to operate satisfactorily because of the lack of proper maintenance for the technology.

A survey of services following birth in five Latin American countries showed that rooming-in was practised in over half of the 20 hospitals covered (Suarez-Ojeda 1986). Other practices consistent with a combined medical and social approach, however, were few. For example, four of the hospitals allowed the father to be present during labour or after birth, six provided breastfeeding assistance and one allowed parents into the neonatal intensive care unit. The report concluded "The incorporation of these basic contents of family neonatal psychology is still very limited and the services show a high degree of rigidity and predominance of surgical criteria concerning delivery and newborn care" (Suarez-Ojeda 1986).

The influence of the social model on services following birth varies considerably even among industrialised countries. According to WHO surveys, it is greatest in Canada, The Netherlands, the United Kingdom, the United States and the Scandinavian countries (WHO 1986). The countries of central western Europe, such as Austria, France and Germany, show somewhat less incorporation of the social model, the southern European countries still less, and the eastern European countries least of all.

In eastern European countries, the length of the hospital stay for the woman and baby after a normal birth is slowing, coming down from 10 to 7 days, and one or two hospitals are just beginning to experiment with rooming-in. All hospitals in eastern Europe have normal newborn nurseries; all babies are taken there immediately after birth and kept for 24 hours before being given to their mothers for the first time. The father is not allowed to visit mother or baby during hospitalisation. All over eastern Europe, fathers can be seen standing in the street outside the maternity hospital in the evenings, calling up to the women who lean out of the windows above them. Neither parent is allowed into neonatal intensive care units, although the most advanced unit in Moscow has a special room in which mothers may nurse their infants if the babies are capable of sucking, or pump their breasts for milk for the weaker infants. This small amount of contact between woman and baby is permitted not for attachment but to provide the best nourishment.

Findings

While some countries have a trend towards adjusting care in the general direction of decreasing the medicalisation of services, all countries east and west, north and south, are continuing a strong trend towards a high-technology approach. More neonatologists are trained, more neonatal intensive care units are built, and more new technology is introduced. These opposite trends are behind the great disparity in types of care following birth between and within countries, as well as the rapid changes taking place.

Principles for policy-making

From discussions on the first day, the participants in the consensus meeting developed some broad principles to guide policy formulation on care following birth. They are prerequisites for the policies that respect and guarantee the preservation of the normalcy of the period following birth. The principles also formed the basis for a number of recommendations.

Respect for cultural practices

Recognition must be given to the importance to every culture of birth and the period following it, and the importance of culture to every birth and family with a new infant. Passage through this period of transition has continued to be aided by rituals. Modern rituals, however, are not collective and social, but medical. Women are segregated from the community in maternity hospitals. The umbilical cord and placenta are burned in the hospital incinerator (or used to generate medical technology) rather than being buried near the place where mother and child live.

The participants agreed that infancy and motherhood belong to the community, not to the medical establishment. The people who assist during and after birth should recognise and respect the autonomous and important functions of parenthood. This requires communication between the health workers, who understand the medical culture, and the family, which understands its community's culture. The participants recommended that:

> *"In any country or region, existing cultural practices in the period following birth should be respected and maintained unless they have been proven harmful. Better communication between women and health workers would improve opportunities to recognise strengths of local traditions, which could then be disseminated to other women."*

Rights of individuals and families

The participants repeatedly suggested that preserving the normalcy of the first month after birth requires the preservation of the sanctity of the individual and family in society. This led to the notion that the approaches used in care following birth and the attitudes of care givers must guarantee certain fundamental rights of the individuals and families concerned. Because of the importance of these rights, they became a preamble to the recommendations.

Women's right to choose

Women have the right to *"choice of place of birth and primary birth attendant"*. This can include a planned home birth or an empirical midwife as the birth attendant. The principle here is not the correctness of the choice, but the right to make it. The care system should honour this choice and provide the necessary support and medical backup. WHO surveys (WHO 1985) and the observations of WHO staff on field visits show that some women and families will choose home birth and/or empirical midwives, regardless of local circumstances or official sanctions.

Arrests of empirical midwives in the United States, for example, show that some American women continue to choose home birth and empirical midwives. Sweden has a highly developed health care system, with universal coverage and no direct costs to the user, and some of the lowest maternal and perinatal mortality rates in the world. The system does not cover home birth, and many health officials believed that the rate of hospital birth was 100%, except for unplanned precipitous births elsewhere. Gradually WHO staff discovered that some families choose home birth, even though it means the loss of child allotment benefits. Although the USSR has an official policy of hospital birth, families in Moscow and elsewhere have chosen birth at home or even in the sea. Further, Turkey has made a major effort to provide every village with a trained midwife. As the local primary health care worker, she is to screen all pregnant women and attend home births for low-risk women, free of charge. Studies show, however, that in many villages over half the women choose an empirical midwife.

In addition, studies show that attempts by the government or the medical establishment to eliminate alternative methods and practitioners have failed (see chapter 6).

The right to choose the place of birth and primary birth attendant also extends to the community. In a number of places in the world (including the entire circumpolar areas of North America and Europe) where small groups of people live in isolation, far from hospitals, government policy has been to fly all pregnant women from their homes to large hospitals where they wait for birth, often for weeks. Certain communities, such as the Inuit Eskimos around Hudson Bay in the Arctic portion of Canada and the Aboriginals in central Australia, have mounted grassroots campaigns to change this policy. These groups feel strongly that the removal of birth from the community erodes their cultures and ways of life. They have taken responsibility for the consequences of a non-transport policy for low-risk pregnant women, and have negotiated with government authorities for change. Demonstration projects are training women chosen by their villages to be empirical midwives and to attend home births in remote areas.

Privacy and physical integrity

Another right is the *"Preservation of physical integrity and privacy for mother and child"*. Such a right can sometimes be difficult to preserve in a crowded hospital. In many hospitals, several women give birth in the same room. They lie side by side, each in the lithotomy position on a surgical table with their bodies exposed to the many staff coming and going.

Simple and inexpensive measures can go a long way towards improving such conditions. For example, partitions can be put between beds or surgical tables. In one London hospital, the simple expedient of putting a lock on the inside of the door to the labour room (when the woman's partner or other companion was present) resulted in staff having to knock and request permission to enter.

Postpartum wards can be arranged to give as much privacy as possible, and, of course, architects can be asked to design new wards that preserve physical integrity and privacy. Staff can make an even more important contribution by always asking permission to approach and to examine the woman and always being careful not to expose the woman's body unnecessarily.

Respect for birth

Third is the right of *"respect for birth as a highly personal, sexual and family experience"*. This view of the nature of birth appeared to be new to many of the physicians at the consensus meeting. In fact, the participants with a medical perspective could quickly be distinguished from those with a social perspective by their answer to the question as to whether birth is sexual. The discussions also tended to break down along gender lines as the sexual nature of birth was more difficult for the male participants to grasp. While consensus came fairly quickly on the idea of birth as a personal and family experience, much discussion, including many examples from women participants' lives, was necessary before agreement was reached on the sexual nature of birth.

The implications of this right for policy on care following birth are fairly straightforward. It is one of the bases for policies that allow:

- women and their families to choose the kinds of birth they will experience;
- the woman to control who will examine her body and sexual organs during and following birth, and to choose her birth attendant;
- family members to be present at birth and to visit freely during any period of hospitalisation afterwards.

Warmth, food and shelter

Society's support for the new infant sometimes ends at the door of the hospital. Thousands of dollars can be spent to save the life of a tiny premature infant in a neonatal intensive care unit, only to discharge the baby to a family without the means to give it adequate food and shelter. The child may later die from an infection precipitated by malnutrition and exposure. This is the reason for the right to *"warmth, food and shelter, especially during the first month after birth"*.

Financial support

A right, which is really part of the preceding one, is *"assurance of financial support adequate for the care of the family"*. The medical services provided during the month following birth must be combined with adequate social and financial benefits. While health personnel are not responsible for systems of social and financial support in the community, they are in a position to document the harmful consequences of inadequate support. Then they can actively advocate the improvement of services for families with infants. This would be another example of the importance of combining medical and social priorities.

Health care

Health personnel can be more directly involved in working to ensure the next right, to *"proper health care following birth"*. Large numbers of people in developing regions of the world are denied this right, and the nature of the health care systems in many industrialised countries gives some groups limited or inadequate access to the system. Barriers may be financial, social, cultural and linguistic. People who provide postpartum care to families need to be involved in efforts to eliminate such barriers.

Protection from abuse and neglect

The last right listed in the preamble might seem to be rather far from the issues surrounding care after birth, namely the right to *"protection of children from abuse and neglect"*. The participants included it because increasing evidence relates events in the period after birth, such as the separation of mother and baby, to abuse and neglect in later childhood. The protection of children should therefore begin with preventive measures including: time for infant and mother to be together the first hour after birth, rooming-in, allowing parents in the neonatal intensive care unit, and liberal visiting hours after birth. These measures are not just nice frills, to be allowed when convenient, but fundamental rights. Ignoring them can have serious consequences.

Focus on the needs of the woman

Because of the tendency for present health services at and after birth to focus on the needs of the infant, sometimes to the detriment of the mothers, the participants also stated in the preamble that:

> *"Becoming a mother is a difficult life transition. The family and its support system of relatives and friends need to understand and be prepared for changes following birth. Health planners and workers must consider the woman's health as well as that of the baby."*

This is part of the principle of preserving the sanctity of the individual and family in society, and a prerequisite for all services following birth.

Social equity

An important element in the rights listed by the participants is social equity, a third broad principle to guide policy formulation on care. This principle is so important that the participants made it the subject of their first recommendation. A fundamental truth that should guide health policy in every country is that poverty is the greatest threat to the health of women and infants. Health professionals and politicians sometimes have difficulty in understanding that infant mortality is not a health problem, but a social problem with health consequences. It is analogous to deaths from traffic accidents: the first priority for reducing them in children is not to build more and better medical facilities, but to change traffic laws and improve the education of drivers and children. The solution is primarily environmental, social and educational. The first priority for reducing infant mortality is not to supply more obstetricians, paediatricians, hospitals or prenatal or well baby clinics; it is to provide more social, financial and educational support to families with pregnant women and infants.

Medicalising the causes of infant deaths has helped to obscure the key role of poverty in infant mortality. A review of babies' death certificates shows pneumonia and gastroenteritis as major causes of death. Careful analysis makes it clear that these deaths are related to poor housing and nutrition, inadequate child supervision and poor social and economic conditions in general. These conditions weaken the infant, who becomes more susceptible to contracting such infections and dies because of inadequate resistance.

Combining the medical and social approaches

Again a combination of the medical and social approaches is needed. Most countries lean far more heavily on the medical approach to lower infant mortality. Even the United Nations Children's Emergency Fund (UNICEF) has sometimes emphasised medical solutions, such as antibiotics given by village health workers to babies with pneumonia, and oral rehydration therapy given by the family to babies with diarrhoea. Such medical magic bullets can indeed save lives and begin the process of lowering infant mortality. These approaches need to be combined with less dramatic but, in the long run, more profound and permanent social approaches, such as improving women's status in society and working to reduce social inequities such as poverty.

All of the countries with the lowest infant mortality rates have government programs that guarantee every family with an infant a certain minimum of financial and social benefits, to ensure the basis for a healthy environment and good supervision and care for infants. The lack of these vital benefits is not limited to developing countries. The United States, for example, is twenty-first in the world in infant mortality. A child born in Hong Kong or Spain has a better chance of surviving its first year than a child born in the United States, and a child born in Czechoslovakia or Bulgaria has a better chance of celebrating its first birthday than a black child born in the United States (Commission on the Prevention of Infant Mortality, US Congress 1990). Data show that the excess mortality among infants in the United States occurs in poor families (Ruzek 1991). The United States is not guaranteeing everyone in its next generation adequate conditions for the best possible start through social and financial support to all families with pregnant women and infants.

It might be difficult to imagine a neonatologist refusing a new piece of equipment and proposing that the money be spent on social care for poor families with infants. Nevertheless, the participants in the consensus meeting (in spite of having a majority coming from a medical background and attending a meeting run by a health organisation) concluded that health services may not be the highest priority for care following birth. In addition, they were concerned not only that resources for health and social care be properly balanced, but that health care reach the people who need it most.

Studies in a variety of countries have shown that the people who need health services most — the socially disadvantaged — have the least access to them. The reasons for this problem are many but the solution requires some fundamental reorganisation of services in most cases. Again, the way in which health policy is formulated plays a role. Perhaps the only way to ensure that the interests of the socially disadvantaged are served is to include such people in the policy-making process. WHO calls this community participation in health care; it is easy to find on paper but hard to find in reality. When it occurs, community participation causes significant changes in health policy and services. In Canada, when the Province of Quebec moved towards local autonomy and local control of health and social services, no-one could have predicted that the results would include a demand from the Inuits (Eskimos) of the Arctic region that their babies be born in their own communities, not 1000 km to the south.

There was enthusiastic consensus in Trieste that, following the preamble, the very first recommendation of the consensus meeting should focus on the principle of social equity:

> *"Poverty is the greatest threat to the health of the woman and the infant. In the absence of concerted measures to promote social equity, little improvement can be expected in maternal and infant mortality and morbidity. Mortality and morbidity rates are higher in socially disadvantaged communities, which may also receive much less in the way of formal health care. Thus (a) in the allocation of resources, nationally and locally, direct spending on health services may not be the highest priority; and (b) services for healthy women and babies should be organized so that those most in need have access to adequate care."*

Self-help and mutual aid

Community participation includes taking part not only in health policy formulation but also in care itself. Organisations such as

Alcoholics Anonymous have existed for a long time and have demonstrated the effectiveness of the self-help and mutual aid approach. This approach consists of a group of lay (i.e. non-professional) people having the same need gathering together to share experiences and give support to each other. But the health establishment has been slow to acknowledge the importance of this approach in the overall health care scheme. When the WHO European Perinatal Study Group looked beneath the official health care rug for alternative perinatal services, it found widespread mutual aid groups in all the countries surveyed, providing assistance to families in the first month after birth (WHO 1985).

These groups offer two functions that official health services lack. First, they remind women, families, health workers and communities that having and rearing a baby is a normal social process, regardless of any medical problems which may befall the woman or the baby along the way. Such reminders are valuable because of their rarity. Second, mutual aid groups help women and families to believe in themselves and their ability to bear and rear children. Building self-confidence and a belief in the ability to cope is fundamental to the mutual aid approach, no matter the issue around which a group forms.

Breastfeeding support groups are an outstanding example of the application of this approach to care following birth. The need for such support was described in a working paper for the consensus meeting:

> "Breastfeeding women need continual encouragement during at least the first four weeks. There are nearly always moments of despair when we think the baby is not getting enough, when our nipples are cracked and sore, when the baby wakes all the time, or when she or he has colic. There are so many moments when it is tempting to think how much easier it would be to turn to the bottle, especially in western countries where bottles and formula are available at the drop of a hat and where there is no lack of people who will heave a big sigh of relief if you give up breastfeeding (it does not really fit in with many people's lifestyles)" (Cottingham 1986).

This need for support starts right after birth; in many countries, the support groups come to the hospitals to offer help. This sometimes precipitates conflict with health professionals. In Israel, for example, breastfeeding support groups have been forbidden to enter hospitals to give advice because their members are not qualified health professionals. It is precisely because they are not professionals that they need to be there.

The lay support groups' fund of knowledge is based on traditional practices, a holistic approach and much experience in successful breastfeeding; this knowledge complements professionals' knowledge about the content of breast-milk and its production. In addition, the members of a postpartum mutual aid group can help each other in other ways:

> "My own experience with a women's support group at the Dispensaire des Femmes (Women's Health Centre) in Geneva was tremendously positive. It can serve as an example of the kind of support women's groups can and do give. The group — which was essentially made up of the same women who had been together in the birth preparation group — met once a week with two workers from the Dispensaire. One of these women was a paediatrician but in many ways this was not important except in so far as she shared her own personal experiences with us. We generally concentrated on one topic per week: vaccination, feeding, sleeping, growth and development, colic, rashes, vomiting, etc. Women in the group chose the topics and very often we came back to feeding and nutrition. All of us shared our experiences — talking of how our babies reacted to this and that, and talking of how we felt as mothers. Each one of us had a different approach, a different kind of baby and a different set of problems. Yet precisely because of this we gained strength and insight into these problems by seeing how others were resolving them. Most importantly, there was a regular contact with people going through the same experience (the weeks following birth). This helped enormously in both cutting down isolation (for me it was like a lifeline to the rest of the world) and in dispelling fears and anxieties which so easily get out of proportion in this period" (Cottingham 1986).

Mutual aid is an important grassroots process that sometimes evolves into a broader social movement. Some health professionals shy away from mutual aid groups because some groups go beyond practical advice and encouragement to community action.

Breastfeeding support groups provide a good illustration of this phenomenon. Groups work to ensure that hospital professional practices and baby food manufacturers' promotion methods favour breastfeeding. An international coalition of many local groups (the International Baby Foods Action Network — IBFAN) played a key role in collaborating with WHO in the formulation and approval by the World Health Assembly of the WHO International Code of Marketing of Breast-milk Substitutes. IBFAN continues to monitor national and local compliance with this Code. The political activism of lay groups is an essential counterbalance to the potential conflicts of interest that accompany collaboration between industry and medical professionals. In building the Code, WHO collaborated actively with both industry and lay groups.

Although health professionals and government agencies must not control self-help and mutual aid groups, they should actively collaborate with and support these groups, to ensure effectiveness. This demands a delicate balance, with mutual respect; the ability of the professionals to recognise the value of the lay role is particularly important. Such a balance is beginning to be struck in a number of countries. Gradually, collaboration with and referral to lay support groups are becoming understood as necessities in bringing the right combination of the medical and social approaches to care following birth. For this reason, the participants agreed that the necessity of complementing professional care with care provided by lay people, through self-help and mutual aid groups, was a fourth principle to guide policy formulation in care following birth. The recommendation states:

> *"Self-help groups should be promoted and funded in local communities to enable parents to meet the responsibilities of infant care. Professionals have a duty to be knowledgeable about self-help groups in the community and they should inform parents about these groups. As one example, breastfeeding support groups in the community provide a valuable form of information exchange and support among women."*

Education

The final principle for policy-making was the need to educate all children and adults on childbirth and child rearing. In particular, the participants felt that the education of children about birth and infancy was inadequate in every country. This problem is more serious in industrialised countries and in the urban areas of developing countries, in which children no longer have extended families to give them a natural opportunity to learn about birth and the care of infants. Because birth involves the sexual organs, schools hesitate to approach the topic in countries with religious or cultural prohibitions. In addition, the medicalised concept of birth and infancy prevailing in industrialised countries may filter down to children, leaving them with fears that they find hard to express or resolve. More carefully planned education is needed in all government-sponsored schools, starting at an early age and emphasising normal birth and infant care as part of family life. The consensus recommendation states:

> *"In societies where young people have little opportunity to learn about childbirth, infant care and the responsibilities of parenthood, education is needed to prepare them for these experiences."*

The education of adults on birth and infancy can be more difficult, as they have already been exposed to much misinformation. It is important for the mass media to obtain balanced, accurate information, rather than just listening to the loudest or most powerful voice. For this purpose, it would be useful to develop mechanisms for better communication between journalists and health workers. Such media resource services have been established in the United Kingdom and the United States; WHO has also begun to organise the distribution of information to journalists. Again, the viewpoints of all interested parties should be included. The media also have a tendency to emphasise more sensational information. One of the participants, the then editor of *Lancet*, a medical journal with wide international readership, stated:

> "This preoccupation with the new, the dramatic, and the potential 'break-throughs' is understandable (I suffer from it myself), but it should not be allowed, anywhere in 'responsible' media, to obscure the importance of redelivering mes-

sages of proven value for mother, child, and the rest of the family" (Munro 1986).

Health professionals have a long history of keeping information to themselves. In the recent movement towards a health promotion approach, such information must be shared with the lay public if birth and the period following it are to remain parts of normal life. The relevant final consensus recommendation states:

"Information about the period following birth which is accurate, clear, attractively presented, of high quality and consistent, should be disseminated widely to parents, schoolchildren, teachers, health professionals and politicians."

Care for the healthy mother and baby

Recently health services following birth all over the world have focused on sick infants, neglecting both healthy infants and in particular the women who have just given birth. Discussions were therefore held to give proper attention to the great majority of mothers and newborn infants who are healthy.

In discussing healthy women having healthy babies, the first consideration must be the transition to motherhood. In the modern world, motherhood as an institution defined by society (and health professionals) is divorced from motherhood as women experience and perceive it. As an institution, it is a sacrosanct ideal:

"When we think of motherhood we are supposed to think of Renoir's blooming women with children at their knees, Raphael's ecstatic madonnas, some Jewish mother lighting the candles" (Rich 1977).

Research has shown, however, a serious discrepancy between women's experience of the ideal and the reality. Motherhood is a rite of passage, often accomplished with some difficulty and substantial personal adjustment.

Support for the new mother

Despite the idealisation of motherhood, society often fails to provide adequate practical support to mothers. Some of the difficulties women face in the transition arise from the social and economic positions of mothers — a reality regardless of the development or political system of the country they inhabit. Material forms of deprivation, such as poor housing, are linked to women's financial dependence on men and disadvantaged position in the labour market. In recent decades, women and children have formed one of the largest social groups living in poverty.

The shift in industrialised societies from the extended to the nuclear family deprives the new mother of traditional forms of adequate social support, and society fails to fill the gaps in economic support. Both these trends combine with the recent redefinition of infancy and infant care to leave the new mother feeling inadequate and overwhelmed. The participants responded to this situation by drafting recommendations to reaffirm the central role of the mother as the essential and most appropriate giver of care to the infant, and to provide her with the proper support to carry out this role. The first of these recommendations addresses the general principle that mothers are the primary and continuing human resource available to sustain optimum infant development and must be given general and specific practical support so that they can carry out this primary role.

Paid parental leave

Practices to support the mother, so the woman and her family can concentrate on and enjoy the new infant, are an old idea in most cultures. The first necessity is to relieve the mother of her usual responsibilities, so that she has the time needed for her new baby. If these responsibilities include paid work, paid maternity leave is essential. Time is something that a woman has to carve out for herself. The help of family and support groups in carrying out her normal tasks can have little impact if maternity leave benefits are inadequate or absent.

Governments need systems that guarantee such benefits. Every industrialised country in the world except one (the United States of America) and many more developing countries guarantee some amount of paid leave for the mother before and after the birth. In most countries in the WHO European Region, the combined period is at least 12 weeks, which is considered by the United Nations to be the bare minimum. Some countries offer a choice between long and short leave, with less money per month for the longer period. Many countries automatically extend the postnatal leave for certain cases such as premature and multiple births. In some European countries the length of postnatal leave grants depends on the size of the family; it increases with the number of children.

Most recently, the Scandinavian countries have led the way in extending these benefits to fathers. The usual pattern is to allow the mother and father to decide which parent will stay home during all or part of the postnatal leave. The participants in the consensus meeting considered that paternity leave was a vital step in fostering a good relationship between father and baby, and providing adequate support to the mother.

Other benefits

Beyond continuing to receive all or part of a salary while on parental leave, mothers and fathers receive other special benefits. Most countries in the European Region provide a grant of money for each child born, to help with expenses. The size of the grant may vary, increasing in some countries if, for example, there are other children in the family, the new baby is sick or disabled, or the mother is breastfeeding or a student. Several countries make payment contingent on attendance at prenatal visits. In addition to the lump sum, many countries also provide a family allowance consisting of regular monthly payments for each child. The amounts vary widely among countries; for two children, the family can receive 2–20% of the average monthly industrial wage. The amount usually increases progressively with each subsequent child.

A number of other social benefits are available. They include special privileges when travelling by public transport, priorities for loans and housing, permission to change jobs, the provision of milk, vitamins and baby equipment free of charge, and special working hours.

Most countries in Europe have laws and regulations on the working conditions of women during pregnancy and after childbirth. Night-time, overtime and dangerous work is often prohibited and women are transferred automatically to a less demanding job. It is important to note that the woman is protected from unfair dismissal because of pregnancy, and in most countries her right to reinstatement after maternity leave is ensured.

If the pregnant woman is sick, European countries give (on medical certification) sick leave with partial or full salary for as long as necessary. If the baby is sick, on the other hand, most countries provide for leave from work for either parent. The amount of time allowed for the care of a sick child varies from five days to six weeks (with partial or full salary). Some countries have unlimited unpaid leave, with job protection, when a child is sick. Many countries provide paid time off work to allow women to make official health care visits during pregnancy. Several also offer paid time off for women (and sometimes men) to attend pregnancy classes.

A final important aspect of working conditions is regulations for women who are breastfeeding. Nursing breaks — from two half-hour breaks to two one-hour breaks — are provided in many countries and counted as fully paid hours of work. In a few countries the breastfeeding mother is entitled to a shorter working day at full pay.

Single mothers — on the increase in most countries — are often eligible for special rights. These include longer maternity leave, increased financial benefits, loans and educational grants and priority for placement of the child in day-care centres.

Home help

Most of the benefits just described are tied somehow to the mother's and father's paid employment. Regardless of whether a woman has a paid job, support and assistance with her unpaid housework is important. Here the Dutch system is an outstanding model. In The Netherlands, women who are trained as maternity home helpers, are considered an essential and integral part of the overall maternity care system. They assist midwives at the 35% of all births that take place at home. Then they continue to spend all day, every day in the homes, for two weeks, to assist with the housework, supervise any other children, and provide the practical support that allows mothers to focus on their new babies.

All these benefits were agreed to form the core of an adequate support system for mothers and their families after childbirth. Ready consensus was reached:

> *"Every woman in employment should have an adequate period of paid maternity leave before and after childbirth. Social security systems should not penalize women for motherhood. Women should also be relieved of unpaid work after childbirth, and home help services should be available. After birth, paid leave should be provided for the father so that he can foster a relationship with the baby and support the mother."*

Mother and baby at home

Consensus was clear on two issues: the importance of keeping sick newborn babies in the hospital and, perhaps surprisingly, the importance of releasing healthy women and newborn babies to the home. The home is in general a much safer place than the hospital for well newborn infants and their mothers. The dangers in the hospital are multiple:

- the concentration of disease-causing micro-organisms;
- high rates of iatrogenic effects;
- a usually inadequate regard for the importance of psychological, social and cultural influences on infant development;
- the medicalisation of infancy and professionalisation of infant care comes naturally in a hospital setting.

The home is a natural remedy for all the dangers just listed. Even in the developing world, homes are much freer of dangerous germs than any hospital; in any case, the breastfed infant receives immunity to the germs in the home and not to the germs in the hospital. The infant must come home sooner or later and confront the germs normally found there. If the baby is healthy and is breastfed, natural immunity will allow the gradual adaptation of the baby to its home. As there are no physicians, midwives or nurses in the home, except for occasional visits, iatrogenic effects are not usually a problem. In addition, visiting health professionals can more easily identify serious psychological, social and cultural deviations by observing the family in the home environment. Home care — that is, the mother and father's care of the infants, with sensitive support from the formal and informal care systems — is the best safeguard for the parents' confidence in the normalcy of infancy and their ability to manage their child.

Some participants argued that women need a rest after childbirth, particularly if they have other children. Other participants replied that the hospital is an expensive as well as a dangerous hotel. The expense to society of keeping mothers and babies in the hospital for several days following birth is enormous. There are strong arguments that spending these funds on the training and provision of maternity home helpers and other home-based support services would realise much greater benefits.

It was also proposed that keeping the woman in the hospital provides an ideal opportunity for educating her about baby and child care. The same arguments applied; the hospital is an expensive and dangerous school. Educational assistance, too, is much more appropriate and relevant when given in the home.

To some extent, the participants' view of the home as the best place for the healthy mother and newborn infant endorses an already significant trend in newborn infant care. In 40% of all births in The Netherlands, mother and baby are discharged from the hospital within 24 hours of the time of birth. Another 35% are born at home, so that 75% of Dutch babies are in their own homes at no later than one day of age. The practice of discharging healthy mothers and babies within 24 hours of birth is rapidly gaining acceptance in many countries in western Europe and North America. The participants made two final consensus recommendations regarding the early discharge from hospital of mother and newborn infant. The first recommendation was drafted after the discussions on the healthy mother and baby; the second was drafted after the discussions on the sick newborn infant.

> *"Mothers and babies should not be kept in hospital beyond the time when they can benefit from further hospital diagnostic or therapeutic measures. If rest or social or educational support are needed, they should be provided in the home.*
>
> *"Discharge from hospital should depend on the wellbeing of the mother and infant, the wishes of the parents, and the availability of home support. In particular, discharge poli-*

cies should not be based on the single criterion of weight and should concentrate on earliest possible discharge."

Both the above recommendations stress the necessity of home support, in part because the participants did not advocate the dumping of mothers and babies into their homes without proper follow-up and home-based support. This concern was largely part of a major principle emerging from the discussions: the care following birth should be characterised by a proper emphasis on services and resources (financial and human) for the home. With the exception of The Netherlands, every other industrialised country in the world, as well as many of the developing countries, has focused the majority of services and resources for postpartum care on the hospital. Working towards a proper balance between hospital and home services was another aspect of the participants' search for the optimal mixture of the medical and social approaches.

In the discussion on home-based family care following birth, as provided by health professionals working within the formal care system, concern was expressed about two problems with professional care provided in the home. First, how can health care professionals visit the home to give support and advice without reinforcing the tendency, which their mere presence implies, towards medicalised infancy and professionalised parenthood? Can the professional and the parent have an egalitarian relationship when only one party in the encounter is considered an expert and paid for the time involved? One way to try to resolve this dilemma is for the health professional to give as much of the control of the visit as possible to the family. The family should decide whether there will be a visit and, if so, when it will take place, who will be present and what will be done. Thus the professional facilitates family and community empowerment and self-reliance.

The second problem is the conflict between society's need to monitor the adequacy of the care provided by the family, and the family's need for support (Mayall 1989). The recent wave of inquiries into deaths from child abuse and neglect has only confirmed many professionals (in their mind and in public expectation) as primarily monitors of child care. Can a visiting professional simultaneously monitor and empower?

Non-professional care givers in home-based care following birth do not have these problems. Their dilemmas are quite different: how to gain credibility and acceptance as legitimate providers of care and support and how to coordinate their services with professional care so that the two systems are complementary. Non-professional providers of care are of two types. They can be people with experience with the situation (such as members of self-care and mutual aid groups) or lay care givers with special skills such as breastfeeding counsellors. Determining the border between these two groups is difficult and perhaps not meaningful; it is important to recognise the full gamut of non-professional helpers and the essential role they play.

The participants agreed on the importance of a system of postpartum care with proper emphasis on the well woman and healthy infant and on home-based services and the use of both professionals and non-professionals to provide them.

> *"For healthy women and babies, support equivalent to that provided in hospital should be made available to all mothers and babies at home.*
>
> *"Resources should be allocated, both in hospital and in the community, to the follow-up of the health of the newborn infant and the woman. Ideally, personnel involved in the birth and in hospital aftercare would make the first home contact with the woman and family to inquire about their wellbeing. Every woman and baby should have the opportunity to receive community-based health care. Home-based care givers should encourage the promotion of health in the woman and her baby."*

Successful breastfeeding

The importance of the successful establishment of breastfeeding cannot be overemphasised. While the importance of breastfeeding in the developing countries is indisputable, evidence for its importance in industrialised countries is also mounting. The contribution of breastfeeding to the optimal psychological and social development of the infant, as well as the optimal development of the immune and other biological systems, is indubitable in all regions of the world. For example, less illness and fewer allergies among breastfed infants are global phenomena (Minchin 1985).

Babies have been carried and nursed frequently for more than 99% of human history. To ensure survival, babies were carried close to the mother's body, to be fed and kept warm. In western society, the Industrial Revolution with its nuclear family and the Puritan ethic with its shame about breasts resulted in the loss of knowledge about breastfeeding among women. Seeing women breastfeeding was no longer a normal part of life for most children. This new gap in knowledge among young women was gradually filled by scientists and physicians who developed a knowledge of breastfeeding based on the medical model. The shift of birth and postpartum care from the home to the hospital helped to complete the medicalisation of breastfeeding. The situation is strange today. The medical model's scientific work has proved the superiority and importance of breast-feeding, and the medical world argues for its promotion, but medical systems jeopardise its chances for success.

Many of the normal practices for feeding newborn infants in hospitals, in place for decades, unwittingly raise barriers. Many hospitals, for example, still bring the baby to its mother for the first breastfeed many hours after birth, in spite of the research showing that such delays increase the likelihood of mothers ceasing to breastfeed within two weeks. (Oakley 1986) It is now strongly recommended that the baby be put to the breast within the first half hour of life. Other hospital practices (including caesarean section, the use of general anaesthesia during birth and babies' admission to special care) have been shown to prejudice the chances of successful breastfeeding.

Another persisting hospital practice in many areas is that of allowing (when the baby is in the nursery) or promoting (with rooming-in) breastfeeding at intervals of 3–4 hours or 6–8 times within 24 hours. The origin of this custom is not clear, but is probably related to the work schedules of the hospital staff. In any case, such practices differ markedly from those observed among hunter-gatherers. Women in these latter groups nurse for a short period 30–40 times in 24 hours. Recent research indicates that the infrequent nursing in the hospital has had several unintended harmful consequences (Kennell & Klaus 1986). Increasing the frequency of breastfeeding in the hospital increased milk output by 40%; increasing the length of each feeding had no effect on milk production. Other studies have shown that increased breastfeeding frequency in the hospital resulted in less breast pain, less nipple soreness and increased success in lactation. The possible relationship of infrequent feeding with iatrogenic jaundice of the newborn is discussed on page 256.

In addition, some biochemical evidence supports more frequent breastfeeding for young infants. In species adapted for long separation (feeding every 4–12 hours), infant animals receive breast-milk with high protein and fat concentrations and reduced water. Infant mammals, who are carried by or follow their mothers and feed almost continuously, receive milk with low concentrations of protein and fat. Human milk is low in fat and extremely low in protein.

In summary, the hospital practice of scheduled breastfeeds 3–4 hours apart has probably had the following unfortunate effects: increased incidence of jaundice in the infant, decreased breast-milk output, increased breast and nipple soreness and increased incidence of lactation failure. There is now sufficient evidence to question whether any breastfeeding mother should be subject to 3–4 hour intervals between feeds.

The participants at the consensus meeting made three recommendations on breastfeeding. The first urged that:

> *"If the mother desires breastfeeding, it should be initiated within the first hour after birth. Practices concerning breastfeeding should follow the resolutions adopted at the Thirty-fourth World Health Assembly in 1981."*

The second recommendation concerned the role of health personnel in promoting breastfeeding. Recent studies have identified the information given and the attitudes expressed by health professionals as a major deterrent. For this reason a final recommendation on the education and training of health professionals for care following birth included the following:

> *"... Regarding breastfeeding, special attention must be given to the training and practices of health professionals who come in contact with women in the postpartum period. Contradictory advice must be avoided. The practice of giving food other than milk during the first months is to be discouraged."*

The third recommendation endorsed the important role of non-professionals in supporting women who breastfeed. Health professionals should recognise the value of such assistance. Health professionals often seem unhappy about such lay initiatives in motherhood, possibly because the advice conveyed is contrary to the professional model and cannot be controlled. It is for this reason that the participants wanted a consensus recommendation on self-help groups to include the following:

> *"Breastfeeding support groups in the community provide a valuable forum of information exchange and support among women."*

It is interesting that 3 years after the meeting in Trieste, WHO and UNICEF initiated a global program to promote breastfeeding. This program focuses on what happens in the hospital after birth because this is where the most serious barriers to promoting breastfeeding occur. The program, called "The Baby Friendly Hospital Initiative", has 10 steps which are strikingly similar to the recommendations from Trieste (WHO 1990).

When discussing the healthy mother and newborn baby at the meeting, participants of many disciplines (anthropology, midwifery, nursing, obstetrics, paediatrics, public health, psychology and sociology) reiterated the principle that the mother and her baby are a fundamental dyad. The existence of the public health specialty called maternal and child health reflects this principle. Although discussions on various topics tended to focus on either the woman or the child, it was clear that any activity that supports the wellbeing of one also supports that of the other. This was most clearly seen in the discussions on contact between the newborn infant and the parents.

Contact between the parents and the baby

The past 25 years have seen an accelerating discussion of a 'new' and extremely important dimension of care following birth: attachment or bonding between parent and infant. This process became visible only when the medicalisation of motherhood made it difficult. Moving birth to the hospital and newborn infants to the centralised nursery placed the usual chances for contact in the first few days under institutional control, where many were lost. A woman becomes a mother by forming a relationship with her new baby. Accomplishing this task in the hospital may not always be easy. Imagine a man in hospital recovering from surgery and suffering from enforced insomnia, being required to take on a new job for which he has had no previous training and also being expected to fall in love at the same time.

Until the discovery of the phenomenon called mother-infant bonding in the 1960s and 1970s, the love new mothers felt for their babies was widely believed to be instinctive and therefore virtually automatic. The usual conditions in the mother's home might have facilitated attachment. Research conducted during the past 20 years suggests two modifications to the understanding of the development of a relationship between a woman and her new baby. First, the speed and intensity of this development varies between dyads; in one study, 41% of the women surveyed said that they first loved their babies during pregnancy; 24% at birth; 27% in the first week after birth; and 8% after the first week (Kennell & Klaus 1986). In addition, the process is strongly influenced by environmental factors such as the amount of time the mother and baby have together, and stresses such as coping with strange surroundings (e.g. a hospital). A study of first-time mothers, giving birth in a modern hospital with typically high obstetrical intervention rates, showed that the predominant reaction of these women on first holding their babies was a relative lack of interest in the child. Their primary feeling was relief at surviving the birth and producing an apparently healthy child. Most said that they felt too physically and emotionally exhausted to relate properly to the baby (Oakley 1986).

Attachment is seldom immediate. Much recent research suggests that attachment involves many processes that operate during the first days of life. It has been shown that contact during the first several days after birth initiates and strengthens the operation of known sensory, hormonal, physiological, immunological and behavioural mechanisms; these probably attach the mother to her infant. After all, it seems unlikely that the establishment of such a vital relationship would depend on a single process. It is now hypothesised that a cascade of interaction occurs during the first several days, locking mother and baby together and ensuring the further development of the attachment.

Research results

A review of 17 controlled studies conducted between 1975 and 1985 compared newborn infants in the hospital who had routine contact with their mothers with those receiving additional contact. In 13 studies the additional contact occurred only during the first hour of life; 9 of these noted significant positive differences in the later behaviour of the mothers towards their infants. In the four studies in which the extra contact extended through the first three days of life, the mother–child relationship was measurably better in quality for the extra-contact infants than for the control infants at one month, one year and two years of age. Increased contact at any time during the first three days after birth (when the mother and baby spend this time in the hospital) produces a long-term improvement in the quality of the relationship between mother and child. Increased contact may in part make up for the marked deprivation that is a part of current routines in modern hospitals. There is some evidence that this, with the additional deprivation of insufficient contact, can have serious consequences for the child — both child abuse and failure to thrive without organic cause are found more frequently in infants who have been separated from their parents immediately after birth (O'Conner et al. 1980a, 1980b, 1981). Since the meeting in Trieste, a more recent review of 29 random control trials between 1972 and 1985 of restrictive versus unrestrictive mother-infant contact in the immediate post-partum period found strong evidence that restricting contact significantly reduced both subsequent maternal affectionate behaviour and subsequent breastfeeding (Thomson & Westreich 1991). Women of lower economic status may be particularly vulnerable to the adverse effects of restricting contact.

> "It may be thought surprising that disruption of maternal–infant interaction in the immediate post-partum period may set some women on the road to breastfeeding failure and altered subsequent behaviour towards their children. Paediatricians, psychologists, and others have debated this issue. This scepticism does not, however, constitute grounds for acquiescing in hospital routines which lead to unwanted

separation of mothers from their babies. In the light of the evidence that such policies may actually do harm, they should be changed forthwith" (Thomson & Westreich 1991, p. 1328).

Separation of the mother and infant after birth can also have serious consequences for the mother (see later section on mother's unhappiness in this chapter).

The understanding of the importance of contact between parent and infant has been deepened by other recent research on the perceptual abilities of newborn infants. Contrary to general belief 25 years ago, newborn infants are known to have extraordinary perceptual abilities. A newborn baby will mimic the facial expressions of an adult and synchronise its movements with adult speech; infants who room-in with their mothers regulate the physiological rhythm of their sleeping and waking cycle to follow their mothers' diurnal rhythms. Research has shown that the infant can discriminate between the voices of a stranger and its mother in the second week of life (Maratos 1986).

Observational and anecdotal evidence suggest that the mother–infant relationship may begin before birth. Advances in ultrasound technology have provoked a rapidly increasing interest in such an attachment. Now that a pregnant woman can be given a photographic print of her fetus, the effects of such a picture on the normal course of attachment could be significant; they require study.

The participants in the consensus meeting readily agreed to recommend close contact between mother and baby from the moment of birth. There is evidence that every parent and infant should be offered the chance for at least 30–60 minutes of contact, in privacy, within the first three hours after birth. If the health of the mother or the infant makes this impossible, then discussion, support and reassurance should help the parents appreciate that they can still establish a good relationship with their new baby although it may require more time and effort. There is also scientific support for a hospital policy that allows the infant to remain with the mother as long as she wishes, throughout the hospital stay. In establishing such practices in hospitals parents must have informed choice about contact. The important recent information on mother-infant contact should not be translated into inflexible bureaucratic procedures. Enforced bonding is as wrong as enforced separation.

Rooming-in

The increasing understanding of the importance of contact has stimulated the rapid acceptance and practice of rooming-in as the most logical, economical and sensible way to guarantee sufficient contact controlled by the mother. Rooming-in is widely practised in western Europe (WHO 1985) and is beginning to be tested in several eastern European countries. All other industrialised countries in the world have options for rooming-in at many if not most hospitals. In developing countries, although rooming-in has come to be seen as an unfortunate necessity due to lack of funds and health personnel, the value of the practice is being recognised. The extra contact guaranteed by rooming-in has been shown to be particularly important when mother or infant have been separated or ill (for example, after caesarean section or other major obstetrical interventions), or if the mother is at the limit of adaptability because she is poor, single or very young, for example. The participants easily agreed to urge the promotion of rooming-in.

The other side of the coin is the closure of the central nursery for newborn infants. There are reasons for replacing nurseries with rooming-in; each is based on scientific evidence.

1. The mother and infant will have an optimal opportunity for contact, and in general this interaction will be controlled by the mother rather than the hospital staff.
2. The mother will become familiar with the baby's early signals, needs and schedules, and thus will be better prepared to meet the baby's needs at home.
3. The baby can nurse frequently, on demand, obtaining a larger volume of milk sooner. The probability of successful breastfeeding increases with all its nutritional, immunological and psychological benefits.
4. The baby will cry less.
5. Mothers detect symptoms and signs of problems earlier than nursing staff.

6. With more frequent breastfeeding, babies will have lower levels of bilirubin and less jaundice, and thus less need for laboratory tests and phototherapy.
7. There will be less risk of infection.

Nevertheless, the possibility of closing the central nursery for normal newborn babies was not unanimously endorsed. Some participants were convinced that the invention of a centralised nursery for normal newborn infants was the single biggest mistake in the history of the care of the newborn in the twentieth century. While all participants agreed on the dangers, however, some argued that the nursery must remain to ensure that mothers have a choice about rooming-in and that babies receive adequate professional observation. Others argued that other alternatives to rooming-in should be found. The discussions showed that such institutional changes are very difficult to make, even when supported by research data, and particularly in an environment dominated by physicians concerned about detecting and treating a variety of rare conditions. While the majority of participants favoured recommending that central nurseries for normal babies be closed, this proposition never achieved consensus. Everyone wanted to mention this possibility, however, so a compromise was reached: *"Thought should be given to abandoning central nurseries for normal babies"*. Since the conference in Trieste a lot of thought has been given to closing central nurseries. This possibility is actively debated in many countries and several large new maternity hospitals have been built in the United States and Canada without any central nursery (Young 1992).

The participants in Trieste were very involved in the issue of parent/infant contact and considered the final consensus recommendation on this subject as one of the most important to come from the meeting:

> "All parents and newborn infants have the right to be in close contact from the time of birth. Closeness between mother and infant should be promoted in all circumstances, including the period after caesarean birth or other medical interventions affecting the woman or infant. Women and babies should not be separated and should be together as much as the mother wishes. Rooming-in should be promoted; and thought should be given to abandoning central nurseries for normal babies. Furthermore, involvement of

parents in the care of the unhealthy newborn should be promoted, including the actual care of the unhealthy infant and participation in decisions about treatment."

Hospital infections

The high frequency of hospital-acquired infection is a serious danger to mothers and their new babies, particularly because the infectious agents most commonly found in hospitals are very virulent and often immune to antibiotics. The connection between hospital birth, newborn nurseries and epidemic infections has already been made. In general the initial solution was to try to eliminate germs from the central nursery by using many disinfectants, frequent hand-washing, increasing the space around each infant bed in the nursery, reducing the contact with the mother (but not the nurses) and eliminating contact with family members. These procedures were never completely successful and often made things worse. "The extent of the problem presented by infection among babies who were apparently healthy at the time of birth has almost certainly been greater than it should have been, precisely because of the measures taken to avoid it" (Rush et al. 1991, p. 1335).

When rooming-in was first proposed as a way to promote mother–infant contact, many feared the practice would increase hospital infection rates. Considerable subsequent research has shown, however, that rooming-in results in far fewer infections in infants than the central nursery system (Rush et al. 1991). As long ago as 1959 research showed lower rates of colonisation of dangerous bacteria and lower rates of infection in rooming-in (Montgomery et al. 1959). Over 30 years later, every time I propose rooming-in Eastern Europe I am told that it cannot be considered because of the danger of infection. An interesting natural experiment with rooming-in occurred in Guatemala (Kennell & Klaus 1986). A very large hospital in that country had a persistent infection morbidity of 17 per 1000 newborn infants in the central nursery. A major earthquake in 1976 destroyed the nursery, forcing a change in hospital policy. Newborn babies were kept in their mothers' beds. Even though these beds were crowded closely together, the morbidity due to infection dropped to 2 to 3 per 1000 infants and remained at this low level.

Postpartum women also have significant problems with hospital-acquired infections. One of the stimuli for a policy of early discharge from hospital for healthy women and newborn infants has been the frustrating results of hospital staffs' heroic efforts to reduce the infection rates for both mother and infant. Moving birth into the hospital created the problem; it seems more and more logical that the solution is to remove the woman and her baby as quickly as possible from the source of the problem: the hospital. The final consensus recommendation on this problem is:

> *"Since hospital-acquired infections are a major threat to women and infants, hospitals should monitor their infection rates and introduce programs for the prevention of such infections. Rooming-in rather than a central nursery can be an important part of such a programme. Early discharge of women and infants would also be part of such programs."*

Evaluation at birth

The participants recommended that every baby should be evaluated at the time of birth for both its condition (vital signs such as breathing and heart rate) and the presence of congenital abnormalities. The person who should make this evaluation was not specified; it will vary with local conditions. For example, midwives evaluate infants in many countries with low perinatal mortality rates, such as Denmark. Clearly the person making the assessment must be trained for the task.

Further, the participants recommended that the initial evaluation should take place in the mother's presence unless the baby's condition is poor enough to require special care immediately. The examination can be done in the room where the birth takes place, preferably next to the mother on her bed, so as not to interfere with contact between the mother and her new baby. This also provides an ideal opportunity to answer the mother's questions about the baby and to teach her how to do her own evaluations. The initial evaluation was seen as not only a preventive check-up but also part of a program to promote mother and child health.

"Every newborn baby should be evaluated initially for vital signs and gross congenital abnormalities. Evaluations should take place next to the mother if possible, in a room at the right temperature and without hazard to baby or woman."

Care for the sick woman

Postnatal depression

When attention turned to the woman who is unhealthy after childbirth, the participants discussed postnatal depression, which can probably be described as a twentieth-century epidemic. One study found that, among first-time mothers in London:

- 84% had experienced postpartum 'blues' — a condition of emotional instability marked by crying and lasting a few days, normally while the mother was still in the hospital;
- 71% felt extremely anxious on first coming home with their babies; 33% felt depressed 'on and off' in the early weeks of motherhood; and
- 24% experienced a more disabling, symptomatic depression that could appear weeks or months after the birth of the child (Oakley 1986a).

Similar rates of maternal unhappiness after birth are found in other studies. A review of the literature has identified three different levels of postpartum unhappiness (Romito 1991). About 80% of women experience some degree of postpartum blues or 'baby blues' (mood instability, anxiety and irritability) in the first days after birth. At the other extreme one or two women in every thousand new mothers has a postpartum psychosis, often requiring psychiatric hospitalisation. In between these two is a catch-all diagnosis of postpartum depression. This phenomenon is elusive and is reported to affect 15–20% of childbearing women (WHO 1991). It has even been suggested that researchers assume postpartum depression exists and their research results inevitably confirm the assumption (Day 1982).

"The variety of conceptual descriptions and definitions of postpartum depression suggest that the phenomenon labelled 'postpartum depression', rather than being an actual entity, is not only defined by, but actually constructed by the instruments used to measure it" (Romito 1991). Such research shows that many or most women have negative feelings about themselves, their babies and their lives as a part of the usual experience of hospital birth and new motherhood in industrialised societies. Unfortunately, data are lacking on women's emotional state after planned home birth.

The normality of such negative feelings is now part of the institution of motherhood in western culture. For example, an analysis of books written by health professionals to advise new mothers showed that normal mothers are married, need medical care and protection (doctor knows best), are rather childish, and ought to be happy but are usually depressed (Oakley 1986a). Further evidence of the institution of unhappiness as part of normal motherhood was contained in an official booklet for health personnel and parents, stating that postpartum depression is normal (United Kingdom Department of Health and Social Security 1977).

There is no evidence that women have always felt depressed after birth. What factors are associated with the depression now prevailing in new mothers? A number of attempts have been made to find hormonal explanations for postpartum unhappiness. These studies are limited to specific aspects of early postpartum biochemistry, however, and most have been negative or inconclusive. On the other hand there is evidence for an association between postnatal depression and psychological and social factors.

One study showed that an ambivalent or negative experience of birth by the woman was associated with a later depressed mood, and the physician's assessment was not (WHO 1991). The same study showed that other important psychological factors were associated with depression included experiencing a greater need for care during pregnancy than other pregnant women, and feeling that the staff of the maternity ward were too busy to give enough support. Another study found that the presence of four social factors — bad housing, a distant relationship with the baby's father and the lack of a paid job and previous experience of babies — appeared to make women highly vulnerable to feelings of depression; all women in the study with these four factors were depressed (Oakley 1986a).

In addition, a large survey found a strong association between depressed mood in the mother and the admission of her baby to a paediatric department (WHO 1991), regardless of the reason for which the baby was referred. An analysis of the data, however, showed that depression increased with the complexity of the treatment of the baby. These results suggest that these feelings probably result from separation from the baby and anxiety about its wellbeing. It approaches common sense to conclude that postpartum women who have had a bad experience during pregnancy or birth, or who have a new baby who is sick, or who have a difficult situation at home will be unhappy. "The medicalisation of unhappiness as depression is one of the great disasters of the 20th century" (Oakley 1986b). Rather than concluding that something is wrong with the women (blaming the victims), hopefully in the future the health care system will recognise the need both to provide appropriate social support to women and also to advocate for a re-examination by society of the impossible burdens often given to new mothers.

The participants felt that postnatal depression should receive more study to clarify the relationship between the way women and babies are treated in the hospital and the later wellbeing of women. One final recommendation included the phrase *". . . an area of research needing high priority is health problems in the women following birth, including postpartum depression"*.

Basic health care

The participants themselves felt depressed while discussing the plight of women who do not receive the most basic health care needed after birth. In developing countries, haemorrhage, infection and pregnancy-induced hypertension are important causes of maternal morbidity and mortality; many places lack the health services to provide effective treatment for women with these conditions. Where services exist, in developing and industrialised countries, financial, cultural, linguistic and geographical barriers may limit access to them. An effective referral and transport system must be part of these basic services. For these reasons all participants, regardless of their country of origin, agreed on the importance of recommending:

> *"Every women should receive basic care immediately fol-*
> *lowing birth. In those parts of the world where haemorrhage,*
> *infection and pregnancy-induced hypertension are impor-*
> *tant causes of maternal mortality and morbidity, every*
> *effort should be made to provide effective treatment and to*
> *prevent long-term sequelae. An effective referral system is*
> *necessary for the woman when complications arise during*
> *pregnancy, birth, or the period following birth. Such a sys-*
> *tem must include free transport where necessary."*

Care of the sick baby

Transport

The importance of the mother-infant dyad also extends to the care of the sick newborn infant. One of the first issues discussed was the transport of the sick infant from the place of birth to the place where adequate treatment is available. The participants quickly agreed that the best transport system is the mother, that is, when the infant is still inside the mother, rather than after birth.

This requires adequate screening and care of the woman during her pregnancy, a prerequisite that demonstrates the indivisibility of care during pregnancy and birth and after birth, and of services for the treatment of sick women and newborn infants. In reality, however, health service systems in all countries tend to make these separations, creating iatrogenic barriers to the functioning of referral systems, the flow of information and smooth transport. The understanding of the importance of contact between mother and infant increases the urgency of eliminating such barriers. In the recommendation on the subject, no such artificial separations were acknowledged:

> *"A woman who becomes seriously ill during pregnancy or*
> *labour or whose fetus is endangered should be provided with*
> *an appropriate level of care, ideally before birth. Transport*
> *must also be available for every unhealthy infant who needs*
> *care elsewhere. Vehicles for the transport of infants should*
> *be equipped with the basic means of maintaining body tem-*

perature and supporting respiration. If she wishes, the woman should be able to accompany her infant. A referral network must be established and understood by all concerned. The infant should be accompanied by the record prepared by the primary care provider. Communication between the different levels of care is important."

Immediate care and resuscitation

Another issue was the immediate care and resuscitation of the infant at the moment of birth. In the decade prior to the consensus meeting, France had launched an extensive new program in perinatal services. When the results were evaluated, the most effective medical strategy to reduce perinatal mortality was found to be the training of midwives and general practitioners, to ensure that such care was immediately available to all newborn babies, not just those considered at risk. It is simple and non-invasive, using equipment available in any local hospital and transportable to home births.

The French experience showed this primary care to be highly cost-effective. Similar experiences in many countries led to consensus that, in every country, the first priority for the treatment of sick newborn infants should be, not specialist care, but guaranteeing high-quality immediate care at the place of birth. The recommendation states:

"A first priority is that every newborn baby, whether born at home or in hospital, should be assessed for breathing difficulties and be given the necessary support to initiate and sustain respiration. Every birth attendant should be trained in and equipped to deal with immediate care and resuscitation of the newborn, including identification of the need for consultation or referral to more specialized care."

Iatrogenic jaundice

The participants discussed jaundice of the newborn infant as an example of iatrogenic problems. A review of the management of the condition pointed out that, although the vast majority of jaundiced full-term infants appear completely healthy, standard textbooks of paediatrics and newborn medicine require diagnostic investigations (to rule out 'pathological' jaundice) in those whose concentrations of bilirubin in the blood exceed a certain level (Maisels 1986). Research has shown, however, no cause for the jaundice in over half the babies with higher levels, suggesting that many of these babies have non-pathological jaundice, for which it is agreed that no investigations are necessary (Berger 1991). Other research has shown that the level of bilirubin during the first few days after birth can be related to many non-pathological factors, such as the induction of labour with oxytocin, maternal diabetes, maternal non-smoking, breastfeeding, the amount of weight lost by the baby after birth and male sex. The increasing jaundice in breastfed infants reported here is associated with 6–8 feeds per day. Increasing the frequency of breastfeeding in the first three days after birth produced significantly lower serum bilirubin levels in infants (high levels are present in infants with jaundice). Frequent feeding probably leads to increasing gut motility. This increases the faecal excretion of bilirubin, thus decreasing its intestinal absorption. If further research proves this hypothesis correct, at least some of the jaundice of the newborn infant is the iatrogenic result of hospital feeding practices.

Present knowledge of jaundice of the newborn is clearly insufficient, justifying a policy of watchful expectancy (do nothing until further cause for alarm appears) for many babies who have borderline bilirubin levels and one or more of the non-pathological factors. It is also clear that current definitions of physiological jaundice have created a class of healthy jaundiced infants who receive a battery of laboratory tests and often treatment with phototherapy, with a high cost in money and iatrogenic parental anxiety.

Proof of this is a retrospective study in The Netherlands of how often phototherapy was given to health babies born spontaneously at home compared to a matched group of healthy babies born in hospital (Van Enk & De Leeuw 1987). Infants in hospital received 7 times more phototherapy than those at home and the surveillance at home was not inferior to that in hospital. The authors conclude: "Being in a hospital has thus become a factor in its own right and determines the frequency of medical interventions. In this case it concerned phototherapy, but it might also apply to the frequency with which many obstetric procedures are carried out, which is at present widely criticised" (Van Enk & Le Leeuw 1987).

The management of jaundice in the newborn infant is an example of diagnostic and therapeutic iatrogenesis. The participants' consensus recommendation states:

> *"Iatrogenesis (harm to the woman or her infant by diagnostic or therapeutic measures) should be avoided, for example harm from treatment of jaundice in the newborn. Jaundice affects many full-term newborn infants, but the vast majority of them are healthy and do not need diagnostic investigation or treatment."*

Neonatal tetanus

The participants found the need for a recommendation on neonatal tetanus to be a sad commentary on inappropriate priority setting in perinatal care. Some participants wondered what kind of policy-making allows the development of a situation in which many otherwise healthy babies die of neonatal tetanus (which can be entirely and fairly cheaply eradicated), while in the same country enormous resources go to extremely expensive specialist care for a very few very sick babies with a high risk of death or permanent disability. At least part of the answer lies in the imbalance of the social and medical approaches to perinatal care.

The eradication of neonatal tetanus involves a more social approach. The work must be done at primary care level by health care workers such as midwives and nurses working in close cooperation with the local community — an unglamorous, tedious and sometimes frustrating effort. If the work is successful, the result is far less dramatic than that of neonatal intensive care; all that can be photographed is a normal, healthy baby who did not get tetanus. It took the participants only a few words to make the recommendation on this issue:

> *"The eradication of neonatal tetanus is a high priority."*

Low birth weight

The care of babies with low birth weight (less than 2500 g) is a major part of services for newborn infants and a profound drain on financial and human resources. Again, low birth weight is the most important factor associated with illness or death in babies around the time of birth. This fact, along with the failure to discover the causes of either type of low birth weight (prematurity or intrauterine growth retardation), leads logically to the two highest priorities for action: research and the immediate use of what is known for prevention. Until further progress is made, the care of low birth weight babies must be seen as a form of rescue medicine.

Research on and preventive action and care programs for low birth weight infants require a combination of the medical and social approaches, as low birth weight is both a medical risk factor and a social indicator. Research must take into consideration the close association of birth weight with socioeconomic status and the medical questions such as the causes of failures in placental functioning, which retard the growth of the fetus. Preventive action must include social programs to control substance abuse (of tobacco, alcohol and both licit and illicit drugs) and to give social support to pregnant women, as well as medical efforts such as family planning, prenatal care and nutrition programs. Care for low birth weight babies involves medical elements (such as neonatal intensive care) and social elements (such as follow-up support in the home).

MANAGEMENT

Because of the subject of the meeting, discussion focused on the management of low birth weight infants, rather than on preventing the condition. The evolution of such care in the past few decades was similar to that of other perinatal and maternal health care programs; an initially medical approach has gradually been modified to incorporate a social approach (Richards 1986). In the 1950s and 1960s, sick babies were moved out of the central nursery into a nursery in which they could receive special care. Very low birth weight infants (less than 1500 g) were included in special care because they almost always need special assistance in feeding, and maintaining body heat and perhaps respiration. Gradually, the babies referred to special care came to include those who were not really sick but needed special observation, such as babies with jaundice or a birth weight of 1800–2500 g. These larger low birth weight babies were included because of the statistical fact that they have a higher perinatal mortality rate, although there was insufficient proof that special observation lowered mortality.

By the end of the 1960s, it was conventional paediatric wisdom that all low birth weight infants should be kept in a special care nursery until they weighed 2500 g. This policy placed a tremendous strain on hospital staff and budgets. The time spent on the care of each of the larger low birth weight infants amounts to about 4 hours per 24 hours (Prudent 1986). The special care units act as feeding stations for these babies, who are at a distinct disadvantage in competing for attention with the truly sick infants. As a result, they are usually fed on schedule rather than on demand, often with a feeding tube as a matter of expediency. Staff seldom have the time to provide a satisfactory amount of fondling and verbal and visual contact with these babies. In any case, such attention depends on the level of activity in the nursery at any given moment and the nurse/baby ratio. Unsatisfactory conditions are more frequent in crowded hospitals in developing countries, although they also exist in some hospitals in industrialised countries.

TRANSITIONAL CARE

In the 1970s, a recognition of this situation and increasing concern about hospital-acquired infection and adequate parent-child contact prompted a reassessment of the management of low birth weight babies. Several alternatives were developed and tried. The central nursery for sick babies was divided into two levels of care: special and intensive. A third level of care (called transitional or intermediate) was also developed, in which babies who were not sick (such as larger low birth weight infants) but considered to need observation were able to room-in with their mothers with special attention from the staff. This also involves providing care where the baby was born rather than moving the infant to another unit or hospital. Experience in both developing and developed countries has shown this level of care to be safe, effective and economical (Richards 1986, Prudent 1986).

EARLY DISCHARGE

Another alternative was early discharge, without waiting for the baby to reach some arbitrary weight. Research studies in Canada, Chile, England, Ethiopia, Jamaica, Tanzania, the United States and Zimbabwe have demonstrated that the length of stay of a low birth weight infant in a special care unit can be significantly shortened if the decision for discharge is based on the condition of the baby (not sick and able to feed well by breast or bottle) and maternal coping ability (Richards 1986). One study demonstrated the feasibility of such a scheme in Argentina (Prudent 1986). A randomised clinical trial in the United States, published in the same month as the consensus meeting was held in Trieste, examined the safety and economic benefits of discharging very low birth weight infants before they reached 2200 g (Brooten et al. 1986). This study showed that the practice was safe, although the babies in the early discharge group went home a mean of 11.2 days earlier and weighed 200 g less than those in the control group. The mean hospital cost for the early discharge group was US$47,520; for the control group it was US$64,940. There were mean savings in hospital costs of US$17,420 per infant and US$1716 in physicians' charges. There was an extensive home support program using a specially trained nurse with a mean cost per infant of US$576. Thus, the savings on every infant discharged early could subsidise home care for 33 infants. A more recent study in the United Kingdom showed that a similar program saved the City of Manchester US$500,000 in one year (Couriel 1988).

All such studies strongly recommend that early discharge be accompanied by a program of home support. Most programs included regular home visits by a nurse and/or other health professionals, easy contact with the home visitor by telephone when necessary, and periodic return visits to the hospital. Such home-based follow-up programs have proved very valuable in providing the continuing support needed by families during the crucial transition of the baby from hospital to home.

The early discharge of low birth weight infants, although consistent with the general trend towards early discharge, has not been readily accepted by the new profession of neonatology. An analysis in the United Kingdom has shown that the best predictor of the use of special care units is the number of places in these units, not measures of need (Richards 1980). A study in Canada found that admission rates to neonatal intensive care units were strongly correlated with availability of cots and physician characteristics but not strongly correlated with clinical need (Campbell 1984). Both studies show that if facilities exist, they are likely to be used. This is partly because if governments severely limit the resources for medical care, a facility must be shown to be widely used to ensure its survival. Another reason for resistance may lie in the fact that this alternative is based on an assumption of the social model, that in general women are competent to care for their babies. This conflicts with the medical notion that babies are fragile and thus need the care of experts.

KANGAROO CARE

The 1980s have seen yet another alternative method of care of otherwise healthy low birth weight infants; it has come to be called kangaroo care. This method of care originated in Bogata, Colombia in 1979 because of lack of incubators (Rey & Gomez 1986). The preterm infant is placed upright, prone and skin-to-skin between the mother's breasts and allowed self-regulatory breast feeding. The mother's body (like a kangaroo pouch) provides heat, touch, movement, breastmilk and maximum skin to skin contact with her infant. The method was publicised by UNICEF in 1984. Early claims of dramatic decreases in infant mortality, morbidity and abandonment were under suspicion because of non-concurrent and non-equivalent comparison groups (Anderson 1992). But because of the publicity, interest developed in the method among several university medical centres in developed countries who began to carefully research the method. A number of studies have taken both repeated as well as before and after physiological measurements of babies receiving kangaroo care (Acolet et al. 1989; Bosque et al. 1988; de Leeuw et al. 1991; Ludington et al. 1991). This research has demonstrated that, compared with lying in cribs and with control infants in incubators, babies receiving kangaroo care have: no increase in infections, adequate oxygen saturation, better temperature regulation, less periodic breathing, fewer apnoeic episodes, better sleep patterns with longer periods of deep sleep, and are more often in the alert state in which eye contact is possible. The research also suggests that mothers lactate longer, produce more milk, infants can leave incubators and move into open air cots sooner, go home sooner and cry less at 6 months (Anderson 1991; Whitelaw et al. 1990).

The results of one research project suggests the extraordinary possibility that thermal synchrony develops between the mother and her baby. The data suggested that the mother involuntarily changes her own temperature in the direction needed to compensate for the trend of her infant's temperature. Further research is needed on this possibility. Random controlled trials on kangaroo care have been conducted in England (Whitelaw et al. 1988), Germany (Schmidt &

Wittreich 1986), and Finland (Tuomikoski-Koiranen 1988). These studies have demonstrated that "babies as small as 700 g who no longer require oxygen, can be safely and enjoyably held naked, except for a nappy, between the mother's breasts for up to 4 hours a day" (Whitelaw 1988, p. 1377). The kangaroo care babies have tended to grow faster, are discharged sooner and are breastfed longer. Preliminary results of most recent research suggests that it is feasible and efficacious to start kangaroo care on preterm infants within the first 30 minutes of birth (Ludington 1992).

Here we have a new perinatal technology which, through careful scientific study, is proven to be efficacious and without apparent risk. Furthermore, unlike most new perinatal innovations, it is cheap and likely to save money. And yet the past 10 years has not seen a rapid proliferation of this method. Individual centres are investigating and taking up this method in a number of countries: Sweden, Finland, Germany, The Netherlands, England, United States, Colombia, Uganda, Peru. But in general the technology has not spread beyond these centres. Why this is so gets to the heart of one aspect of the birth machine. The experience of one neonatologist is illustrative. When I urged Professor Schmidt in Germany to mount research on kangaroo care, he visited the hospital in London where a random control trial was in progress. Impressed, he returned home to start a similar trial. The doctors and nurses in his hospital were strongly against such a 'risky' method, insisting it was unethical to take babies out of incubators. It was necessary for Professor Schmidt to first replicate some physiological measurements to demonstrate its lack of risk. The hospital staff finally relented and the trial began. Before the trial was completed, however, the hospital staff wanted to stop the trial because it was clear that the experimental group with kangaroo care was doing much better and the staff felt it was unethical to deny the control babies kangaroo care (Schmidt 1986).

The slow spread of kangaroo care is clearly because doctors and nurses have considerable resistance to it, even though the babies are in the hospital under close observation. The approach needs further evaluation, but few are interested. Trust in a new type of mechanical medical technology seems sufficient to justify a study, while a method that clearly relies on a woman and her body is suspect and difficult to examine. In addition, much more scientific proof of value is needed for the kangaroo method than for the more mechanical methods before diffusion and acceptance by the medical profession.

Transitional care at the place of birth, early discharge and the kangaroo method require a combined medical and social approach. The participants endorsed this trend in their recommendations on the management of low birth weight.

> *"Low birth weight, which correlates strongly with both perinatal mortality and morbidity, should receive high priority for research into causes and prevention. Meanwhile, however, some actions seem to reduce the incidence of low birth weight and other causes of perinatal mortality and morbidity. Services should be developed with such actions in mind and the public should be fully informed of the reasons for and importance of these actions, which include: family planning (to avoid a large number of children and too short intervals between children); prenatal care to identify possible risks to the fetus and woman and to treat any diseases or conditions developing during pregnancy; nutritional and social support during pregnancy; avoidance of cigarettes, alcohol and drugs during pregnancy; and appropriate care during labour and delivery.*
>
> *"Discharge from hospital should depend on the wellbeing of the mother and infant, the wishes of the parents, and the availability of home support. In particular, discharge policies should not be based on the single criterion of weight and should concentrate on earliest possible discharge.*
>
> *"Low birth weight is both a risk factor and a social indicator. A decision to refer a low birth weight infant for care in another unit should take account not only of the infant's condition and the ability to care for him or her locally, but also the need to avoid separation of families.*
>
> *"Two areas of research needing high priority are: fetal growth and its retardation and the prevention of low birth weight infants"*

Neonatal intensive care

A major impetus to organising the consensus meeting was the results of the WHO Perinatal Study Group survey of neonatal intensive care services in 22 European countries, showing how the problems and issues surrounding the birth machine extend beyond birth (WHO 1985). The rapid proliferation of special care nurseries soon led to further specialisation and the proliferation of neonatal intensive care units.

This development did not result from a systematic health care policy based on rational evaluations of the need for and efficacy of the services. In fact, government policy, if it existed at all, was made after the services were already in existence and tended simply to endorse or legitimise them (WHO 1985).

Of the 22 European countries in the WHO survey, only 11 were able to provide basic information on the organisation of neonatal intensive care services. Only three had any special legislation on such care. Only ten had generally accepted definitions of the care; most of these had been generated by non-governmental professional organisations. While eight countries had criteria for designation of a newborn intensive care unit, these came from the government in only two cases. The survey showed that in many countries the health care system had an active periphery with a number of uncoordinated and technological clinical initiatives in neonatal intensive care. The health authorities were less active, limiting their role to attempts to register the existing situation, and lacked a comprehensive policy or official guidelines.

DEVELOPMENT

Physicians' belief in the efficacy of emergency intervention and intensive care provided the basic impetus for hospital support for high-technology care for newborn infants. The trend began in the larger teaching hospitals, where the development of knowledge of the physiology of the fetus and newborn infant appeared to offer an ideal situation for the clinical application of this knowledge in the new scientific discipline of neonatology. Technology — such as better incubators and machines for artificial ventilation and monitoring breathing — quickly evolved. The existence of specialised units stimulated further research and the development of a new clinical practice, not least because they made clinical problems more visible. These events were simultaneous with the shift in medical priorities from maternal to perinatal mortality and with large epidemiological surveys showing the close association between low birth weight and perinatal mortality. While medicine could do little to prevent low birth weight, the establishment of neonatal intensive care units was seen as a way to increase the chances of survival of small babies when they were born.

Observation, not experimental data, convinced the clinicians working in these units that this special care was effective. This gradually led to the notion that this life-saving new care should be available to everyone (small towns, rural areas and developing countries). In the absence of measures of need and effectiveness, the argument for equality of access is often the rationale for a policy of universal provision at the level of the best-endowed teaching hospitals.

Once neonatal intensive care units were established, attention focused on determining the need for the care. In the 1960s, 1970s and 1980s some governments organised expert committees of paediatricians to consider the provision of facilities for small and sick newborn babies.

An example is the working party report of the British Royal College of Physicians, published in 1988 (Royal College of Physicians 1988). The report made a plea for additional resources for neonatal intensive care when funds were short throughout the National Health Service. When the report was released, journalists were told by the College that 2000 of the 3500 babies who die each year in the neonatal period could have been saved if adequate resources for neonatal intensive care were available. Nothing in the report justified this figure. The report did not discuss the existing literature on the balance of supply and demand nor what was known of the benefit of neonatal intensive care. An editorial in the *Lancet* was quite critical of the report and did use the literature to make the key point about the need for neonatal intensive care: "As supply increases beyond a certain point, overall benefits tail off as fewer and fewer appropriate patients receive care (Bunker et al. 1977). Moreover, increased supply of neonatal services would lead to more research and technological advances and therefore generate more patient demand and the need for additional resources. The ongoing spiral of resources leading to research leading to demand leading to resources is almost limitless" (*Lancet* 1988, p. 1345). This editorial concludes with a statement which, unfortunately, would apply to most governmental and non-governmental working parties in most countries making recommendations regarding perinatal technology: "The opinions of the working party are perhaps not surprising — it was composed almost entirely of neonatologists and representatives from allied clinical and nursing groups, but there was little sign of the resource experts such as perinatal epidemiologists, community medicine specialists, health economists, or even general managers. What is perhaps more worrying is that reports such as these are often viewed as special pleadings by a self-interested group, and debase the medical profession's role in providing a balanced view on the provision of medical care" (*Lancet* 1988, p. 1346).

Other groups in other countries have also calculated need on the basis of demand on the existing neonatal intensive care units, extrapolated to the entire country, or on the assumption that all newborn infants weighing less than 2500 g at birth or born of difficult births would require special care. Both methods produced quite high rates of need: 15–25% of all newborn babies would require special care.The fallacy in such calculations has been clearly documented (Richards 1980, 1986; Campbell 1984). Hospitals vary widely in admission rates for neonatal intensive care — in one study in the United Kingdom, from 6% to 30% (Campbell 1984). These variations were not found to be correlated with rates of perinatal mortality or low birth weight, but with the availability of cots and the personal characteristics of physicians. For example, physicians who were female or had specialist training in neonatology were less likely to admit babies to intensive care.

In the absence of reliable information on the need for neonatal special care, there is general agreement that 7–20% of all newborn babies will show some sign that is judged to require paediatric observation and possible treatment. This estimate, however, is not particularly useful for health policy-makers and planners. There is reasonable agreement, on the other hand, that very few newborn babies (about 2%) actually require specialist care in a neonatal intensive care unit. Because of this a study by the American Academy of Pediatrics showed that the United States has enough neonatologists. They conclude: "Increasing the number of neonatologists beyond that needed may result in a disturbance of the paediatrician's role in newborn care and in more fragmented and inconsistent care of the sick newborn" (American Academy of Pediatrics Committee on Fetus and Newborn 1985).

PUBLIC ATTITUDES

Neonatal intensive care is essentially the product of deep societal ambivalence about death and reproduction (Guillemin 1986). Societies have left education about pregnancy and birth largely to individuals, as if birth and the death or illness of newborn babies had only private consequences. Instead of programs to promote more healthy pregnancies and greater sensitivity to the risks of chronic disease and disability in children, societies have spent their money on incorporating the newborn into the framework of adult, disease-oriented hospital services. The rapid development of technology for neonatal intensive care accurately reflects the high value that the public places on 'magic bullet' solutions in medical care, particularly for high-risk patients.

The development of neonatal intensive care in the 1950s and 1960s was thus characterised by a medical approach, similar to that characterising care at birth and for normal newborn babies. More resources were devoted to hospital and specialist care for sick or nearly sick infants, to the neglect of primary care for all infants. The 1970s saw the beginning of a reassessment of neonatal intensive care, also similar to that for care at birth and for normal babies. Although these reassessments were in part stimulated by an increasing appreciation of social factors, there were three additional stimuli to a new look at neonatal intensive care: extremely high cost, questionable benefits (particularly in care for very small low birth weight infants) and iatrogenic effects.

COST

The economic considerations arising with the recession of the 1970s were particularly important in evaluations of neonatal intensive care because of its extraordinary costs. These costs have another worrisome characteristic: the smaller the baby, the higher the cost and the lower the benefit (Mugford 1986). As a result cost-benefit and cost-effectiveness analyses of neonatal intensive care raise real questions. For example, one United States study evaluated the cost-effectiveness in reducing neonatal mortality of a variety of interventions including: teen-age family planning programs; supplemental food programs for women and babies; community health centres for treating women and babies; abortion services; prenatal care; neonatal intensive care (Joyce et al. 1988). The study found prenatal care and food programs the most cost-effective in reducing neonatal mortality. On the other hand they found that "Neonatal intensive care, although the most effective means of reducing neonatal mortality rates, is one of the least cost-effective strategies" (Joyce et al. 1988, p. 348).

Neonatal intensive care follows the same law of diminishing returns that we have found with so many other parts of the birth machine: as the indications for use expand and it is used in more marginal cases, neonatal intensive care becomes more expensive and its impact on neonatal mortality declines. For this reason, some argue that the application of neonatal intensive care may have reached the point of severely diminishing returns (McCormick 1985). The importance of recognising this is made by one of the Trieste participants:

> "The reformulation of medical care for the newborn will be directed by a changing consciousness of the limits of intensive care. Until that change is evident, we can count on heavy and rising costs in the medical management of neonates" (Guillemin 1984, p. 133).

The majority of funds for most neonatal intensive care units goes for the care of very low birth weight infants, who represent only about 1% of the newborn population. In most industrialised countries, the average cost for neonatal intensive care is estimated to be US$50,000–100,000 per infant weighing less than 1500 g. Further, the care of even a few extremely small infants (under 1000 g) can place a great strain on the financial resources of a hospital or community. A Swedish study found the cost per survivor of level 3 and 4 neonatal intensive care to be US$48,650 (Ewald 1991). As a result one-third of all money spent in Sweden for care of all newborns, goes to the care of the few babies who end up in level 3 or 4 intensive care. And the cost doesn't stop when the baby is finally discharged from the neonatal intensive care unit. A study in the United States followed neonatal intensive care survivors for 3 years and found that, because of their vulnerability to serious illness as well as handicap, "Children with and without neurodevelopmental deficits after neonatal intensive care unit discharge have significantly higher medical costs than children without" (Shankaran et al. 1988).

Because of inflation, even these high cost figures are soon underestimates. More recent figures show "The average cost of care nationally [in the United States] for an infant weighing less than 1 kg was over $100,000 in 1987 (US Congress 1987) (more costly than a heart transplant) and this particular infant's charges would now easily exceed a quarter of a million dollars. The cost for caring for a severely handicapped child is even greater, more than $22,000 per year in 1982 dollars, or as much as a million dollars in a lifetime. (US Congress 1988)" (Paneth 1992).

BENEFIT

The issue of the benefits of neonatal intensive care is contentious. The core of the issue is the fate of low birth weight babies (Bennett 1984). The first major benefit is clear; fewer low birthweight babies die shortly after birth. The past 10–15 years have seen a significant reduction in neonatal mortality, particularly for very low birth weight infants. In the 1960s, about two thirds of all babies born weighing less than 1500 g died in the first month of life; by the end of the 1980s this mortality rate had dropped to about one third. While some of this improvement was certainly due to social factors, neonatal intensive care played a significant role.

The optimism rightly engendered by this reduction in mortality is somewhat dimmed by what is known about what can happen to the survivors: death, illness or disability. Sadly, the post-neonatal infant mortality rate (deaths occurring between one month and one year of age) for infants discharged from neonatal intensive care is high — in one study babies surviving neonatal intensive care were 5 times as likely to die before their first birthday as other children. (Allen et al. 1989) Other studies substantiate this increased mortality (Heinonen et al. 1988; Denmark National Board of Health 1992). Major causes of this mortality include sudden infant death syndrome, congenital malformations and chronic lung disease.

In addition, research shows increased illness found in very low birth weight babies who survive the first month of life. One study (Morgan 1985) found that 53% of survivors of neonatal intensive care re-entered hospital one or more times before their first birthday, as compared with 10% of the control group of full-term infants. The additional hospital stays of the very low birth weight babies were repeated and long, resulting in a sixteen-fold increase in the number of in-patients, an eightfold increase in surgical procedures and a twofold increase in outpatient clinic visits. Other studies showed similarly high rates of hospital and clinic care for survivors of neonatal intensive care, with high medical costs (Shankaren et al. 1988; McIlwaine et al. 1987; Denmark National Board of Health 1992).

The most hotly debated aspect of the issue of the benefits of neonatal intensive care is whether decreasing mortality has meant an increase in the production of a permanently disabled population. Many neonatologists have argued that, while some of the earlier forms of intensive care in the 1960s and early 1970s might have failed to reduce the incidence of disabled survivors, more recent follow-up studies suggest that current care is more successful. Nevertheless, research in the 1980s in Sweden (Hagberg et al. 1982) and Australia (Kitchen et al. 1987) and in the 1990s in Denmark (Denmark National Board of Health 1992) reports increases in the cerebral palsy rates. Perhaps the most cautious verdict on this issue is that the modest increase in disability prevalence results from the presence of more survivors, rather than increased rates of disability among them.

Whether the incidence of disability among surviving low birth weight infants is going slightly up or down, the overall rates of disability are the most important consideration in judging the benefits of neonatal intensive care. More and more follow-up studies of the survivors of neonatal intensive care are being done; the data are quite good and reasonably consistent. A review of the literature has brought together and summarised the neurodevelopmental outcome of low birth weight infants (Bennett 1984). The findings are as follows: among the major neurological and developmental disabling conditions, cerebral palsy is the most common in very low birth weight infant survivors, the current incidence being 7–12%. Mental retardation alone is found in 5% of survivors, and when they reach school age, these children have a significantly lower mean IQ (85–95) than normal birth weight children, even after controlling for social class. Progressive hydrocephalus (water on the brain) is found in 1–3% of very low birth weight infants.

The scientific review also found permanent and significant sensory disability in neonatal intensive care survivors (Bennett 1984). Severe hearing impairment — requiring amplification, special education and non-vocal communication — is found in 2–4% of very low birth weight infants and 5% of extremely low birth weight infants. An added 6–8% of small infants will have mild to moderate hearing loss related to nerve damage, and a high incidence (20–30%) of chronic middle-ear infection and intermittent hearing loss has been reported. The tragic story of retrolental fibroplasia as an (at least partly) iatrogenic cause of sight loss in low birth weight infants has been well described (Silverman 1980); 2–4% of very low birth weight infants (and 5–10% of extremely small babies) have major visual impairment as a result of retrolental fibroplasia.

As the studies of neonatal intensive care survivors follow children to older ages, more data are revealing a number of long-term minor disabling conditions. The early, subtle developmental delays and differences in development and behaviour are not necessarily out-grown but may lead to problems in school. Various studies have shown minor neurological and developmental problems (minimal brain dysfunction) in 15–25% of very low birth weight survivors and, like the major disabilities, these minor disabilities increase with decreasing weight and gestational age at birth, with the severity of illness after birth and in male survivors (Bennett 1984). This important group of neurological effects is likely to be missed if outcome is assessed before school age.

When the major and minor disabilities found among the survivors are considered, the total prevalence of abnormality found at school age among a low birth weight population approaches 50%. In a study of school children 7 years old whose birth weight was 1500 g or less, 54% required special education or special help of some kind (Vohr & Coll 1985). A literature review of 20 years experience with neonatal intensive care with very low birth weight infants raised serious concern for the problems encountered when these children enter school (McCormick 1989). Of 100 babies born alive weighing less than 1500 g, 30 will die by the age of 12 months; of the 70 survivors, 35 will have a permanent major or minor disability and 35 will be normal. This picture of mortality and morbidity among survivors of neonatal intensive care, combined with the costs of the care, has provoked wide discussion of its value.

THE SITUATION IN DEVELOPING COUNTRIES

Reassessment of the provision of neonatal intensive care services in the past 15 years has largely been limited to the industrialised countries. As with birth services, earlier trends in neonatal intensive care services have trickled down to the developing countries. As a result, neonatal intensive care units are scattered through the major cities of developing countries. They are not rationally distributed:

"The current situation in Argentina and many other [developing] countries results in the highest quantity and quality of medical care being offered to the middle and upper social economic classes who are the lowest risk members of the population" (Prudent 1986).

This inequity in distribution was illustrated in a paper pinpointing the location of the neonatal intensive care units in ten Latin American countries: 45 units are found in private hospitals, 47 in university hospitals and 22 in the social security hospitals serving the poorest segment of the population (Moreno 1986).

Developing countries urgently need to reassess their neonatal intensive care services to develop rational health policies. Numerous problems complicate this task (Moreno 1986). Data are lacking on morbidity, mortality, and the use of services and technology, for example. The studies and evaluations in developed countries are not always relevant in developing countries with different epidemiological profiles and health systems. Decision-makers are often unreceptive to the type of analysis necessary. The structure of health services may be chaotic, which hinders the applicability of the findings of reassessment. For economic reasons, expensive technology, however effective, may not be available to all the high-risk groups for whom it is most needed. The follow-up of infants discharged from neonatal intensive care is extremely difficult. Finally, the indicators used to measure the outcome of medical treatment are particularly sensitive to marked variations in social factors; this can confound research results.

Until neonatal intensive care is reassessed and policy changes in developing countries, the present inappropriate allocation of resources for high technology (including specialist neonatal intensive care) will continue. A review of the economics of neonatal intensive care summarised this situation very well:

"For the wealthier countries of the world, neonatal intensive care could be seen as a rational decision, where considerable resources are already committed to the health and wellbeing of all childbearing women and their babies. Although there is a lack of research on the subject, it seems likely however that cost-effectiveness studies would indicate that many aspects of maternal and neonatal health care should precede the introduction of many neonatal intensive care techniques in countries where comprehensive maternal and child health services do not already exist" (Mugford 1986).

The participants in the consensus meeting were concerned that, when money for health care is handed out in countries, the public and policy-makers should have a clear picture of the costs and benefits of neonatal intensive care. The participants recommended that decisions for resource allocation for neonatal intensive care be made on the basis of many considerations, including need, efficacy, cost, benefits, resource availability, and moral and ethical standards.

"The allocation of health care resources to intensive life support systems for the newborn should be determined nationally. That decision must be informed by research findings, socioeconomic factors, and moral and ethical considerations. It should be based on consultation among care providers and representatives of parents and the community as a whole. It should include the establishment of minimum standards and requirements for staffing, equipment, and the siting of units for the newborn."

IATROGENIC EFFECTS

The growing awareness of the extent of iatrogenic effects was a particularly sharp spur to the reassessment of neonatal intensive care in the 1970s and 1980s. The range of iatrogenic effects causes special concern:

"Advances in understanding neonatal physiology and the technologies to deal with its dysfunctions have produced an environment for the newborn that is only peripherally concerned with the infant's overall wellbeing. This environment has developed largely, and unwittingly, to serve those instruments and techniques and the needs of physicians, nurses, and technicians to employ them. The actual practices of intensive infant care, as in so much of medicine, have caused iatrogenic diseases of serious dimension" (Sisson 1985).

Further evidence is given in a book that lists some seven 'proclaimed' treatments that led to disaster in perinatal medicine (Silverman 1985). The tragic effects of the use of diethylstilboestrol (called DES) to prevent miscarriage are perhaps the best known. The idea occurred to neonatologists that the continued hustle and bustle in the neonatal intensive care unit might itself affect the wellbeing of the babies. Careful analysis of the environment in the neonatal intensive care unit began (Gottfried et al. 1984). It revealed that the infants are bombarded 24 hours a day with sensory stimulation — visual, auditory and tactile — with no daily variation or rhythm. In one random controlled trial on preterm infants the experimental group had reduced intensity of light and noise between 7 pm and 7 am in the nursery while in the control group the intensity of light and noise was not reduced. The experimental group spent longer sleeping, less time feeding and gained more weight. At 3 months of age the experimental infants were on average a half a kilogram heavier ($p < 0.02$) (Mann et al. 1986). At the same time, the units are startlingly non-social environments; almost all contact the infants have with human beings comes through treatment procedures.

The participants welcomed the increase in concern about iatrogenic effects among health professionals and the public. New regulations for the management of newborn babies, particularly those in intensive care, should acknowledge their vulnerability to over-treatment, as well as neglect.

CHANGES IN CARE

The reassessment of neonatal intensive care has brought to light the need for certain fundamental changes in the services, which reflect a movement towards combining the social and medical models. The participants were convinced of the need for a series of uniform new policies for neonatal intensive care that would take account of the needs of the newborn infant and those of the infant's family and community. Such new policies are needed if the interests of the infant, family and community are not to yield to professional and institutional goals. Although the inappropriate referral and treatment of newborn babies involves no malice from any decision-maker, they have tremendous negative repercussions for infants, family and society.

MINIMUM STANDARDS

The WHO European Perinatal Study Group's survey of neonatal intensive care in 22 countries showed that very few countries have minimum standards of care (WHO 1985). Such standards must ensure that proper staff and facilities are available 'around the clock' to the infants who need intensive care. The standards must also reflect social criteria such as giving parents a role in decision-making about care and in the provision of care. If a country has or wants a regionalised system with different levels of neonatal intensive care, each level must be carefully defined and standards of care established. Because in the United States some hospitals refuse to admit infants to neonatal intensive care units if families cannot pay, the participants from that country asked for an additional sentence in the recommendation to address the problem.

> *"Ideally, unhealthy infants requiring intensive care should receive it in special units within maternity hospitals. In these units, paediatric and specialised nursing staff should be on duty 24 hours a day. The minimum acceptable facilities for life support, including biochemical tests and radiology, should be available. No institution providing tertiary care should be permitted to refuse to accept a case presenting at their facility, at least for assessment, stabilisation and referral."*

CONTINUOUS EVALUATION

Another necessary policy should require built-in and continuing evaluation of neonatal intensive care. The WHO survey showed that, of 22 countries, 15 have no statistics on neonatal intensive care services, 16 have made no attempt to determine the cost of the care, 10 have no audit of perinatal deaths, and 6 have no system to follow up the babies discharged from intensive care (WHO 1985).

Determining the effectiveness and efficiency of the care is thus very difficult. Making such judgements requires a detailed knowledge of the needs of each category of baby, how appropriate care might be efficiently provided, and the size of the gap between the existing system and the ideal. Several working papers reported attempts at evaluation in France, Italy and Latin America. The final recommendation on program evaluation addresses not only neonatal intensive care but all care following birth.

"Care following birth should be evaluated on a population as well as in an institution. The basic requirements are knowledge of: the population for whom care is being provided; the services available for unhealthy women and unhealthy newborn infants; which women and which infants receive what kinds of service and their outcomes, including mortality and short-term and long-term morbidity; the satisfaction of the parents with the service and the satisfaction of those who work in the services; and financial costs. This evaluation should be done in the context of overall evaluation of perinatal care."

INCLUSION OF PARENTS IN CAREGIVING

The recent incorporation of the social model into neonatal intensive care is nowhere better illustrated than by the issue of the role of parents in neonatal intensive care (which was the subject of several consensus meeting recommendations). Ironically it is medical science which is providing much of the ammunition for this. Swedish research showed that sucking and touching release hormones that facilitate the growth and maturation of low birth weight infants (Uvnas-Moberg 1987). Earlier in this chapter we discussed the research showing the importance of carrying and touching in the survival and development of babies (Hunziker & Barr 1986; Field et al. 1986). Similar results appear in research from Third World countries; when mothers were permitted to live in a crowded neonatal intensive care unit in Ethiopia the unit could care for three times as many infants, survival increased 500%, infants were discharged earlier and breastfeeding increased (Prudent 1986). This and other work shows that it is essential for parents to be present in the neonatal intensive care unit, not only to provide contact but also to participate in the care (Guillemin 1988). Nevertheless, according to the WHO survey, only 10 countries admitted the mother to the neonatal intensive care unit and only 8 also admitted fathers (WHO 1985). Surveys of parents who have experienced having a baby in a neonatal intensive care unit reveal that the parents have differing beliefs about causes of low birth weight in general as well as the cause of their own babies' low birth weight (Rajan & Oakley 1990). While parents are easily intimidated by neonatal intensive care unit staff, nevertheless at least 78% prefer to stay in the hospital with their newborn (Bolton et al. 1991).

The parents of a baby in intensive care must also be involved in the decisions about the care. All the participants felt strongly that unit staff should both educate parents about the care and integrate them more fully into the decision-making on the course of medical treatment.

If the parents' choice conflicts with the judgment of the staff, an ethical dilemma results. The ethical issues involved in neonatal intensive care are many and difficult, and could not be fully discussed at the consensus meeting. Nevertheless, the participants felt that these issues needed to be highlighted and brought into the final recommendations. For example, a crucial question is who should make the decision to start or stop the treatment of a very sick or extremely small newborn baby? In addition to the informed choice of the parents, consensus seems to be growing on the value of reviewing such decisions in a group whose membership is wider than the family and the neonatal intensive care unit staff. All sorts of social, psychological, ethical and economic factors are involved and ways must be evolved to make choices that embody as far as possible the wishes of the community at large. Various experimental review bodies are being tried out. They must be evaluated and the development of other such experiments encouraged to provide a variety of models for adaptation to local conditions.

To enable parents to fulfil their roles in the neonatal intensive care unit, they should be provided with temporary quarters in or near the hospital. These have been established in a number of countries. For example, a hospital in Argentina has a 'home for parents' giving women the opportunity to live in rooms adjoining the neonatal intensive care unit (Prudent 1986). This allows them to receive continuing education and support from the staff, participate in care and decision-making, breastfeed and have other contact with their babies, and give and receive mutual aid.

There was ready and strong consensus for several final recommendations regarding the role of parents in the care of sick newborn infants:

"Furthermore, involvement of parents in the care of the unhealthy newborn should be promoted, including the actual care of the unhealthy infant and participation in decisions about treatment.

"Health care personnel should support efficacious and safe technologies, but they should not impose them on women and families. When the desire of parents is judged to go against the good of the infant, then a formal advisory system for solving these problems must be implemented in each health care facility.

"Parents have the right to early active involvement in the care of their unhealthy infant: early and free visits to the special infant care unit; encouragement of feeding and skin-to-skin contact, whether or not the infant is connected to monitoring systems; facilities where parents can live while the infant is in special care; and participation in decisions regarding diagnosis and treatment."

LINKING THE HOSPITAL AND THE COMMUNITY

Recent efforts by neonatal intensive care unit staff to discharge babies earlier and follow them up at home has forged important links between hospital and home. These efforts have been matched by the interest of community groups in reaching into the hospital. The number of families with experience of a neonatal intensive care unit is growing annually. These experiences are multiplied and communicated with increasing frequency through the mass media. This collective community testimony, not always positive, forms the basis for public support of neonatal intensive care. The realities of care must be clearly communicated to the community, lest people's faith in technology (augmented by dramatic photographs in newspapers and on television) blind them to the realities of nature and the limits of medical intervention. Mechanisms must be developed for determining the community's views to guide policy on neonatal intensive care in at least two areas: resource allocation and ethical issues. The consensus recommendation on such new policy states:

"Staff in every special care unit for the newborn must be aware of the wishes and attitudes of the community it serves. Communication with the community is vital. Policies of special care units must be consistent with the community's values."

EXPERIMENTAL TREATMENT

Closely tied to the need for new policies on the roles of parents and the community in neonatal intensive care is the need for a new policy on experimental treatment. It has been too easy for medical staff, particularly in hospitals, to try out new diagnostic methods or treatments without proper controls. In many hospitals and countries, the use of properly identified experimental procedures is subject to clear guidelines, requiring the procedures to be reviewed by hospital research committees, and the informed consent of the patient or the patient's family. However, in Eastern Europe such guidelines do not exist and in Latin America they are found in only a few countries. Unfortunately, clinicians who are not researchers often see these safeguards as nuisances or barriers to progress and efficient care. New procedures are thus simply identified as accepted practices in the hospital. This circumvention of the controls can create a justifiable and serious backlash from the family and community if the use of the new procedure is later associated with death or disability. This has frequently been a problem, particularly in the persistent treatment of extremely small and severely abnormal infants (Stinson & Stinson 1983).

It is easy to see why neonatal intensive care treatment has been extended to ever smaller and sicker infants. The application of improved knowledge and techniques to babies to whom earlier methods had little or nothing to offer is understandable and desirable. Nevertheless, mortality and morbidity remain very high among the smallest infants and there must be some point at which the chances of survival are so remote that treatment should not be attempted. In addition, experience suggests that stopping treatment is harder than starting it. Attempts to treat extremely low birth weight infants inevitably contain an element of experimentation. While such attempts are essential to the development of new methods of treatment, the participants in the consensus meeting recommended that they always be identified as experimental, not as part of routine care, so that full ethical approval is obtained. The final recommendation for this new policy is:

"All countries should develop criteria by which to determine whether or not certain treatments for the newborn should be regarded as experimental. Examples of 'experimental' treatment, in present circumstances, include the management of

extremely premature infants and serious congenital defects. Guidelines should be formulated for the selection of infants for whom maximum intensive care and surgery are justified. The possibility of short-term and long-term negative consequences of such treatment should be fully communicated to the parents."

CARE GIVERS

The application of a more social approach to neonatal intensive care has prompted a number of new policy recommendations focusing on the people who receive the care — newborn infants and their families and communities. The social flashlight can also be turned on care givers, to illuminate their needs. Every day, physicians and nurses in neonatal intensive care work with babies who are ill or disabled and those who die. Further, the care provided is very labour-intensive, placing nearly constant demands on staff running from crisis to crisis. Coping with such a work environment can be most stressful and the turnover in the staff of intensive care units can be quite high, particularly if there are not sufficient staff for the job. The WHO survey of neonatal intensive care revealed a wide range of recommended numbers of staff in industrialised countries: 7 countries provided figures of 2–18 neonatal intensive care beds per physician; 8 countries recommended 0.2–4 nurses per bed (WHO 1985).

The participants stressed the need for people training or working in neonatal intensive care to receive information on the stresses of this work and how to cope. The final recommendation on staff training contains the sentence *"Training of all health care staff should make them aware of the stresses and anxieties that both care receivers and givers may undergo"*. A second recommendation on staff training states:

"Those working in special care units face infants with severe illness, handicap and often death, so they must be oriented to the implications of such stresses and how to cope with them, and they should receive emotional support."

FINDINGS

It seems fair to say that we are probably approaching the limits of the benefits of neonatal intensive care as a technical art for reducing death and disability. Clearly services should be maintained in the parts of the world where they are appropriate (in view of available resources) and have the consent of the community. Neonatal intensive care needs continuing refinement; here, the development of rational, clear policy is most important.

As one example, the government of Denmark has begun the process of developing policy for the management of low birth weight babies. In 1990 a national consensus conference on extremely preterm (before 28 weeks gestation) newborns and their treatment was held (Denmark National Board of Health 1990). One of the results of the conference was the recognition of the need for better data on which to make policy. Accordingly a follow-up study of these extremely preterm infants was organised using the national birth register, the national death register, the national hospital register, and the national congenital malformation register.

A report (Denmark National Board of Health 1992) found that the mortality rate of extremely preterm infants, which is 50% in the first week of life, does not reach the level of full term infants until babies are 3 years old. The hospitalisation rate was 2.5 times greater for the first 6 years of life. The cerebral palsy rate is 8 to 10 times higher, both for babies born before 28 weeks and also for babies born between 28 weeks and 32 weeks. The Danes will now use this data to set further policy on the management of low birth weight babies.

Another approach to setting policy for neonatal intensive care is that tried in Oregon State in the United States. All possible forms of medical care were ranked by the community in order of priority and then available public funds spent according to these priorities. Because of the great expense and poor outcomes of neonatal intensive care for extremely preterm infants, the treatment of newborn infants under 500 g received a priority of 708 out of a possible 712 treatments on the list. This means public funds would not be used for this purpose.

No single policy can fully address this complex type of care. Policies must be made at several levels: at the unit level (including, for example, the designation of experimental cases); at the hospital level (including, for example, hospital review committees); and at the government level (including, for example, regulations to prevent harm to human beings — including infants — from the unknown risks of experiments). Finally, while the refinement of neonatal intensive care continues, it is essential that new policies shift the highest priority in newborn care away from specialist hospital treatment to primary services for the prevention of low birth weight and the management of all infants at the moment of birth.

Services following birth

Organisation

Resource allocation was a primary topic in the consideration of the organisation of services. In addition to recommending that spending on social rather than health services might be the most important way to improve the health of women and babies, the participants strongly believed that services for women and infants have been short-changed in the allocation of money for health care. While politicians may win popularity by extolling the importance of the family, women and babies are not a vociferous or powerful group demanding their piece of the economic pie. For this reason the participants recommended that:

> *"If the goal of health for all women and newborn infants is to be achieved, resources must be equitably reallocated from overall health care funds, making the care of this vulnerable group a priority."*

Vigorous debate arose over the issue of the appropriate role of commercial interests in health systems for care following birth. The potential conflicts of interest have already been discussed. The participants' experience with and attitudes to commercial interests in health care varied with their national background. For the participants from eastern European countries, for example, the issue essentially does not exist as there have been until very recently few or no commercial elements in their health systems. At the other end of the continuum were participants from some Latin American countries, who said that, without funding from companies making drugs or medical equipment, little research and very few meetings of practitioners and researchers would be possible. In general, the participants from Scandinavia and the United Kingdom had strong ethical objections to commercial influences, while the North Americans tended to be much more sanguine about them. Such diversity of opinion made consensus difficult.

Another source of possible conflict in the organisation of care involves the needs of the providers and users of services. The WHO survey of neonatal intensive care showed that standards for practice in many European countries were set by the professional organisations of health workers alone (WHO 1985). These efforts may be a welcome start where standards do not exist, and the participation of professional organisations in the process is certainly appropriate. The public (care receivers) and their representatives (the government) should also participate, however, to ensure that everyone's needs are considered. The participants felt that the solution to any danger arising from vested commercial or professional interests lies in bringing these issues under public scrutiny and control.

> *"The structure of health care systems and the way they operate are influenced by commercial interests and by the needs and perspectives of professionals and others who work in them. When such influences are strong, they need to be publicly recognised and, if necessary, controlled."*

The participants were convinced that governments — through planning, setting policy and establishing guidelines with mechanisms for their implementation — should have a central role in the improvement of care following birth. Considerable evidence was presented to demonstrate that many countries did not take such a rational approach. After much discussion, the participants agreed that such an approach begins with a clearly defined process for health planning, taking place at both the central and local levels. The key to the success of this planning process is the contribution at both levels of all interested parties: parents, health professionals, health care planners and administrators, community groups, other related sectors (such as education and industry) and policy-makers and politicians. Representative committees need to be formed to involve such a varied group in planning. These committees would generate the basic policies for services and review and approve any guidelines drafted to ensure that they translate policy into reality. In carrying out this mandate, committees and the drafters of guidelines must have access to information from evaluations of the existing system of care following birth. The guidelines should outline mechanisms for including services, users and the community in decision-making on the content of care. These mechanisms can include, for example, multidisciplinary ethics committees and review boards in local hospitals and communities, which allow the community to assess care.

In addition to working out the basic principles for a system to plan and monitor health services following birth, the participants wished to emphasise that these services should facilitate not only the prevention of illness and the treatment of disease but also the promotion of the health of women and babies. Although health promotion means many things to many people, enhancing the wellbeing of the woman and her new baby is the basic purpose or an additional benefit of many of the policies contained in the recommendations, such as those for: breastfeeding, rooming-in, early discharge with a focus on home care, parent-infant contact and parental participation in neonatal intensive care.

When birth and care following birth lose their medical nature and families are encouraged to care for their new babies, a pattern of life-long and inappropriate dependence on the health care system can be avoided, which would benefit the child, the family and society. The planning, policies, guidelines and mechanisms involved in care following birth should be based on a conscious recognition of the importance of this form of health promotion. The relevant recommendations are:

> *"The improvement of care following birth must be a collaboration between: parents, health professionals, health planners, health care administrators, other related sectors, community groups, policy-makers and politicians. Policies and mechanisms should be developed which will guide decisions about the care of women and babies — for example, multidisciplinary committees on ethics and review boards for the assessment of the care of the newborn. Communities must examine how far their attitudes and practices support or obstruct the opportunity for women and babies to receive the best available care.*

> *"All countries need a systematic process of health planning, including resource allocation for the care of women and babies. This process would ideally be both local and national, and it would reflect the views of a broad cross-sec-*

tion of professionals and interested groups in the community. Planning for the health of women and babies must go beyond an approach based on potential risks to the physical health of the woman, fetus and newborn infant; a positive effort is called for to involve the entire society in the promotion of health.

"All governments should appoint a broad-based representative committee, including health care providers and the users of health care, to establish guidelines and recommendations for the care of mothers and infants. These guidelines should be based on a continuing evaluation system and should be widely distributed and frequently revised. Such guidelines should include minimum standards for equipment and care practices following birth."

The organisation of health services includes the keeping of records. Despite the reluctance of health professionals to share information with the woman and her family, such sharing would:

- allow the family to make informed choices about care;
- educate the family on health and health care;
- honour the egalitarian nature of the relationship between family and health professionals;
- facilitate parents' confidence in the normality of infancy and their ability to manage their child;
- improve the informal health care given in the family; and
- ensure the optimal flow of health information on the individual woman or baby between health care providers and the family, and between different groups of health care providers and health care facilities.

Believe it or not, all this can be accomplished through the simple act of giving the health record to the family to keep at home. This is why the participants recommended the home-based record so strongly, and why WHO has developed model home-based health passports for women during pregnancy and birth and following birth and for babies. A few participants worried that home-based records might be lost; research, however, has shown that fewer records are lost at home than in the clinic or hospital. Such studies reinforce the social model's confidence in the integrity and reliability of women. Keeping a record at home means that the information is always at hand for visits to any health facility and home-based care.

> *"Every baby should have its own record from the moment of birth, which may include data about pregnancy and birth. This record, or at least a copy of it, should be kept at home by the woman. It would include data about growth, development, nutrition, immunization and medical history. It can form a basis for communication among givers of health care and with the woman. The woman should also have her own health record in her home. Confidentiality of these records must be protected."*

Access to basic care was another issue in the organisation of services. In developing countries, the access problem is mainly one of whether basic care services actually exist. Here the solution lies in changing priorities and policies to build a primary health care system making basic services available to every family. In industrialised countries, the infrastructures are usually in place but access may be hindered by economic, linguistic, social and cultural barriers. Creating universally easy access to basic health services is a complex problem and finding means of doing so was beyond the scope of the consensus meeting. Nevertheless, the participants insisted on stating the right of everyone to have ready access to basic care in a recommendation:

> *"Every woman and infant should have access to a basic level of care regardless of whether the birth takes place at home or in a primary or secondary health care setting."*

Content

Three recommendations addressed specific issues in the content of care following birth. The first of these urged the development of home-based alternatives to hospital technology. Home-based care is well established in developing countries and increasing in industrialised countries. It is therefore extraordinary that so little effort has been directed towards developing simple portable equipment or equipment with long-range monitoring capabilities (using, for example, the telephone, radio or television) for home care.

> *"Home-based alternative technologies for women and babies, such as portable phototherapy for neonatal jaundice,*

should be developed to allow expansion of coverage to the population that lacks access to hospital care. Such innovations should be evaluated just as rigorously as complex hospital technology."

The second recommendation addressed both immunisation and screening tests; they were considered together because both are universally applied and therefore need the same safeguards and controls. In the WHO survey of perinatal services in Europe every responding country had a variety of immunisation and screening programs for women and babies (WHO 1985). Experience with both types of program has shown that they must be carefully evaluated before universal application. Since the incidence of certain detectable diseases (thalassaemia, phenylketonuria, etc.) varies and since the chances for follow-up and treatment vary between countries, each country must evaluate and determine its needs for these programs. Further, the efficacy and safety of certain routine practices, such as the preventive administration of vitamin K and eye drops, are still actively debated; thus, existing universally-applied technology sometimes needs re-evaluation.

"All women and newborn infants should receive immunisation and screening tests in accordance with the recommendations of their own countries, whether at home, in a clinic or in a hospital. Before screening of women or babies is contemplated, it must be evaluated by random controlled trials, examining not only efficacy and safety but also psychosocial costs and benefits. Each country should evaluate the relevance of particular screening procedures to its own particular needs or resources. The means of administration of vitamin K and the type of eye prophylaxis in the newborn infant need further evaluation. When indicated, immunisation with anti-D is recommended for the woman."

The third recommendation suggested the inclusion of family planning services in care following birth. The presence of representatives of the social approach at the meeting guaranteed that this discussion stressed the principle of informed choice and the need for the care giver to be sensitive to the social and emotional needs of the woman. In addition, participants from the developing countries and the inner cities of industrialised countries pointed out that the period just after birth may be one of the few times the official health care system is in contact with people most in need of family planning, such as poor families.

> *"The period following birth may be an important time for making family planning advice and services available to both parents. The person giving such information to women should be someone in whom they have confidence. In many contexts, the best person will be a nurse or midwife. Information should be given on a variety of contraceptive techniques, so that women can make informed choices."*

Staffing

As events immediately following the moment of birth (such as examining the baby and giving resuscitation if necessary, and allowing immediate contact between mother and baby) are crucial to the future of the mother and baby, the participants recommended that one birth attendant (whether physician, midwife or empirical midwife) be in charge.

> *"At every birth, wherever it takes place, one attendant should take overall responsibility for the woman and infant."*

Further, in industrialised countries, some women will always want to use alternative practitioners, such as empirical midwives (WHO 1985). Again, these alternative care providers are important in developing countries (DeSouza 1986). Most empirical midwives extend their care to include assistance in the home in the weeks following birth. They help establish breastfeeding, advise on infant care routines, and assist in the postpartum care and adjustment of the woman and referral to the official health care system when necessary. Indeed, they often accompany the woman to the clinic or hospital to give continuing support. By supporting the provision of postpartum care by alternative practitioners and facilitating collaboration between them and professionals working in the official system, governments guarantee families the best of both worlds, social and medical.

> *"Government agencies should support the provision of health care by alternative providers, such as empirical midwives. The role and efficacy of these alternative providers should be systematically evaluated."*

288

Changes in the nature of care following birth, arising from the combination of the social and medical approaches, require changes in the attitudes and approaches of staff giving the care, which must begin with changes in their basic training. Most training in medical schools is based solely on the medical model. Many nursing and midwifery schools have tried to strike a more balanced approach but, as these schools are dominated or controlled by physicians, this is often an uphill struggle.

> "WHO *should be active in ensuring that appropriate courses in public health, with special emphasis on maternal and child health, are taught at universities and schools of medicine, nursing and midwifery.*"

Further, the participants urged that initial and in-service professional training be based on the needs of women and babies and linked to local community services. This suggests that health care workers need to gain experience outside the walls of the hospital. Such workers also need a new type of training more closely allied to the medical approach: training in research methodology and the interpretation of results. Many physicians and nurses and most midwives have received little or no such training methodology and thus cannot benefit from the research literature. Without such knowledge, they are too easily influenced by peers' unfounded statements or commercial interests. A cadre of practising doctors, nurses and midwives — knowledgeable about the latest findings in their field and able to analyse statements from colleagues, pharmaceutical or equipment sales people and the scientific literature — would be a major deterrent to the inappropriate use of the birth machine.

> "*For staff working in hospitals or home health services, initial and in-service training should be based on the needs of women and babies and be linked to local services, so that training is realistic and relevant. Training should include the ability to conduct research and/or interpret research findings. All professionals should receive the lists of relevant random controlled studies.*"

Research

Three issues in research were considered the most urgent: changing priorities, improving the quality of investigations and using the results.

New priority topics

The great majority of research on women and infants following birth has focused on clinical management. The history of the development of neonatology is the history of the generation of a new clinical specialty, based in part on clinical research. Such research is certainly important; unfortunately, equally important research has been seriously neglected. To correct this imbalance, priority should be given to research on: health services, preventive techniques, technology assessment, long-term follow-up of care after birth and systems for routine continuous surveillance.

> *"Most research on women following birth and on infants has focused on clinical management. Priority should now be given to research on: the organisation and overall content of services; preventive services; assessing the appropriate use of technologies; and the long-term future of women and infants. This research should include surveys of the views of parents and the community."*

The first priority — health service research includes the organisation of services, the content, cost and benefit, and the attitudes of service users. A paper suggested that such research could be begun by going into the community and asking families with new babies about their views (Sterky 1986). Using simple questions can begin the formulation of questions that studies can be designed to address. If the simple questions have not been asked or attempts to ask them are thwarted, the researchers can turn to studying the reasons for resistance in the research establishment. The vested interests of a political, industrial or professional group, for example, may be so strong that the questions cannot be posed. Changes may require studying the actors and delineating their powers. This can be one type of health service research.

Other issues need the attention of health service researchers. An important and poorly researched area is the study of the optimal mixture of staff for various parts of the system of services following birth. Starting such studies may not be easy, as strong professional and labour union interests are usually at stake and people's willingness to experiment with their jobs is minimal (Wagner 1987b). Nevertheless, the biggest part of health care costs is usually salaries for personnel. With the differences in the salaries of physicians, nurses, midwives and auxiliaries, the staff mixture is of fundamental importance for health care costs.

Routine procedures also need study. As pointed out earlier, only about 10% of routine obstetrical procedures have been studied adequately, but there is a similar lack of research on routine procedures performed on the baby after birth. Most of these procedures have not been assessed scientifically. A case in point is the Apgar score; although it has been used religiously for over 25 years, several studies have shown it to be of limited value in identifying infants at risk of developing neurological handicap (Sterky 1986). The appropriateness of the Apgar score should be re-examined in the light of more recent knowledge about the causes of birth asphyxiation and the feasibility of the method in some cultures and settings. A modified score, based only on respiration and heart rate, may well be more useful (Sterky 1985).

In most places in the world, health service research does not have the prestige, and consequently the funding, now enjoyed by biomedical research. Public concern and political will are needed to change these priorities. In Denmark, for example, the government decreed that at least 10% of all government-funded medical research must focus on services.

"In improving care following birth research on the services themselves, including relevant social science research, can help to change both individual practices and policy. This type of research lacks funding and institutional support now enjoyed by biomedical research. Health workers should be encouraged to inquire into their own performance with the support of a competent team with expertise in study design, analysis of data, and dissemination of results."

A second major but neglected priority for research is the study of possible preventive measures in postpartum care. Neonatologists are growing tired of practising rescue medicine and damage control; they are becoming more and more interested in preventing the problems they must now try to treat, such as low birth weight and the respiratory distress syndrome. They are also becoming more interested in preventing iatrogenic effects by more careful evaluation of new technology.

Another major research priority, then, is technology assessment — a subject already dealt with at some length. The need for such assessment is acute in care following birth. A senior statesman in neonatology has written:

> "Like weapons in the modern arsenals of war, therapies have become increasingly powerful and the potential for harm on a very wide scale has escalated accordingly. Spectacular therapeutic disasters have made it clear that informal, let's-try-it-and-see methods of testing new proposals are more risky now than ever before in history. Since there are no certainties in medicine, it must be understood that every clinical test of a new treatment is, by definition, a step into the unknown" (Silverman 1985).

The consensus in Trieste on this recommendation was strong:

> *"Any technology used in care following birth should undergo evaluation before its introduction for general use. Such evaluation should include efficacy and safety, economic implications, and cultural acceptability. The results of technology assessment should be widely disseminated to professionals and the general public.* WHO *should continue to promote and expand a network of technology assessment centres to assist countries in selecting new technologies and assessing them. This network will constitute a focal point for the dissemination of information."*

The importance of long-term follow-up studies has already been reviewed. Perinatal mortality has been the principal measure of the outcome of care, but the emphasis must shift to morbidity (psychosocial as well as physical). This means longer follow-up, at least up to school age.

The final research priority is the establishment of permanent perinatal surveillance systems. An entire chapter of *Having a Baby in Europe* (WHO 1985) is devoted to the importance of such systems, their status in countries and how they can be established. A perinatal surveillance system demands a good national or regional statistical system for reliable recording of vital events such as birth, death and birth weight. More and more such systems incorporate data on services (such as rates of obstetrical intervention and referral to neonatal intensive care), making it possible to evaluate regional variations in services and relationships between services and outcomes.

> *"All countries should make an effort to improve perinatal records. Birth and death certificates should include birth weight, and they should be linked whenever possible. A good statistical system is essential, beginning with registration of all births and deaths. Permanent perinatal surveillance systems are needed at the national level."*

Improved quality

The participants in the consensus meeting were concerned about the poor calibre of many current studies and sought ways to improve the quality of research. As with obstetrical research, most neonatal research is observational, non-experimental and carried out on unrepresentative populations. Another weakness is the widespread lack of objectives for care; these are necessary to decide which outcomes to measure in service evaluations. Many countries have general policy statements that the researcher must translate into measurable outcome variables to conduct meaningful research.

Another problem with today's research is the uncontrolled nature of so many clinical observations, as candidly described by a neonatologist at the conference:

> "When neonatologists decide to ventilate an infant with hyaline membrane disease at a rapid rate with low pressure or at a slow rate with higher pressure, they are performing experiments — uncontrolled experiments to be sure — but experiments nevertheless. If they are convinced of the benefit of their particular mode of treatment, these physicians will almost always object on 'ethical grounds' to a clinical trial which might determine if their therapy is, in fact, helpful or

harmful. It does not occur to them that the treatment itself is unproven by any scientific rationale and, indeed, may be causing serious harm. When I say 'them' I include myself — indeed all of us — because every day we simply must make therapeutic decisions for which we have little scientific basis. Our enthusiasm for the latest fashion in treatment should be tempered, however, by our experience with the therapeutic disasters — treatments that were believed to do good but, in fact, caused considerable harm. Given this experience we would do well to heed the advice of workers in fireworks factories: 'It is better to curse the darkness than to light the wrong candle'" (Maisals 1986).

An added problem connected to the quality of research is the interpretation of the results by the investigator. It has been said that nothing improves the performance of an innovation as much as the lack of controls in the experiment (Silverman 1985). A review of 53 studies of a particular surgical procedure, for example, found marked enthusiasm for the treatment in most of the studies that used uncontrolled observation and moderate or no enthusiasm in well controlled trials (Silverman 1985). Another example, closer to home for people interested in care surrounding birth, is an enthusiastic report on how the use of a specific protocol reduced the incidence of premature birth over a 12-year period (Papiernik et al. 1985). In fact, the effectiveness of the protocol cannot be known, as time bias cannot be eliminated from such historical controlled studies.

After considering these problems, the participants emphatically endorsed the use of the strongest possible research designs. In most cases, the best method is the randomised controlled trial. Both people and health care units can be randomly assigned to experimental and control groups. The particular advantages and difficulties of such trials are described elsewhere (Silverman 1985; Maisals 1986). Despite the outstanding successes of this approach, less than 2 of every 100 papers published in reputable paediatric journals report randomised controlled trials. For these reasons, the final recommendation states:

> *"All research should use the strongest possible design. In the assessment of any technology, this design is a randomised controlled trial, probably a multi-centre collaborative trial that can achieve adequate sample size. Community-based*

research, organised by community groups and assisted by relevant experts, should be encouraged."

Use of results

In services following birth, as in all health services, there is a serious gap between correct clinical practice as shown by research and the actual practices of the majority of clinicians. Researchers and clinicians must take responsibility for this gap and work together to close it.

A proven strategy is to involve the users of the technology under examination in all phases of the study; this has the added advantage of training clinicians in performing and evaluating research. A promising strategy is also to involve the people on whom the technology is used: women, families and community groups (Wagner 1987b, 1988). In addition, the scientific method can be used to test different strategies for information diffusion, measuring the changes in clinical practice resulting from each. This approach is being used in studies of regional variations in medical and surgical practices. It is also the final step in the consensus approach.

In the past, professional duty did not require the researcher to accept responsibility for the diffusion and use of results, or the clinician to be involved in, understand and critique relevant research (Wagner 1987a). Both groups are slowly taking on these duties, however; nowhere is this change more welcome than in care following birth.

The participants made a recommendation to demonstrate their commitment to work to bridge the gap between what is known (and recommended) and what is practised.

> "WHO *and its regional offices should institute a regular program of meetings with journalists, media and public relations leaders, and editors of professional journals to familiarize them with the recommendations of* WHO *meetings and other issues affecting maternal and child health.* WHO *should promote the implementation of the recommendations of the Trieste meeting and the two earlier meetings."*

The WHO Regional Office for Europe accepted the challenge of this recommendation and the final chapter 8 describes the action taken to promote the implementation of the recommendations made by the consensus meeting. Experience with these subsequent activities suggests that the proper balance in care — between medical intervention and nature, between care provided by health professionals and by the family, and between hospital and home — is not yet fully known. Nevertheless, the swing of the pendulum towards nature, family and home is most likely a desirable trend, steering the birth machine towards an optimal blend of the social and medical approaches to care following birth. A participant wrote:

> "The physiological expressions of womanliness such as pregnancy, birthing and nursing should be paid respect and reverence not only by authors and artists but even by society at large and in particular by the health care system" (Sterky 1986).

References

Acolet D., Sleath & Whitelaw A. 1989, 'Oxygenation, heart rate and temperature in very low weight infants during skin-to-skin contact with their mothers', *Acta Paediatrica Scand*, vol. 78, no. 2, pp. 189–93.

Allen D., Buehler J. W., Samuels B. N. & Brann A.W. Jr. 1989, 'Mortality in infants discharged from neonatal intensive care units in Georgia', *Journal American Medical Association*, vol. 261, no. 12, pp. 1763–1766.

American Academy of Pediatrics Committee on Fetus and Newborn 1985, 'Manpower needs in neonatal pediatrics', *Pediatrics*, vol. 76, no. 1, pp. 132–135.

Anderson G. 1991, 'Current knowledge about skin-to-skin (kangaroo) care for preterm infants', *J Perinatology*, vol. 11, pp. 216–26.

Bennett F. 1984, 'Neurodevelopmental outcome of low birth weight infants', in *Practice of Pediatrics*, ed. V. Kelley, Harper & Rowe, Philadelphia.

Berger H. 1989, 'Clinical Examination of the Newborn Infant', in *Effective Care in Pregnancy and Childbirth*, eds I. Chalmers, M. Enkin & M. Kierse, Oxford University Press, Oxford.

Bolton K. 1991, 'Maternal attitudes to prematurity', unpublished manuscript, c/o Prof. B Chalmers, School of Psychology, University of Witwatersrand, South Africa.

Bosque M. 1988, 'Continuous physiological measures of Kangaroo versus incubator care in a tertiary level nursery', *Pediatric Research*, vol. 23, no. 4, part 2, p. 402A (Abstract 1204).

Brooten D., Kumar S., Brown L.P., Butts P., Finkler S.A., Bakewell-Sachs S., Gibbons A. & Delivoria-Papadopoulos M. 1986, 'A randomised clinical trial of early hospital discharge and home follow-up of very-low-weight infants', *New England J of Medicine*, vol. 315, no. 15, pp. 934–93.

Campbell D. 1984, 'Why do physicians in neonatal care units differ in their admission thresholds?', *Soc Sci Med*, vol. 18, no. 5, pp. 365–374.

Commission on the Prevention of Infant Mortality, *US Congress 1990 Report of Findings*, Washington DC.

Cottingham J. 1986, 'Women's support groups in care following birth', paper at the WHO Consensus Conference on Appropriate Technology Following Birth, Trieste.

Couriel J. & Davies P. 1988, 'Cost and benefits of a community special care baby service', *British Medical Journal*, vol. 296, pp. 1043–1046.

Day S. 1982, 'Is obstetric technology depressing?', *Radical Science Journal*, vol. 12, pp. 17–45.

de Leeuw R., Colin E., Dunnebier E. & Mirmiran M. 1989, 'Physiological effects of kangaroo care in very small preterm infants', *Biology of the Neonate*, vol. 59, no. 3, pp. 149–155.

Denmark State Health Science Research Committee and State Hospital Institute 1991, *Consensus Report: Extremely early born infants.*.

Denmark National Board of Health 1992, *Extremely early born children, a register study.* Copenhagen.

DeSouza P. 1986, 'Nonprofessional resources in neonatal care', paper at WHO Consensus Conference on Appropriate Technology Following Birth, Trieste.

Doyle L. 1987, 'Experience in the neonatal intensive care unit at Monash Medical Centre', paper given at WHO meeting on Appropriate Perinatal Technology, Melbourne, Australia.

Ewald U. 1991, 'What is the actual cost of neonatal intensive care?', *International Journal of Technology Assessment in Health Care*, vol. 7, supplement 1, pp. 155–161.

Field T., Schanberg S. M., Scafidi F., Bauer C. R., Vega-Lahr N., Garcia R., Nystrom & Kuhn C. M. 1986, 'Tactile/kinesthetic stimulation effects on preterm neonates', *Pediatrics*, vol. 77, no. 5, pp. 654–658.

Gottfried A. & Hodgman J. 1984, 'How intensive is newborn intensive care? An environmental analysis', *Pediatrics*, vol. 7, no. 2, pp. 292–294.

Grant A. & Sleep J. 1989, 'Relief of perineal pain and discomfort after childbirth', in *Effective Care in Pregnancy and Childbirth*, eds I. Chalmers, M. Enkin & M. Kierse, Oxford University Press, Oxford.

Guillemin J. 1984, 'Priceless Lives and Medical Costs: The case of newborn intensive care', *Research in the Sociology of Health Care*, vol. 3, pp. 115–134.

Guillemin J. 1986, 'Intensive care for newborns in the United States: the question of policy', paper at WHO Consensus Conference on Appropriate Technology Following Birth, Trieste.

Guillemin J. 1988, 'The family in newborn intensive care', in *Childbirth in America*, ed. R. Michaelson, Bergin & Garvey, Massachusetts.*.

Hagberg B., Hagberg G. & Olow 1982, 'Gains and hazards of intensive neonatal care: an analysis from Swedish cerebral palsy epidemiology', *Developmental, medicine and child neurology*, vol. 24, pp. 13–19.

Hagberg B., Hagberg G. & Olow I. 1984, 'The changing panorama of cerebral palsy in Sweden', *Acta Paediatr Scand*, vol. 73, pp. 433–440.

Hagberg B. & Hagberg G. 1987, 'Epidemiology of cerebral palsy and other major neurodevelopmental impairment relation to perinatal events', in *Early Detection and Management of Cerebral Palsy*, ed. J. Galjuard, Martinius Nijhoff, The Netherlands.

Heinonen K., Hakulinen A. & Jokela V. 1988, 'Survival of the smallest: Time trends and determinants of mortality in a very preterm population during the 1980s', *Lancet*, vol. II, no. 8604, pp. 204–207.

Hunziker U. & Barr R. 1986, 'Increased carrying reduces infant crying: a randomised controlled trial', *Pediatrics*, vol. 77, no. 5, pp. 641–648.

Jarvis S., Holloway J. & Hey E. 1985, 'Increase in cerebral palsy in normal birthweight babies', *Arch Dis Child*, vol. 60, pp. 113–121.

Joyce T., Corman H. & Crossman M. 1988, 'A Cost-Effectiveness Analysis of Strategies to Reduce Infant Mortality', *Medical Care*, vol. 26, no. 4, pp. 348–360.

Kennell J. & Klaus M. 1986, 'General Overview on care of the normal newborn infant', paper at WHO Consensus Conference on Appropriate Technology Following Birth, Trieste.

Kitchen W. 1987, 'Cerebral palsy in very low birthweight infants surviving to two years with modern perinatal intensive care', *American Journal of Perinatology*, vol. 4, no. 1, pp. 29–35.

Lancet 1988, Editorial: Medical Care of Newborn Babies, vol. 2, no. 8624, pp. 1344–1346.

Ludington-Hoe S. 1991, 'Physiological responses to skin-to-skin contact in hospitalized premature infants', *J Perinatology*, vol. 11, pp. 19–24.

Ludington-Hoe S. 1992, personal communication.

Maisels J. 1986, 'Jaundice in the healthy newborn infant', paper at WHO Consensus Conference on Appropriate Technology Following Birth. Trieste.

—— 1986, 'Perspectives on perinatal research', paper at WHO Consensus Conference on Appropriate Technology Following Birth, Trieste.

Mann N., Haddow R., Stokes L., Goodley S. & Rutter N. 1986, 'Effect of night and day on preterm infants in a newborn nursery: randomised trial', *British Medical Journal*, vol. 293, pp. 1265–1267.

Maratos O. 1986, 'The newborn infant: his needs for care and interaction', paper at WHO Consensus Conference on Appropriate Technology Following Birth.

Mayall B. 1989, *Child Health Care--Living with children, caring for children*, Heinemann, London.

McCormick M. 1985, 'The contribution of low birth weight to infant mortality and childhood mortality', *New England Journal Medicine*, vol. 312, p. 82.

McCormick M. 1989, 'Long-term follow-up of infants discharged from neonatal intensive care units', *Journal American Medical Assoc*, vol. 261, no. 12, pp. 1767–1772.

McIlwaine G., Skeoch H., Skeoch C., Rosenberg K. & Turner T. 1987, 'Very low birthweight survivors: illness and readmission to hospital in the first 15 months of life', *British Medical Journal*, vol. 295, pp. 579–580.

Minchin M. 1985, *Breastfeeding Matters*, Alma Pub., Australia.

Montgomery T. et al. 1959, 'A study of staphylococcal colonisation of post-partum mothers and newborn infants: Comparison of central care and rooming-in', *Am J Obstet Gynecol*, vol. 78, pp. 1227–1233.

Moreno E. 1986, 'Economic aspects of neonatal assistance in Latin America', paper at WHO Consensus Conference on Appropriate Technology Following Birth, Trieste.

Morgan M. 1985, 'Late morbidity of very low birthweight infants', *British Medical Journal*, vol. 291, pp. 171–173.

Mugford M. 1986, 'A Review of the economics of care for sick newborn infants', paper at WHO Consensus Conference on Appropriate Technology Following Birth, Trieste.

Munro I. 1986, 'Role and responsibility of the media in promoting change in technology in the health care field', paper at the WHO Consensus Conference on Appropriate Technology Following Birth, Trieste.

Oakley A. 1986a, 'Technology following birth', paper at WHO Consensus Conference on Appropriate Technology Following Birth, Trieste.

—— 1986b, 'Beyond the Yellow Wallpaper, or taking women seriously', in *Telling the Truth About Jerusalem*, ed. A. Oakley, Blackwell Pub., Oxford.

O'Conner S., Vietze P. M., Sherrod K. B., Sandler H. M. & Altemeier W. A. 1980a, 'Reduced incidence of parenting inadequacy following rooming-in', *Pediatrics*, vol. 66, pp. 176–182.

O'Conner S. 1980b, 'Quality of parenting and the mother-infant relationship following rooming-in', in *Parent-Infant Relationships*, ed. P. Taylor, Grune & Stratton, New York.

—— 1981, 'Responsivity of mother-infant interaction after extended postpartum contact', *Pediatric Res Abst*, vol. 15, p. 484.

Paneth N. 1992, 'Tiny babies—Enormous cost', *Birth: Issues in Perinatal Care*, vol. 19, no. 3, pp. 154–5.

Papiernik E., Bouyer J., Dreyfus J., Collin D., Winisdorffer G., Guegen S., Lecomte M. & Lazar P. 1985, 'Prevention of preterm birth: a perinatal study in Haguanau, France', *Pediatrics*, vol. 76, no. 2, pp. 154–158.

Prudent L. 1986, 'Early discharge and follow-up of low birth weight infants', paper at WHO Consensus Conference on Appropriate Technology Following Birth, Trieste.

Rauan L. & Oakley A. 1990, 'Low birth weight babies: the mother's point of view', *Midwifery*, vol. 6, pp. 73–85.

Rey Sanabira E. & Gomez H. 1986, 'Rational handling of the premature infant', paper given at the WHO consensus conference, Trieste.

Rich A. 1977, *Of Woman Born*, Virago, London.

Richards M. 1980, 'Is neonatal special care overused?', *Birth & Family Journal*, vol. 7, no. 4, pp. 225–233.

—— 1986, 'Patterns of care of sick and low birth weight newborn infants', paper at WHO Consensus Conference on Appropriate Technology Following Birth, Trieste.

Romito P. 1989, 'Unhappiness after childbirth', in *Effective Care in Pregnancy and Childbirth*, eds I. Chalmers, M. Enkin & M. Kierse, Oxford University Press, Oxford.

Royal College of Physicians of London 1988, *Medical care of the newborn in England and Wales*, a report of the College, London.

Rush J., Chalmers I. & Enkin M. 1989, *Care of the New Mother and Baby*, in *Effective Care in Pregnancy and Childbirth*, eds I. Chalmers, M. Enkin & M. Kierse, Oxford University Press, Oxford.

Ruzek S. 1991, 'Women's Reproductive Rights: The Impact of Technology', in *Women and New Reproductive Technologies: Medical, Psychosocial, Legal and Ethical Dilemmas*, Lawrence Erlbaum, New Jersey.

Schmidt E. & Wittreich G. 1986, 'Care of the abnormal newborn: a random controlled trial study of kangaroo method of care for low birth weight newborns', paper given at WHO Consensus conference, Trieste.

Shankaran S., Cohen S. N., Linver M. & Zonia S. 1988, 'Medical care costs of high-risk infants after neonatal intensive care: a controlled study', *Pediatrics*, vol. 81, no 3, pp. 372–378.

Silverman W. 1980, *Retrolental Fibroplasia: A Modern Parable*, Grune & Stratton, New York.

—— 1985, *Human Experimentation: a Guided Step into the Unknown*, Oxford University Press, Oxford.

Sisson T. 1985, 'Editorial: hazards to vision in the nursery', *New England Journal of Medicine*, vol. 313, no. 7, pp. 444–445.

Stanley F. & Watson L. 1988, 'The cerebral palsies in Western Australia: Trends 1968–1981', *Am J Obstet Gynecol*, vol. 158, pp. 89–93.

Sterky G. 1985, 'Breathing and warmth at birth: Judging the appropriateness of technology', *Sarec Report*, R:2, Stockholm.

—— 1986, 'Future research in care following birth', paper at WHO Consensus Conference on Appropriate Technology Following Birth, Trieste.

Stinson R. & Stinson P. 1983, *The Long Dying of Baby Andrew*, Little, Brown & Co., Boston.

Suarez-Ojeda 1986, 'Health services in the neonatal period in Latin America', paper given at WHO Consensus Conference on Appropriate Technology Following Birth, Trieste.

Thomson M. & Westreich R. 1989, 'Restriction of mother-infant contact in the immediate postnatal period', in *Effective Care in Pregnancy and Childbirth*, eds I. Chalmers, M. Enkin & M. Keirse, Oxford University Press, Oxford.

Tuomikoski-Koiranen P. 1988, unpublished manuscript available from Anna Maria Laine, University Hospital of Rurku, Department of Pediatrics, 20520 Turku, 52 Finland.

United Kingdom Department of Health and Social Security 1977, *Reducing the risk: safer pregnancy and childbirth*, H. M. Stationary Office, London.

US Congress, Office of Technology Assessment 1987, *Neonatal Intensive Care for Low Birthweight Infants: Costs and Effectiveness*. OTA–HCS–38, Washington, DC.

—— 1988, *Healthy Children: Investing in the Future*, OTA–H344, Washington, DC.

Uvnas-Moberg K., Widstrom A. M., Marchini G. & Winberg J. 1987, 'Release of GI hormones in mother and infant by sensory stimulation', *Acta Paediat Scand*, vol. 76, no. 6, pp. 851–860.

Van Enk A. & de Leeuw R. 1987, 'Phototherapy: the hospital as risk factor', *British Medical Journal*, vol. 294, pp. 747–9.

Vohr B. & Coll C. 1985, 'Neurodevelopmental and school performance of very low-birth-weight infants: a seven-year longitudinal study', *Pediatrics*, vol. 76, no. 3, pp. 345–350.

Wagner M. 1987a, 'The epidemiology of ourselves: a light in a dark tunnel' *Pediatric & Perinatal Epidemiology*, vol. 1, no. 1, pp 14–16.

—— 1987b, 'Is epidemiology for us or them?' *Pediatric & Perinatal Epidemiology*, vol. 1, no. 2, pp. 139–140.

—— 1988, 'Whose data is it anyway?', *Pediatric & Perinatal Epidemiology*, vol. 2, no. 1, pp. 7–10.

Whitelaw A. & Sleath K. 1985, 'Myth of the marsupial mother: Home care of very low birth weight babies in Bogata, Colombia', *Lancet*, May 25, pp. 1206–1208.

Whitelaw A. 1986, 'Skin-to-skin contact in the care of the very low birth weight babies', *Maternal & Child Health*, vol. 7, pp. 242–246.

Whitelaw A., Heisterkamp G., Sleath K., Acolet D. & Richards M 1988, 'Skin to skin contact for very low birthweight infants and their mothers', *Archives of Diseases in Childhood*, vol. 63, pp. 1377–1381.

Whitelaw A. 1990, 'Kangaroo baby care: just a nice experience or an important advance for preterm infants?', *Pediatrics*, vol. 85, pp. 604–5.

World Health Organisation 1985, *Having a Baby in Europe*, Public Health in Europe no. 26, WHO Regional Office for Europe, Copenhagen.

—— 1991a, *Maternal Mortality Rates and Ratios*, Third Edition, Safe Motherhood Program, WHO Geneva.

—— 1991, *Postnatal Depression: A Review*, European Regional Office, Copenhagen.

World Health Organisation/UNICEF 1990, *Protecting, Promoting and Supporting Breast-feeding: The Special Role of Maternity Services*, Geneva.

Young D. 1992, 'Family centered maternity care: is the central nursery obsolete?', *Birth: Issues in Perinatal Care*, vol. 19, no. 4, pp. 183–4.

Chapter 8

Spreading the word: action and reaction

We who are fighting
To realise dreams
Ask for the task
Of uniting extremes.

Piet Hein

The telephone call from the United Kingdom whose description began this book was only one of many received by WHO Regional Office for Europe on the consensus recommendations expressing either strong opposition or support. This chapter will summarise the actions taken by WHO to promote the consensus recommendations, the reactions to the recommendations, both positive and negative, and what seems to be the way forward.

Action

Normally WHO issues reports, sends them to ministries of health and moves on to something else. The consensus process, however, demands a final step: presenting the recommendations to all relevant parties (including the public) for consideration and discussion. Such debate must take place at the national and local levels, to become part of the political process that determines health policy. The consensus process has often met with little success and it is probably because this last step often is ignored. To bridge the gap between what is known to be good medical practice and what is done, it is necessary to bridge the gap between scientific data and policy and between policy and practice. These two latter bridges are too rarely crossed, by governments, by professional organisations, by WHO.

Thus, WHO began an unprecedented effort to spread the news of the three consensus conferences as far and wide as possible so that they could become part of the final step of policy formation and change in practice. We had recently had good success with the book *Having a Baby in Europe*, published in the four working languages of the Regional Office (English, French, German and Russian) and written in a style such that anyone could understand it. It had proved a useful promotional tool with a variety of groups and became one of the World Health Organisation's best sellers. We searched for other strategies.

The final recommendations on care during pregnancy made in the first consensus meeting in Washington were sent to all ministers of health or their equivalents, in the European and American Regions, but there was no reaction. It was like dropping something into a well and never hearing it hit the bottom. To promote discussion, the recommendations of the second and third consensus meetings were published in a prominent international medical journal, the *Lancet*. (WHO 1985, 1986) As will soon be seen, this precipitated considerable reaction.

Birth conferences

In addition to the use of the printed word, national and local 'birth conferences' were organised. Their purpose was to bring together as many of the interested parties as possible (local politics permitting) for discussion in the light of the WHO recommendations, and, it was hoped, to stimulate the process of making new health policy. The success of the first of these meetings in achieving these goals was a revelation that convinced WHO that it needed to continue its efforts at disseminating the policy recommendations.

This first birth conference was organised in Denmark by the Danish midwifery and obstetrical organisations and the WHO Regional Office for Europe. Held at the Regional Office in Copenhagen it was attended by parents, physicians and midwives. Representatives of the mass media also attended and extensively covered both the meeting and the conflict between the medical and social approaches.

The Minister of the Interior (responsible for health matters), a woman with two children, followed the media discussion with interest. The month after the meeting, the Minister received new draft guidelines for perinatal services from the National Board of Health. (When finally approved, such guidelines are distributed to the counties, where they are influential.) The National Board of Health had consulted professors of obstetrics on the new guidelines for perinatal services and based them solely on the medical model. After reviewing the draft guidelines, the Minister of the Interior realised that they were a far cry from what had been discussed in the media at the time of the birth conference. She was concerned and asked the opinion of WHO Regional Office staff. They responded with a short written statement and then, at the request of the Minister met with her and recommended an approach that combined key dimensions of the social as well as the medical model of birth.

The Minister returned the draft guidelines to the National Board of Health, asking that a number of opinions (including those of Danish women) on the draft be secured, as well as more information and ideas on what the guidelines might include. The Danish Institute of Clinical Epidemiology surveyed all the women giving birth in one month in Denmark; 3280 (or 81%) answered an extensive questionnaire. After careful data analysis, a report described the women's experiences during pregnancy and birth and following birth. Meanwhile, the draft guidelines were sent to a number of different groups for critique, including local health officers, medical associations, consumer groups and a women's research group. The National Board of Health asked the women's research group to make suggestions for new guidelines. The group urged a more social approach in its new draft, which incorporated the principles of informed choice, in collaboration with health personnel, on the nature of care, and continuity of care.

The final guidelines, as approved by the Minister of the Interior and published by the National Board of Health, incorporated ideas from all of these sources and were presented to the counties. What were some of the social model elements in the guidelines? As one example, the guidelines proposed that there be neighbourhood midwifery centres staffed by three midwives. All routine prenatal care is provided by these three midwives who are then on call at the local hospital to attend the birth of their own clients, either at the hospital or at the birthing woman's home according to the woman's wishes. Postnatal care is again in the same neighbourhood centre so that true continuity of care is achieved. Each county is now using a multidisciplinary group to adapt the guidelines to its perinatal services. Some plans have already been completed and adhere more or less to the national guidelines.

The impact of the Danish birth conference on health policy for birth prompted WHO to promote similar meetings in other countries. The experience also underscored the importance of the media and the crucial role top policy-makers play. Gradually the initiative for organising these conferences passed to local health officials, professional, and lay groups. The idea's time has come: in the past five years over 40 birth conferences have been held in 24 Eastern and Western European countries as well as in the United States, Canada, Australia and China.

These birth conferences are always held in the local language. The only outsiders are a few WHO representatives, serving as resource people. The discussions are open and intense and sometimes heated. At a Greek meeting, for example, a perinatal survey was discussed; it showed, among other things, that about 50% of all Greek women are given a general anaesthetic during labour and birth. A woman asked a professor of obstetrics the reason for such a practice. When the obstetrician suggested that Greek women might not cope as well as others with the pain of childbirth, there was an outburst of angry responses from many women in the conference hall.

Other meetings

WHO staff have also promoted the consensus recommendations through participation in a wide variety of international, national and local meetings at which the recommendations have been discussed. These meetings have been organised by associations of health professionals, lay groups or a combination of the two, and have proliferated to a point that WHO staff cannot attend them all.

A special series of meetings has been held in Canada and the United States to address an issue of great importance to birth care in North America: midwifery. About 100 years ago, the profession all but disappeared from these two countries. Midwifery became illegal throughout Canada and in many of the states of the USA. For this reason, health professionals and the public have only a vague idea of what midwifery is. WHO has collaborated in organising meetings and media events to educate the public and promote the re-establishment of the profession in North America. Health authorities are gradually realising that midwives are an essential option in a balanced maternity care system.

Contact with the mass media

WHO has established new contacts with the mass media to promote the recommendations on perinatal policy. WHO staff have been interviewed on television in many countries, and articles and interviews have appeared in a large number of newspapers and popular magazines in Australia, eastern and western Europe, and the Americas.

Urgent research

In addition, WHO has proposed, encouraged and sometimes launched the type of research that the consensus recommendations indicated was urgently needed. For example, on discovering the wide variations in rates of obstetrical intervention and the little or no relationship they have to birth outcomes, the Regional Office for Europe decided to approach a number of national obstetrical organisations, to seek their collaboration in launching an international study of obstetrical intervention. Most obstetrical organisations were pleased to collaborate and the result is the study involving twelve countries which was discussed in some detail in chapter 6 (Stephenson 1992).

Because the role played by midwives in maternity services is so important to the appropriate use of technology, WHO decided to launch a study of midwifery in industrialised countries. A questionnaire was given to midwives and obstetricians in a number of countries to compare their approaches to technology and birth care. The result is the book *Helpers in Childbirth: Midwifery Today,* co-published by WHO (Oakley & Houd 1990).

WHO has not always been successful at launching research. We have repeatedly proposed in many countries a clinical trial to test a self-help model for prenatal care. Women found to have no problems at the first prenatal visit would be randomly assigned to two groups. The control group would receive the usual medical prenatal care now available in their communities. The experimental group would receive self-help prenatal care as described earlier. The experimental and control groups would be compared on a number of outcome measures including: the babies' birth weights, rates of medical complications arising during pregnancy and birth, obstetrical intervention, referral of infants for special observation or neonatal intensive care, breastfeeding and postpartum depression; and levels of satisfaction with the experience of pregnancy and birth. The fate of this proposal is described later under reactions.

Models for policy

It was also expected that WHO could promote the implementation of the recommendations through promoting more balanced birth policies. But a problem arose. There are many examples of a purely medical approach to birth, but few if any perinatal policy statements with a purely social basis. It was important to generate a policy document based on the social model, to see what it would look like, to compare it with medical policy documents and to use it as a guide to further policy development which would combine the medical and social approach. Two meetings (in Esalen, California in North America and in Berlin in Europe) were organised by WHO at which small groups drafted such a document. All the participants were committed to and had experience with health policy or birth care with a social orientation. The groups included formally trained and empirical midwives, representatives of user groups, social scientists, health administrators, obstetricians, paediatricians and epidemiologists. Drafting the document was an interesting experiment: although the common denominator was a social orientation, non-practitioners such as health administrators and social scientists were thrown together with practitioners who give birth care every day. As a basis for discussion, a number of the practitioners were asked to prepare case reports from their countries, outlining the present realities in birth practices. The final policy document *Health promotion and birth: a social model for birth* was presented and discussed at WHO's first international conference on health promotion held in Canada in 1987. It is also included in the appendix and a careful reading provides a clear idea of how the social approach to birth care differs from the more typical medical model. This report certainly illustrates the degree to which birth care is medically based and how far we must go if we are effectively to apply social-based health promotion principles to birth. The document also includes strategies to be used in promoting the changes proposed. Although the document is based on the experience in industrialised countries and the proposals are most readily applied there, many principles and strategies are also relevant to developing countries.

Reactions

Whether negative or positive, reactions to the recommendations have been strong.

Negative responses

AT THE LOCAL LEVEL

It is not surprising that most of the negative reactions to the content and promotion of the consensus recommendations have come from the medical establishment in various countries; present perinatal policy in these countries is based for the most part on the medical model and physicians are in control. For example, no location has yet been found for the proposed research project on self-help prenatal care. An experienced midwife in England was eager to participate, some of the funds were available and cooperation was obtained from the local midwives' group and health authority. No consulting obstetrician in the area, however, was willing to cooperate, and thus the project had to be dropped.

When visiting hospitals, WHO staff have been given a long list of reasons why the recommendations cannot be implemented there. The danger of infection is frequently used to explain the exclusion of fathers from the hospital and the absence of rooming-in. Physicians and nurses accuse each other of resistance to change. Change at the local level therefore requires pressure from key leaders in the community or new policy guidelines from central authorities. Without these, change will not take place.

AT THE NATIONAL LEVEL

The publication of the Fortaleza and Trieste recommendations in the *Lancet* provoked strong negative reactions from national obstetrical societies. The Hungarian obstetrical society discussed each of the Fortaleza recommendations and categorically rejected most. The society stated that physicians alone are qualified to make decisions about birth care, and that decisions about caesarean section in particular can only be made on a case-by-case basis; therefore cumulative statistics on birth practices were of no value. In short, the Hungarian obstetricians entirely rejected the epidemiological approach which is central to providing obstetrics with a scientific knowledge base.

The national obstetrical societies of Austria, the Federal Republic of Germany and the United Kingdom also went on record as opposing the Fortaleza recommendations. Angry letters to WHO from obstetrical organisations in these three countries prompted an invitation to each group to send a representative to an informal consultation at the WHO Regional Office. During intense day-long discussions, many misunderstandings were cleared up and disagreements at least partially resolved.

Some of the reactions from the mass media were quite negative. In an hour-long debate on the recommendations that were broadcast on Austrian national television, a professor of obstetrics stated that the recommendations were only applicable to the third world and that in any case, WHO was about to change the recommendations. It was necessary for the WHO Regional Office to inform the Austrians of the applicability of the recommendations to all countries, and our continuing support for their content.

AT THE INTERNATIONAL LEVEL

Strong negative reactions were also expressed at the international level. When a WHO staff member discussed the recommendations at a training course for obstetricians from several countries held in the Alps, some participants were hostile, and wrote angry letters to WHO executive management. When a WHO staff member, speaking to several hundred obstetricians at the opening of a meeting of a European Perinatal Society in Leipzig, suggested that policies for routine ultrasound scanning needed re-evaluation, the obstetrician who spoke next repeatedly described this statement as nonsense.

Another example of deep divisions of opinion arose when the International Federation of Gynaecology and Obstetrics (FIGO) formed a committee to draft guidelines for the use of the electronic fetal monitor during birth and invited WHO to participate. FIGO insisted on recommending routine electronic monitoring of all women during labour, WHO insisted that the scientific evidence did not justify such a recommendation. Despite prolonged negotiation, common ground could not be established, and WHO withdrew its participation.

Additional negative reactions arose inside WHO. Mention has already been made of the opposition of some staff to the consensus meetings. Others disliked some of the recommendations and their publication. There has also been opposition to the publication of this book.

Positive responses

AT THE LOCAL AND NATIONAL LEVELS

Not surprisingly, most of the positive reactions have come from the public sector, from consumer groups, politicians and the mass media. Nevertheless, many obstetricians in many countries see a necessity for change in perinatal services. Thus, as described earlier in this chapter, when staff from the WHO Regional Office proposed a collaborative research project on obstetrical interventions, national obstetrical societies in a number of countries agreed to participate.

There has been considerable positive reaction from both the medical press and the mass media in many countries. Positive articles discussing *Having a Baby in Europe* and the WHO consensus recommendations have appeared in professional medical journals in over 20 countries (e.g. *British Medical Journal* 1987, *Lancet* 1987). Positive articles have also appeared in newspapers and popular magazines, and television programs and interviews with WHO staff and others have been shown. Actually, the tone of an article or program is less important than the fact of its appearance, which brings the issue to the public and increases awareness of the importance of public involvement in decisions about birth care.

One positive reaction began as a grassroots initiative in Italy and has spread to other countries. Over 20 Italian women's groups met to draw up a common agenda. After several days of fruitless debate, one participant brought up the Fortaleza recommendations, which she had recently seen in the *Lancet*. All of the groups quickly agreed to use the recommendations as a basis for collaboration. With WHO approval and financial assistance, the women created a poster listing 15 recommendations. Thousands of these posters were put up in health facilities all over Italy, creating widespread discussion and debate.

A women's group in the United Kingdom learned of the Italian effort and printed and distributed similar posters in English. A French midwife saw one of the English posters on a visit to London, and soon a French translation was widely distributed. Consumer groups in the United States and Finland organised their own poster campaigns. In Australia, the United Nations Centre together with the Royal College of Obstetricians and Gynaecologists, the Australian College of Midwives and the lay organisation, Maternity Alliance, put together a kit based on *Having a Baby in Europe* and the three consensus conferences. The kit includes posters, summary reports of these meetings and other relevant material. It has attracted considerable media attention and discussion. Women have found that being able to quote from the poster has been helpful in discussions with physicians and hospital staff about their right to exercise informed choice about their birth experience. A circle has been completed as the campaign has spread to Brazil. There, where some of the recommendations were generated, Dr Araújo's widow learned about it at a conference in London. The global dissemination of these recommendations reflects the seriousness of the issues raised in these meetings.

The consensus recommendations have become part of the political process in many countries. Mention has already been made of their relevance to the passing of the new legislation on midwifery in New Zealand. In Italy, the recommendations were first used to develop new perinatal guidelines in the Lombardy Region. Next they were used for the development of new guidelines in the District surrounding Milan. Most recently they have been quoted extensively in the national Italian Parliament when new national legislation was drafted. In fact, the recommendations have been so widely used in policy formation that is not possible to track these usages. They are part of the public domain.

Their effects in particular regions have varied. For historical, cultural and political reasons, it can reasonably be said that the news about maternity services in the countries of eastern Europe is both good and bad. The good news is that obstetrical intervention rates are much lower than those in western Europe; the bad news is that no account is yet taken of the social, psychological and family needs related to birth. One of the recommendations — which were, of course, translated and circulated among health authorities and health professionals in these countries — has led to some change. In most of these countries, a few hospitals are beginning to experiment with rooming-in. Although these hospitals have not changed in other respects (they still, for example, exclude fathers), it is hoped that these experiments with rooming-in may be the beginning of greater awareness in this part of Europe of the crucial non-biological aspects of birth and birth care.

After years of negotiations, the first birth conference was held in the former Soviet Union shortly before the change in government. It was an all-union conference with doctors and midwives from many Republics. There were no non-medical professionals nor lay representation as there was simply no precedent for such participation. After the WHO recommendations had been presented and discussed, a group sat down and went recommendation by recommendation, accepting, rejecting or modifying each so as to make them appropriate to the Soviet situation.

The Soviet experience was an extraordinary process. Many of the recommendation were at first rejected out of hand by the obstetricians in the group. After the scientific documentation was brought forth for discussion under the leadership of a strong clinician and public health official from the USSR, the Soviet group accepted most of the WHO recommendations. The group report was then presented to the entire conference for discussion and acceptance as a consensus document. Two months later the Soviet modification of the consensus recommendations were published in the influential journal that is sent to all physicians, nurses and midwives in the former USSR.

As there is no longer a Soviet Ministry of Health to promote their consensus recommendations, the next task is to approach each new government formed out of the old Republics, to start the process again. Two consensus meetings have already been held in the new

Russian Republic, one in St. Petersburg in 1992 and one in Vologda in 1993, to make recommendations for reorienting maternity services. In 1993, the President of Russia gave maternity services highest priority in health care and asked the Ministry of Health to draft new guidelines for maternal care. The WHO recommendations are being used in drafting these guidelines.

The recommendations have had an important effect in Canada, where midwifery did not officially exist. Midwifery was illegal in all provinces of Canada, but a few formally trained and empirical midwives illegally attended home births nevertheless. Recently the jury at an inquest in Toronto heard evidence from a WHO staff member concerning the essential role of midwifery in European countries, and the relevant consensus recommendations. At the end of the inquest, the jury recommended the legalisation of midwifery to the legislature of the Province of Ontario. As a result, a Provincial task force was formed and collaborated with WHO in gathering information on midwifery in Europe. The outstanding final report by the task force, summarising the reasons for legalising midwifery in Ontario and starting a school of midwifery there, was presented at a large birth conference in Toronto, at which the consensus recommendations received further discussion. New legislation has legalised midwifery in Ontario and a new school of midwifery will soon open. Subsequently the Province of British Columbia has legalised midwifery and the Province of Quebec has started the process of legalisation. There is evidence that other Provinces in Canada may follow suit fairly soon.

AT THE INTERNATIONAL LEVEL

In 1988, the European Parliament adopted a resolution on a charter on the rights of women in childbirth. The WHO consensus recommendations were used during the drafting of the charter and the charter is extraordinarily consistent with the consensus recommendations. This charter is included in the appendix.

Positive reactions also appeared within WHO. Because the activities that were described here to promote consensus recommendations are new to WHO, this approach created considerable discussion. Each year when all countries in the world gather at WHO headquarters to discuss the work of the Organisation, there is always a technical discussion on a chosen topic. At the World Health Assembly in

1990, the technical discussio...
document prepared for the d...
studies illustrating how to brid... the gap...
Making. The work of the Europea... Re... promoting its
recommendations on appropriate perinatal te... was one of
the successful case studies chosen (v... 1990). T... ch is now
recognised as providing an importan... new strate... to use
particularly in work with countries th... need to re...
health services that are provided across...

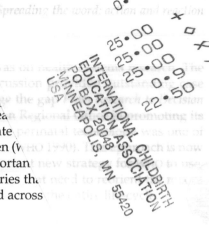

The way forward

Problem

The problem is that the birth machine is out of con... ... Technology is used inappropriately and excessively before, during and following birth. This use of perinatal technology, in large part, is not based on either scientific proof of value nor on valid medical indication. The determinants are, rather, such non-medical factors as habit, convenience, fear and financial gain.

A good example of habit as a determinant of perinatal technology use is the forceps. Doctors continue to use forceps instead of vacuum extraction in spite of good scientific evidence to the contrary. When confronted with this, they do not appear to be concerned, and concern precedes voluntary change.

There are many examples of convenience as a determinant of technology use during birth, all documented in chapter 6. Caesarean section, even emergency caesarean section, has been shown scientifically to occur more frequently at times convenient to the doctor. The widespread use of induction of labour at times convenient to doctors has also been confirmed. Surveys have shown that doctors like the convenience of epidural anaesthesia. The only explanation for the continuing use of the lithotomy position at birth, in the face of so much evidence favouring other positions, is for the convenience to the birth attendant.

It is extraordinary how doctors are so ready to admit that their own fear is an important determinant of their use of birth technology.

The well known professor of obstetrics, Dr. O'Driscoll, wrote: "there is a subtle influence in obstetrics that operates to absolve a doctor who intervenes in the course of a normal pregnancy and which, by implication, exposes a colleague to censure when an infant is born dead. This places a premium on intervention as a form of personal insurance for the doctor, although the consequences are detrimental to some patients" (O'Driscoll et al. 1975).

A survey of British obstetricians found that fear of litigation was the second most common reason given for their increased use of caesarean section (Maternity Alliance 1983). In other words, they openly admitted to picking up a scalpel and cutting open women's bodies out of fear of litigation. The fact that 85% of British obstetricians have been sued at least once, and 65% have been sued twice, has precipitated considerable discussion and analysis (Capstick & Edwards 1990; *Lancet* editorial 1991; *British Medical Journal* editorial 1991). About 60% of American obstetricians have been sued at least once and in New York, half of the obstetricians have been sued on 3 or more occasions (American College of Obstetricians and Gynecologists 1984). As a result of fear of being sued, American obstetricians admit to: increased use of diagnostic tests, increased electronic fetal monitoring during labour, increased use of caesarean section, refusal to take on 'high risk' cases for care. (Fortunately for the rest of the world, this refusal to treat someone in need, which goes against the oath of Hippocrates taken by physicians in the United States as elsewhere, is a uniquely American phenomenon).

There can be no doubt that "the increasing prominence [of legal influences] as determinants of clinical practice is not in the best interests of either present or future users of the maternity services" (Chalmers 1985). An American obstetrician has written that obstetricians "should do their best in pursuit of the interests, health and welfare of their patients consistent with good medical practice. They should not be concerned with the risk of civil liability because, by virtue of the incongruence between the law and truth and justice, one may be sued no matter what one does" (Fribourg 1983).

In chapter 6 we also found how perinatal technology use can be determined by economic considerations. In both Brazil and the United States, there is increasing use of interventions such as caesarean section with the increasing ability of the woman to pay for it. With the growing trend of doctors in a number of countries to increase their private practice, this could become an increasing problem. In the United States, it is already difficult to find doctors who are willing to care for lower-income patients.

Solutions

In searching for solutions to the serious overuse of birth technology, it is important to look at the past record. Do recent events suggest that we can expect the organised medical profession to be part of the solution? Sadly, the answer to this question must be an emphatic 'no'. It is not reasonable to expect a profession to want to change when it already has high status, nearly all of the power and is reaping financial gain. So doctors too often blame lawyers and selfish mothers for the present state of affairs. A few examples will illustrate how the profession is part of the problem, not the solution.

At the international level, we described earlier how the International Federation of Gynaecology and Obstetrics and pushed to recommend routine electronic fetal monitoring of all birth in spite of the scientific evidence that fails to support such a policy. When the European Society of Obstetricians and Gynaecologists met recently in Athens, they learned of the extreme overuse of general anaesthesia and induction during birth in Greece. They admitted to being shocked, but when they were urged to confront their Greek colleagues during the meeting, they did not do so. After the meeting, WHO and Greek perinatal epidemiologists urged the society to publish a statement condemning these practices, but this was not done.

At the national level, the American College of Obstetrics and Gynecology in the United States, for the most part, has been passive in the face of the epidemic of caesarean births. The conservative and self-serving stance of this organisation is illustrated by an extraordinary statement made recently by the former president of this College: "Home birth is child abuse in its earliest form" (*Los Angeles Times* 1992). Earlier in this book we saw the Royal College of Obstetricians and Gynaecologists in the United Kingdom persist over many decades in trying to outlaw home birth despite the evidence of its safety. In 1991, the German Society of Obstetricians and Gynaecologists wrote to their national government demanding that all home birth be outlawed. When WHO suggested a joint meeting with the

Society, the government and WHO to discuss home birth, the German Society refused to meet.

At the local level, examples of the monolithic medical establishment's resistance to change abound. A few examples here illustrate the range and depth of resistance. When two Austrian doctors opened the first free standing birth Clinic in that country and were soon thereafter taken to court, no Austrian doctor would support them. Several leading Austrian obstetricians condemned in court some of their practices which are routine and fully accepted in many other countries. The court refused to accept testimony from outside Austria.

Hospitals in Australia, Canada, the United States have denied hospital privileges to midwives and to general practitioners who provide backup to midwives. In Australia, the United States, Canada, Germany, France, Britain, Italy, Austria, midwives and doctors who take a less technological approach, for example supporting women to have vaginal birth after caesarean section, have had a variety of sanctions applied by the local medical establishments. In Germany, local doctors have applied pressure to have the health insurance system refuse to reimburse women who have birth in alternative birth clinics.

Not only can it not be expected that the medical profession will lead the way to more appropriate perinatal technology, there is also good evidence from past events that it will resist proposed change in technology use. All too often the medical indications and scientific data are ignored and overwhelmed by non-medical factors. Thus the politics of medicine give the science of medicine short shrift. There is growing recognition of this reality. For example, health service researchers Lomas and Enkin point out:

> "In trying to understand and influence current obstetric practice we must utilize our existing limited knowledge on the determinants of clinical practice. It is clearly not good enough to assume that the publication of research results will automatically change practice patterns to match the new evidence. If inappropriate and wildly variable practice patterns are to be made more appropriate and more uniform we must pay attention to the non-medical factors that appear to

have such a powerful influence over practice patterns"
(Lomas & Enkin 1991).

The work of Lomas and Enkin and many others show that, generally speaking, peer review is not an effective means of altering technology use. Hospital review committees can occasionally be helpful
in controlling extreme incompetence among practitioners, such as
alcoholism, but are not effective in reducing inappropriate technology use.

Solutions must be found to the negative impact that litigation has on
obstetrical technology use. Nearly everything which has been written on this has taken the perspective of the doctor and his role as victim. To find solutions, we need also to focus on the perspective of
the woman who brings these law suits. Women give up much going
to the hospital to give birth but, for the most part they are willing to
do so because they have been promised that it is 'safe' there. So
when a woman has a hospital birth which involves complications or
poor outcomes, she feels deceived. It is in part the feeling of betrayal
which motivates the woman to bring the law suit to establish what
happened and to make sure that it does not happen again to someone else. The root of the feeling of betrayal are the promises of the
obstetrician for a risk free hospital birth, promises that can not in
fact be made. In some countries such as the United States, lawsuits
are also the only means many women have for securing funds to
pay for medical care that is needed as a result of medical complications. Betrayal and fear of not being able to get more medical care
drive the women's perceived need to sue.

If the woman turns to the hospital or the local health authority to
complain, she discovers she has absolutely no power and that the
complaints procedures are controlled by doctors. The main weakness of the complaint procedure in most systems is that "it leaves a
doctor (the Regional Medical Officer) to decide whether or not to
initiate a formal investigation of a complaint. Like the police, the
medical and other health professions must recognise that if they
wish to retain the public's confidence they must strengthen their
investigatory and disciplinary procedures by greater involvement
of individuals from outside their ranks. Although there is no way of
knowing for certain what effect a more open and less defensive
stance by the health professions would have on litigation, the professions should have the courage to implement complaints proce-

dures which leave them less open to charges of conspiratorial cover-up" (Chalmers 1985). Although the above statement is from the United Kingdom, it is equally applicable in nearly every country. So what alternatives are available to a woman who feels powerless and betrayed and suspects a medical cover-up? Her only recourse is to turn to the only non-doctor controlled complaints procedure which exists — the courts. If she does so, she is condemned as the source of the 'litigation problem'. This is a clear example of blaming the victim.

Understanding the woman's perspective allows us to see certain policy solutions. An interesting temporary expedient might be to encourage women to bring suit for unnecessary obstetrical intervention. In other words, instead of suing doctors because they didn't do something, doctors could be sued for doing something, for example a baby dies from respiratory distress syndrome following a repeat caesarean section in which the woman was refused the opportunity to try vaginal birth. If the woman is as likely to bring a successful suit for excess intervention as failure to intervene, it should make any obstetrician (whose fear of litigation inappropriately affects clinical judgement) think twice. But this solution only addresses issues that are symptomatic of the larger problem. Symptomatic solutions must be viewed as temporary and accompanied by more profound solutions that are directed at the underlying causes of excessive lawsuits.

There are several ways to address underlying causes of lawsuits. Doctors need to stop trying to sell themselves, the hospital and its technology as a guarantee of safety. Instead they need to help the public regain awareness of the reality that it will always be true that some babies have imperfections or die, partly because nature is not perfect and partly because doctors are not perfect. Governments need to provide adequate medical care and assistance to families with handicapped children, and no one should need to determine if anyone is 'at fault' so that they can get needed care.

New complaints procedures which are not doctor controlled need to be found and implemented. Sadly, in the past the medical profession has fought against such efforts as happened in Britain when recommendations for an improved complaints procedure were made (Committee on Hospital Complaints Procedure 1973). Denmark earlier had a non-doctor controlled complaint procedure, but recent legislation has returned the control to doctors.

The final suggestion for solving the problem of litigation as a determinant of technology use is what might be called 'community maternity care'. The idea is simple — the community is given all of the information on its own maternity services and the power to monitor and control them. This solution addresses the most important factor behind this problem: the imbalance of power between the providers of health care and the consumers of this care. This solution also addresses the unreasonable promises of obstetricians and the secretive 'club like' nature of medical practice.

If the medical establishment cannot be counted on to lead the way towards more appropriate perinatal technology, what about the public health establishment? Ministries of Health, District Health Departments, local health or medical officers are all in place, first and foremost, to protect the health of the people. While this public health establishment is much weaker than the medical establishment in nearly every country, the record indicates that, in general, they have carried out their responsibly to the people adequately with one exception. Again and again if an issue demands a confrontation with the medical establishment, the public health establishment protects the doctors rather than the people. Unfortunately, bringing control into the birth machine will demand, as we have clearly seen, that at times actions are taken which will not be popular with doctors. A few examples will illustrate how the public health establishment protects itself by protecting doctors.

Mention has already been made of how the Minister of Health in Austria asked me to provide him with the documentation as to why routine screening of every pregnant woman with ultrasound was not scientifically justified. He explained that he wanted to resist the pressure from doctors to order government subsidy of two scans. Although he received the documentation, very shortly thereafter, the subsidy for routine ultrasound scans was ordered.

When the recommendations from the conference in Fortaleza were published in the *Lancet*, the Royal College of Obstetricians and Gynaecologists in Britain complained to their Department of Health that the recommendations did not reflect British obstetric practice. The Department of Health contacted the Regional Director of WHO in Europe to complain. I was asked, together with my immediate Director, to visit the Department in London. At the meeting in London, a representative from the Royal College complained to us, and the members of the Department of Health who were present did everything possible to support the Royal College. It was only with great difficulty that we brought the discussion around to the scientific basis of the recommendations and their relevance to the women of Britain. More recently in Britain, when the Health Committee of the House of Commons held hearings on the maternity services, in preparation for drafting new recommendations, it was the Department of Health which, together with the Royal College of Obstetricians and Gynaecologists, resisted any progressive suggestions (Flint & Jenkins 1992).

WHO has had similar difficulty in engaging the support of the public health community in the United States. For example, the State of Alaska in the United States has many isolated communities with no doctors. There is also a serious shortage of midwives and little public awareness of the value of midwives in maternity care. For these reasons, the Maternal and Child Health Unit at the WHO European Office wrote to the Governor of Alaska outlining for him why WHO recommendations include the use of midwives. We also urged him to support pending legislation to strengthen midwifery in that State. Shortly thereafter, the Deputy Surgeon General of the United States Federal Government wrote to the Director General of the World Health Organisation referring to the letter to the Governor and complaining that WHO was meddling in United States internal affairs. The Director General of WHO, in turn, wrote to his Regional Director in Europe asking him not to allow such letters. The Regional Director for Europe, in turn, wrote to the Deputy Surgeon General in the United States apologising for the letter that had been sent to the Governor of Alaska. In none of the correspondence within WHO or between WHO and the United States Federal government was there a single word about the serious problems in maternity care in the United States, the large numbers of poor women who receive no prenatal care, the many doctors who refuse to give poor women maternity care, the ways in which more midwives could help, or the special needs of the women of Alaska. Many doctors and politicians in the United States are against changing the current system of maternity care. In this case, the international and national public health establishments protected themselves from criticism by invoking adherence to formal protocol and bureaucratic procedures that in fact undermined the mission of WHO to disseminate its own policy recommendations. Women's and children's health issues were quickly abandoned under pressure.

One can only hope that in the future, the public health establishment will lose its fear of the medical establishment. The potential for public health professionals to help in the reorienting of health services is enormous. Because WHO staff need not be afraid of sanctions from hospitals, professional organisations, local or national governments, they are in a unique position to promote such things as appropriate technology use and quality assurance. But the WHO staff need for their leaders to have the vision and courage to pursue the WHO mission. Hopefully the profession of public health, at the local, national and international level, will become stronger in the future.

Can we expect the scientific establishment to be part of the solution? Again, sadly, the answer, in general, must be 'no'. Scientists see their role as providing scientific facts which are reported in the scientific literature. They define themselves as 'objective', and most avoid getting involved in policy and practice, both of which require subjective decision-making. Such a stance is certainly safe and comfortable personally and professionally. But it leaves too many decisions in the hands of those who do not really grasp the scientific evidence, or who understand it too well and prefer to ignore its policy implications.

Recently, some scientists have started to apply the scientific method to evaluating medical practices, the use of medical technology and the health care system in an area referred to as health service or health systems research. Even here, many researchers do not feel that their responsibility goes beyond publication of results. This may be partly because there is resistance among doctors to the growth of this type of research. Pressure may be applied to the researcher or to the research funding agencies to stop research which may give results that are unfavourable to some doctors. In chapter 5 we described some important research results from Finland concerning the place in which prenatal care occurs (Hemminki 1990). In a separate paper, the scientists describe how this project "raised opposition from clinical experts, even though increased use of hospital services had caused financial and practical problems. Attempts to prevent our project from taking place came from ethical committees and through expert statements: this opposition changed the original study design" (Hemminki & Kojo-Austin 1989). Health service research is not for the timid or faint of heart.

Some clinicians not only try to block research but also resist the results when published. In 1992 a new journal, the International Journal of Obstetric Anaesthesia, was to be launched. The new editor asked a well known and highly respected perinatal epidemiologist and health service researcher at the National Perinatal Epidemiology Unit to review the scientific literature on the technology which is the bread and butter for this new specialty — epidural anaesthesia. The review was carried out and published in the first issue of the new journal (Howell & Chalmers 1992). The article, as quoted in chapter 6, was quite critical of the paucity of research on this technology. However, in the same issue of the new journal, an editorial stated: "We are taken to task by the [United Kingdom] National Perinatal Epidemiology Unit for having carried out so few randomised control trials of epidural analgesia in labour. The views expressed are those of the authors, the editors being only too aware that most mothers would not take kindly to receiving epidural analgesia on a random basis!" (*International Journal of Obstetric Anaesthesia* editorial 1992). Having asked for a scientific assessment, they then disassociate themselves from it.

If the solution to the inappropriate use of birth technology does not lie with the medical, public health or science establishments, where does it lie? Recent events shows that it lies with the public. Again and again, the record shows that when key members of the public become aware and fully informed of what is happening with the birth machine, they will join forces with selected doctors, midwives, public health officials, scientists and politicians to demand, and often secure, change.

In every country it is possible to find courageous and forward thinking professionals who are willing to stand up and be counted on to help promote change in the use of perinatal technology. The testimony of key obstetricians, midwives and general practitioners to the Health Committee of the House of Parliament in the United Kingdom was essential to the successful outcome with a truly progressive set of recommendations.

Within WHO, some have tried to block activities directed toward the evaluation of perinatal technology out of fear of antagonising doctors. But it was because of the complete support of the then Director General, Hafdan Mahler, and European Regional Director, Leo Kaprio, that this work began in 1979. As long as these two outstanding and fearless public health doctors were in place, the work went forward without compromise.

Scientists can also be fearless and recognise their responsibility to help bridge the gap between their results and policy and medical practice. When the editors of the new *International Journal of Obstetric Anaesthesia* disassociated themselves from the scientific review article on epidural anaesthesia in their own journal, and said that controlled research could not ethically be done on the single most important new technology in their field, the scientist who had done the review immediately wrote a letter to the *Lancet* which concluded:

> "Perhaps the reason that they (the editors of the new Journal) are so confident that women would not take part in properly controlled trials is that they and other anaesthetists are less forthcoming than they should be about disclosing evidence that epidurals may have important adverse effects. Obstetric anaesthetists give the impression that they are not living up to their responsibilities, either as researchers or as clinicians" (Chalmers 1992).

Improving perinatal technology and services also demands courageous politicians. They, too exist everywhere and, not surprisingly, are often women. In 1991 two outstanding women politicians in two state legislatures in the United States (California and Iowa) have led the way to bring more midwives and better maternity services to their States.

But the critical players in the change process are still largely consumer activists. In the consortiums that bring about change in perinatal practices, perhaps the most important of all are those who organise and lead the way for the public. In many countries, including France, Germany, Denmark, the United Kingdom, the United States, Canada, Australia, New Zealand, Switzerland, Austria, Italy, Hungary, I have been privileged to know these consumer advocates and grass roots organisers. It is they who have been the catalyst for bringing the birth machine under at least some control. Although in almost all cases they are not health professionals, they are extraordinarily knowledgable about perinatal technology and the scientific literature. Their ability to bring together disparate groups of people for a common purpose and to organise effective campaigns and public actions are extraordinary. They are the unsung heroes of the change process.

Those who want to work towards combining the best of the medical and social approaches to perinatal care must employ several strategies to succeed. First, it is essential to redefine the issues. Those who define the problem control the solution. To date, the issues have been defined by doctors. The two great enemies that doctors define are pain and death. Most of the discussions on perinatal services focus on the issue which is a favourite of the medical establishment — safety, i.e. "making sure" that the woman and baby will not die. This focus allowed doctors, for a time, to convince the public that they are the safest birth attendants and in this way maintained nearly complete control of the perinatal services. This focus, as we have seen, has backfired and had deleterious consequences. There is no such thing as a guaranteed safe birth, and promoting the concept of completely safe hospital birth has landed obstetricians in court. They are paying a big price for their control. So is society.

The other enemy of doctors is pain. Interestingly, it is doctors, not birthing women, who for many years have been talking about painless childbirth. This issue, like safety, is a double edged sword which, while attracting some women, has sooner or later lead to serious complications. For example, the last act of the epidural drama has yet to be played.

On the other hand, there are several issues in the controversies over the birth machine that are fundamental but have remained largely hidden. The first and most important is the issue of freedom. Does the woman and family have the freedom to have the experience of their choice during one of the most important events in their lives? Who has ultimate control over what happens to a woman's body? Who controls human reproduction? Who controls reproductive services? Who is responsible for the control of the care of the fetus, the newborn? Who controls the information on the birth services, on an individual's birthing? In a recent article, Stephenson (1993) discusses these questions and the role of physicians as agents of social control. The reason why discussions of home birth are always so heated is simple — in the hospital the doctor controls all of the above while in the home the family has the control. A patriarchal society, in order to control women, must control their bodies, their reproduction, their birthing. Health professionals are often agents of this control. But politicians in democratic countries recognise the importance of the freedom issue. This is why, for example, the German government would not agree to the demand of their Obstetrical Society to outlaw home birth. This is why the birth consumer groups who recognise this issue often have been successful. No one can argue against the freedom of the individual and family in such a personal matter, particularly when no compelling scientific evidence can refute its relative safety.

Another fundamental issue in birth care is equity. Equity, like freedom, is something everyone must agree to but the reality is often hard to achieve. Gender equity is a most contentious issue in birth care. While the great majority of obstetricians in the former Soviet Union are women, the great majority of professors of obstetrics are men. In every industrialised country it is men who control birth and women who give birth.

Racial equity is also an issue. Racial minorities find it difficult if not impossible to find birthing support which is consistent with their own cultural traditions: the Inuits in Canada, the Aborigines in Australia, the Gypsies in Eastern Europe, to name a few.

Economic equity is an issue that no one likes to discuss. Doctors make much more money than midwives in most countries. In Greece, obstetricians have the highest income of all doctors. Where the possibility of private practice exists, two standards of birth care exist. Even in Eastern Europe when there was no private practice, it was standard practice for a family to give a doctor an under-the-table payment in order to insure good birth care. In the United States, wealthier women get more obstetrical interventions even though they need them less than economically disadvantaged women. Current political trends toward privatisation in Eastern Europe will probably make the economic inequities of perinatal services greater than they are at present. Whether the United States will equalise access even to basic birth services remains yet to be seen. Currently some members of the public health establishment are moving to support equity, but health reform in the United Steates appears still to be dominated by vested interests.

The Regional Office for Europe of the World Health Organisation has a series of targets to reach Health for All by the Year 2000. The first target is equity. Although the countries in the Region voted in favour of this target, it is not a popular target and no country is happy with the data showing the inequities in the health status of various groups in their countries and in their health services. Equity, like freedom, usually gets only lip service. Nevertheless, efforts must be made to bring these two issues to the forefront of discussions of birth care.

Another issue, largely hidden from the public, is professional control. For 300 years doctors and midwives have been struggling for control of birthing. For over 50 years obstetricians and general practitioners have had a similar struggle. All too often in these struggles, the needs of the professional groups tend to obscure the needs of the pregnant and birthing women.

A second strategy that will be essential to bring the birth machine under control is the use of science. The importance of using science in making recommendations for perinatal technology use has already been stressed. When promoting recommendations, it is important to stress their scientific basis. Because of the gap between what is known scientifically and what is believed and practised, clinicians are often uncomfortable with recommendations which are not consistent with what they are doing. A common response is to discredit the recommendations. When this happens, their scientific basis must be emphasised.

When the recommendations from Fortaleza (see chapter 6) were published in the *Lancet* in 1985 (WHO 1985), the President of the British Royal College of Obstetricians and Gynaecologists wrote in a letter to a Director in WHO: "The guidelines used in the *Lancet* are mostly unacceptable and represent a very radical view which is not reflected in general British obstetric practice." In a more recent paper (Chalmers 1992) the scientific validity of the Fortaleza recommendations (guidelines) were compared one by one with the concluding recommendations from an important and influential book (Chalmers, Enkin & Kierse 1991) that reviewed randomised control trials of perinatal technology. The paper, which ironically appears in the *British Journal of Obstetrics and Gynaecology*, concludes: "The recommendations of WHO for appropriate technology at birth, developed through survey research, discussion and debate, are strongly endorsed by the findings of carefully controlled and critically evaluated randomised control trials". One can only hope that since 1985, British obstetric practice has evolved in the direction of the WHO recommendations that were so vigorously opposed when they first appeared.

In the future, the light of science will be turned more and more on who uses birth technology, why they use it and how to control it.

> "There is an urgent need for quantitative research on the effects of women's expectations and demand, fear of malpractice, increased use of technology, different remuneration mechanisms, the deskilling of practitioners in techniques such as vaginal breech delivery, and the training of the practitioner. In a more general sense, we need to do research to improve our understanding of the determinants of clinical policies — how they come about, what influences them, how they can be changed and the relative contributions of their various determinants" (Lomas & Enkin 1991).

The difficulties described earlier with conducting research on the system of services extends to doing research on the behaviour of those who provide the services. This area of research has been neglected, and yet is obviously necessary if we are to do what Lomas and Enkin have suggested above. It is not to be expected that providers are comfortable as research subjects. Furthermore, and probably more importantly, the perspective of providers, which locates problems in women's attitudes and behaviours, is dominant among the people and groups who control access to research funds (Macintyre 1984). "This means that it can sometimes be difficult to obtain access to service providers for research because those in control do not see the relevance of such studies" (Chalmers 1985). It will not be easy to get this essential research funded, conducted, or taken seriously in policy arenas.

Using science to promote changes in medical practices is in its infancy. So far, only the pharmaceutical companies have been really effective in modifying individual physicians' practices. Using scientific methods to measure the effectiveness of various strategies to change practices is a new idea. The basic methodology is straight forward: select a technology; measure the level of use; apply a strategy to promote change; measure any change in level of use.

A country can choose a technology which is particularly problematic for them (forceps in New Zealand, repeat caesarean section in the United States, induction in Greece) Research data on that intervention can be given to national and local health authorities, obstetrical societies (and, through them, individual practitioners), and consumer groups and the public. Profiles of desirable levels of that technology can be developed (here is where the WHO recommendations are relevant) and measured against the actual levels in local hospitals and for each practitioner. Comparisons can also be made between practitioners and with the regional, national and international levels. Then strategies for change can be selected. These will vary according to the nature of the system, local custom, etc. For example, where relevant economic incentives can be used, such as ceasing to pay obstetricians more for a caesarean section than a normal birth. Then using the chosen strategy, health authorities, practitioners and the community (through the mass media) can launch campaigns to improve the rate of use of that technology. Measuring the resultant changes in the rates will show the effectiveness of the campaigns and the chosen strategy. This method, sometimes called quality assurance, is beginning to be discussed in one form or another in a number of countries and will undoubtedly be implemented soon.

With or without the aid of scientific studies, the use of money is an important strategy for the control of the birth machine. The increasing limitations of financial resources everywhere, the increasing appreciation of the waste of money through the overuse of expensive birth technology, the decentralisation of authority for financing health services, all contribute to the strategy of using money as a carrot and/or stick for technology control. As examples, mention has already been made of: a local health authority in England may have contracts with hospitals based on rates of technology use; the State of Oregon in the United States may only reimburse those technologies with proven efficacy and cost benefit. This is also a quite new field and reaching consensus on what to cover is difficult. We can expect more creative solutions to these problems in the future.

Using the strategies described, important success have been achieved in a number of countries. A prime example is the new recommendations for maternity care in the United Kingdom. The effort involved politicians, doctors, midwives, scientists, public health professionals, consumer representatives all working together. Neither organised obstetrics nor organised public health succeeded in stopping the process. The implementation of the report will undoubtedly be long and difficult, but the way forward has been clearly defined.

The strengthening of midwives, a key element in the control of perinatal technology, is happening in many countries. The Royal College of Midwives in the United Kingdom played a strong role in the report mentioned just above. Midwives in New Zealand got organised and succeeded in having a new law passed giving them more independence. A decision in Spain to stop training midwives, after several years in effect, has been reversed, and Schools for midwives will reopen there. Physicians in Germany tried to change a law requiring a midwife at every birth. This woke up the midwives, who got organised and succeeded in keeping the law in place. A group of younger midwives in Austria wanted to organise a birth conference. They went to their midwife organisation who declined to participate. So they organised the conference anyway, knowing that if fewer than 200 of the over 1000 Austrian midwives showed up, they would be deep in debt. Over 500 midwives came from all over Austria and Germany as well.

Hopefully, these successes are on the path to an emerging solution: community maternity and perinatal care in which the community is given all of the information on its own services and the power to monitor and control them. They can use the quality assurance methods mentioned above. Thus, caesarean section rates per hospital and per clinician are available along with all other obstetrical intervention rates. The community is given the information necessary to compute their own perinatal mortality rate, low birth weight rate, etc. They can compare how they are doing with neighbouring communities. Professionals are called in to the community to present data and debate both sides of issues like home birth, routine ultrasound scanning during pregnancy, etc. All of this is fed to the local media for reporting and discussion. No decisions about services are made behind closed doors. The community decides which issues should be researched and the community has access to all research results. The community, through its representatives, has the control of the resources, financial and human, of its own perinatal services. It is the community which decides if the hospital needs a new piece of birth technology.

Such a solution is neither radical nor new. It is part of what WHO calls community participation. It was suggested by WHO in the 1970s as an essential part of primary health care. When WHO surveyed the countries, all said they have primary health care and yet not one has a system which approaches that described above. The Regional Office for Europe of WHO reasserted the importance of community participation in its targets for Health for All, put forth in the 1980s. Unfortunately, WHO itself does not always set a good example (Stephenson 1993b). In the early 1980s the European office set a policy to always invite consumers to their meetings, an essential ingredient in community participation. With a few exceptions, this policy died out through lack of continuing support from the administration.

Community maternity and perinatal care is, of course, a long range solution. But it is not fantasy. We are slowly moving in that direction. In the United States, hospital statistics are now in the public domain. In the United Kingdom, the community health council is a feeble start in this direction. The recent re-evaluation of perinatal services in Denmark and Britain involving a wide variety of input including service users is a strong step forward.

Returning to the three WHO consensus conferences and their recommendations on appropriate technology before, during and following birth, follow-up actions and reactions continue. More and more countries see birth conferences, professional meetings, action from consumer groups, and articles and programs in the mass media in which these recommendations play a part — which is the last step in the consensus process and precisely what the recommendations were meant to stimulate. Although the struggle continues between the champions of the medical and the social approaches to birth, there is more and more encouraging evidence that people are attempting to combine the best of both approaches.

Final mention can be made of one further action to promote the consensus recommendations -the writing and publishing of this book.

This has not been an easy task. At one point a publication committee at WHO Headquarters in Geneva demanded to see the book proposal. Upon review of the proposal they wrote that "the title is gratuitously aggressive and controversial" (the latter word apparently pejorative in WHO language). Nevertheless the preparation of the book continued because it is essential that all parties interested in birth and birth care know where these recommendations came from, who was involved, what scientific information was used, and how and why the recommendations and the consensus emerged. There should be no closed doors, including in WHO. Only when the wider public understands the policy-making process can the recommendations be made part of the process of ensuring the freedom of fully informed choice by individuals, family, health professionals, policy-makers and society. It is my hope that these recommendations will in fact contribute to the search for the most appropriate ways in which to use the birth machine for the optimal benefit of the woman and her baby.

References

American College of Obstetricians and Gynecologists 1984, '"Donaghue" probes views on professional liability', *Newsletter*, vol. 28, no. 8, p. 6.

British Medical Journal 1987, 'Editorial: European contrasts in obstetrics', vol. 294, p. 990.

British Medical Journal 1991, 'Editorial: Obstetric litigation', vol. 302, p. 1487.

Capstick J. B. & Edwards P. J. 1990, 'Trends in obstetric malpractice claims', *Lancet*, vol. 336, p. 931.

Chalmers B. 1992, 'WHO Appropriate Technology for Birth revisited', *British Journal of Obstet and Gynaecol*, vol. 99, pp. 709–710.

Chalmers I. 1985, 'Schizophrenia in obstetric practice: not intervening is negligence, intervening is assault', paper given in Milano, Italy.

——— 1992, 'Ethics, clinical research, and clinical practice in obstetric anaesthesia', letter to the editor, *Lancet*, vol. 339, p. 498.

Committee on Hospital Complaints Procedures 1973, *Report of the Department of Health and Social Security and Welsh Office*. H. M. Stationary Office, London.

Flint C. & Jenkins R. 1992, personal communication.

Fribourg S. 1983, 'Professional liability', *American Journal Obstet Gynecol*, vol. 146, pp. 227–228.

Hemminki E. & Kojo-Austin H. 1989, 'Problems of mutidisciplinary research in health care — the case of birth services', *Acta Sociologica*, vol. 32, no. 3, pp. 253–260.

Hemminki E., Malin M. & Kojo-Austin H. 1990, 'Prenatal care in Finland: from primary to tertiary health care?', *International Journal of Health Services*, vol. 20, no. 2, pp. 221–232.

International Journal of Obstetric Anaesthesia 1992, editorial, vol. 1, p. 59.

Lancet 1987, 'Editorial: having a baby in the United Kingdom', April 25.

Lancet 1991, 'Editorial: worried obstetricians', vol. 337, p. 1597.

Lomas J. & Enkin M. 1989, 'Variations in operative delivery rates', in *Effective Care in Pregnancy and Childbirth*, eds I. Chalmers, M. Enkin & M. Kierse, Oxford University Press, Oxford.

Los Angeles Times 1992, 'Midwives to leave home', April 28, p. E1.

MacIntyre S. 1984, 'The attitudes of obstetricians and midwives – a neglected area of study', paper presented at the Royal Society of Medicine, London.

Maternity Alliance 1983, *One birth in nine: caesarean section trends since 1978*, Maternity Alliance, London.

Oakley A. & Houd S. 1990, *Helpers in Childbirth: Midwifery Today*, Hemisphere Publishing Corp., New York.

O'Driscoll K., Carroll C. J. & Coughlan M. 1975, 'Selective induction of labour', *British Medical Journal* vol. 4, pp. 727–729.

Stephenson P. 1992, *International differences in the use of obstetrical interventions*, World Health Organisation Regional Office for Europe, Copenhagen.

Stephenson P. & Wagner M. 1993a, 'Reproductive rights and the medical care system: a plea for rational health policy', *Journal of Public Health Policy*, vol. 14, no. 2, pp. 175–182.

Stephenson P. & Wagner M. 1993b, 'WHO recommendations for invitro-fertilization: do they fit with Health for All?', *Lancet*, vol. 341, pp. 1648–9.

World Health Organisation 1985, 'Appropriate technology for birth', *Lancet*, vol. 2, pp. 436–437.

—— 1986, 'Appropriate technology following birth', *Lancet*, vol. 2, pp. 1387–8.

—— 1990, *From research to decision making: case studies on the use of health systems research*, World Health Organisation Headquarters, Geneva.

World Health Organisation consensus conference participants

[Author's note: the participants at the three WHO Consensus Conferences agreed that their titles would not be listed, to promote equality at the meetings.]

Washington DC

Partcipants from the American region (AMRO)

ARGENTINA

Amanda Elisa Pérez de Galli
Fernando Luis Leonfanti
Maria Luisa Ageitos

BARBADOS

Peggy Inniss

BRAZIL

José Galba Araújo
Anibal Faundes
Ronney B. Panerai
José Aristodemo Pinotti

CANADA

Murray Enkin

CHILE
Nelly Chang
Jorge Torres Pereyra

COLOMBIA
Jairo Barragán

CUBA
Ubaldo Farnot

GUATEMALA
Edgar Kestler

JAMAICA
Hugh Hastings Wynter

MEXICO
Samuel Karchmer

PERU
Johan Duncan Pederson

UNITED STATES OF AMERICA
Betty Berryhill
Queta Bond
Charlotte Catz
Doris Haire
Neil Holtzman
Woodie Kessel
Margaret Marshall
Brain McCarthy
Robert Sokol
Norma Swenson
Stephen B. Thacker
José Villar

URUGUAY
Roberto Caldeyro-Barcia

Participants from the European region (EURO)

CZECHOSLOVAKIA
Zdenek Stembera

GREECE
Olga Maratos

THE NETHERLANDS
J. M. L. Phaff

NORWAY
Leif Bakketeig
Per Bergsjø

SWEDEN
Göran Sterky

UNITED KINGDOM
Beverley Beech
Ann Oakley

Participants from the World Health Organisation

REGIONAL OFFICE FOR THE AMERICAS
George Alleyne
David Banta
Rubén Belitzky
Gloria Coe
Angel Gonzalo Diaz
Ricardo Horacia Fescina
Elsa Moreno
Jorge Peña Mohr
Marilyn Rice
Ricardo Schwarcz
Elbio Suarez Ojeda

REGIONAL OFFICE FOR EUROPE
Susanne Houd
Marsden Wagner

HEADQUARTERS, GENEVA
Richard Guidotti

Fortaleza

Particpants from AMRO

ARGENTINA
María Luisa Ageitos
Olga Alicia Dobner
Amanda Elisa Pérez de Galli
Gisela Rubarth

BARBADOS
Peggy Inniss

BOLIVIA
Mario Pommier

BRAZIL
José Galba Araújo
Lorena Araújo
Manuel de Carvalho
Silvio Luiz Conter
Hesio Cordeiro
Anibal Faundes
Helenice Ferraz
Humberto Gazi Lipi
María Andrea Loyola Leblond
Moyses Paciornik
Angela María Magosso Takayanagui

Joao Yunes

CANADA

Gilles Bibeau
Murray Enkin

CHILE

Nelly Chang
Francisco Mardones-Restat
Cecilia Moya
Jorge Torres Pereyra

COLOMBIA

Francisco Pardo
Sonia Pazmino de Osorio

CUBA

Ubaldo Farnot

GUATEMALA

Edgar Kestler
José Villar

JAMAICA

Carmen Bowen-Wright

PERU

Luz Marina Ponce de León

UNITED STATES OF AMERICA

José Carneirio
Doris Haire
Al Haverkamp
Linda Holmes
Barbara Janowitz
Marshal Klaus
Norma Swenson

URUGUAY
Roberto Caldeyro-Barcia

Participants from the European region (EURO)

GREECE
Olga Maratos

NORWAY
Leif Bakketeig

PORTUGAL
Maria da Puificaçao Costa Araújo

SPAIN
Isabel Alvarez Baleriola

SWEDEN
Göran Sterky

TURKEY
Ayse Akin

UNITED KINGDOM
Beverley Beech
Ann Oakley

Participants from the World Health Organisation

REGIONAL OFFICE FOR THE AMERICAS
Rubén Belitzky
Antero Coelho Neto
Tracy Enright
Ricard Horacio Fescina
Florentino García Scarponi
German E. Mora
Johan Duncan Pedersen
Alberto Pellegrini

Jorge Peña
Marilyn Rice
Carlos Serrano
Elbio Suárez Ojeda

REGIONAL OFFICE FOR EUROPE

Susanne Houd
Marsden Wagner

HEADQUARTERS, GENEVA

Richard Guidotti

Trieste

Participants from the American region (AMRO)

ARGENTINA

Luis Prudent

BRAZIL

Conceicao Segre
Maria A. Souza

CANADA

Murray Enkin

CHILE

Jorge Torres Pereyra

COLOMBIA

Edgar Rey

CUBA

Enzo Duenas

UNITED STATES OF AMERICA

Jeanne Guillemin
John Kennell
M. J. Maisels
Norma Swenson

URUGUAY

José L. Diaz-Rossello
Miguel Martel

Participants from the European region (EURO)

BULGARIA

Venelin Angelov Valov

DENMARK

Sue Shila Frening
Susanne Houd

FEDERAL REPUBLIC OF GERMANY

Eberhard Schmidt

FRANCE

Paul Vert

GREECE

Olga Maratos

ITALY

Sergio Nordio

THE NETHERLANDS

David Banta
Rineke van Daalen

PORTUGAL

Maria da Purificaçao Araújo

SPAIN
Juana Llavers

SWEDEN
Göran Sterky
Vivian Wahlberg

SWITZERLAND
Jane Cottingham

TURKEY
Ayse Akin

UNITED KINGDOM
Iain Chalmers
Shirley Goodwin
Miranda Mugford
Ian Munro
Ann Oakley
Martin Richards

USSR
A. G. Antonov
E. A. Chernukha

Participants from the World Health Organisation

REGIONAL OFFICE FOR EUROPE
J. E. Asvall
Marsden G. Wagner

REGIONAL OFFICE FOR THE AMERICAS
Jorge Peña
Ricardo Schwarcz
Carlos V. Serrano
Nestor Suarez-Ojeda

HEADQUARTERS, GENEVA

Richard Guidotti
Barbara Kwast
G. P. Mandruzzato

WHO Consensus Conference on Appropriate Technology for Birth

Fortaleza, Brazil, 22–26 April 1985

The Regional Office for Europe and the Regional Office for the Americas of the World Health Organisation held a joint Conference that was attended by over 60 participants from North and South America and Europe, representing midwives, obstetricians, paediatricians, health administrators, sociologists, psychologists, economists, and service users. The Conference made a number of recommendations based on the principle that each woman has a fundamental right to receive proper prenatal care; that the woman has a central role in all aspects of this care, including participation in the planning, carrying out and evaluation of the care; and that social, emotional and psychological factors are decisive in the understanding and implementation of proper prenatal care.

General recommendations

1. Health ministries should establish specific policies about the incorporation of technology into commercial markets and health services.
2. Countries should develop the potential to carry out co-operative surveys to evaluate birth care technology.
3. The whole community should be informed about the various procedures in birth care, to enable each woman to choose the type of birth care she prefers.

4. Women's mutual aid groups have an intrinsic value as mechanisms for social support and the transfer of knowledge, especially with relation to birth.

5. Informal perinatal care systems (including traditional birth attendants), where they exist, must coexist with the official birth care system and collaboration between them must be maintained for the benefit of the mother. such relations, when established in parallel with no concept of superiority of one system over the other, can be highly effective.

6. The training of people in birth care should aim to improve their knowledge of its social, cultural, anthropological and ethical aspects.

7. The training of professional midwives or birth attendants should be promoted. Care during normal pregnancy and birth, and following birth should be the duty of this profession.

8. Technology assessment should be multidisciplinary and involve all types of providers who use the technology, epidemiologists, social scientists, and health authorities. The women on whom the technology is used should be involved in planning the assessment as well as evaluating and disseminating the results. The results of the assessment should be fed back to all those involved in the research as well as to the communities where the research was conducted.

9. Information about birth practices in hospitals (rates of caesarean section, etc.) should be given to the public serviced by the hospitals.

10. The psychological well-being of the new mother must be ensured not only through free access to a relation of her choice during birth but also through easy visiting during the postnatal period.

11. The healthy newborn must remain with the mother, whenever both their conditions permit it. No process of observation of the healthy newborn justifies a separation from the mother.

12. The immediate beginning of breastfeeding should be promoted, even before the mother leaves the delivery room.

13. Countries with some of the lowest perinatal mortality rates in the world have caesarean rates under 10%. Clearly there is no justification in any specific region to have more than 10–15% caesarean section births.

14. There is no evidence that a caesarean section is required after a previous transverse low segment caesarean birth. Vaginal deliveries after a caesarean should normally be encouraged wherever emergency surgical capacity is available.

15. There is no evidence that routine intrapartum electronic fetal monitoring has a positive effect on the outcome of pregnancy. Electronic fetal monitoring should be carried out only in carefully selected medical cases (related to high perinatal mortality rates) and in induced labour. Countries where electronic fetal monitors and qualified staff are available should carry out investigations to select specific groups of pregnant women who might benefit from electronic fetal monitoring. Until such time as results are known, national health care services should abstain from purchasing new monitoring equipment.

16. There is no indication for pubic shaving or a predelivery enema.

17. Pregnant women should not be put in a lithotomy position during labour or delivery. They should be encouraged to walk about during labour and each woman must freely decide which position to adopt during delivery.

18. The systematic use of episiotomy is not justified. The protection of the perineum through alternative methods should be evaluated and adopted.

19. Birth should not be induced for convenience, and the induction of labour should be reserved for specific medical indications. No geographic region should have rates of induced labour over 10%.

20. During delivery, the routine administration of analgesic or anaesthetic drugs, that are not specifically required to correct or prevent a complication in delivery, should be avoided.

21. Normally rupture of the membranes is not required until a fairly late stage in the delivery. Artificial early rupture of the membranes, as a routine progress, is not scientifically justified.

Implementation of recommendations

1. Governments should identify, within the structure of their health ministries, units or departments to take charge of pro-

moting and co-ordinating the assessment of appropriate technology.

2. Funding agencies should use financial regulations to discourage the indiscriminate use of technology.

3. Obstetric care services that have critical attitudes toward technology and that have adopted an attitude of respect for the emotional, psychological and social aspects of birth care should be identified. Such services should be encouraged and the processes that have led them to their position must be studied so that they can be used as models to foster similar attitudes in other centres and to influence obstetrical views nationwide.

4. The results of the assessment of technology used in birth care should be widely disseminated, to change the behaviour of professionals and give a basis to the decisions of users and the general public.

5. Governments should consider developing regulations to permit the use of new birth technology only after adequate evaluation.

6. National and local birth conferences that include relevant health provides, health authorities, users, women's groups and the media should be promoted.

WHO Consensus Conference on Appropriate Technology following Birth

Trieste, 7–11 October 1986

Summary Report

The Regional Office for Europe and the Regional Office for the Americas of the World Health Organization held a joint Consensus Conference attended by over 40 participants from North and South America and Europe, representing obstetricians, paediatricians, health administrators, sociologists, psychologists, economists, epidemiologists, medical journalists and service users.

Certain rights are fundamental to attitudes and approaches in care following birth. For example, the right to:

(a) choice of place of birth and primary birth attendant;

(b) preservation of physical integrity and privacy for mother and child;

(c) respect for birth as a highly personal, sexual and family experience;

(d) warmth, food and shelter, especially during the first month after birth;

(e) assurance of financial support adequate for the care of the family;

(f) proper health care following birth; and

(g) protection of children from abuse and neglect.

Becoming a mother is a difficult life transition. The family and its support system of relatives and friends need to understand and be prepared for changes following birth. Health planners and workers must consider the woman's health as well as that of the baby.

The Symposium formulated the following recommendations.

Public policy

1. Poverty is the greatest threat to the health of the woman and the infant. In the absence of concerted measures to promote social equity, little improvement can be expected in maternal and infant mortality and morbidity. Mortality and morbidity rates are higher in socially disadvantaged communities, which may also receive much less in the way of formal health care. Thus (a) in the allocation of resources, nationally and locally, direct spending on health services may not be the highest priority; and (b) services for healthy women and babies should be organised so that those most in need have access to adequate care.

2. If the goal of health for all women and newborn infants is to be achieved, resources must be equitably reallocated from overall health care funds, making the care of this vulnerable group a priority.

3. The structure of health care systems and the way they operate are influenced by commercial interests and by the needs and perspective of professionals and others who work in them. When such influences are strong, they need to be publicly recognised and, if necessary, controlled.

4. The improvement of care following birth must be a collaboration between: parents; health professionals; health planners; health care administrators; other related sectors; community groups; policy-makers and politicians. Policies and mechanisms should be developed which will guide decisions about the care of women and babies — for example, multidisciplinary committees on ethics and review boards for the assessment of the care of the newborn. Communities must examine how far their attitudes and practices support or obstruct the opportunity for women and babies to receive the best available care.

5. All countries need a systematic process of health planning, including resource allocation for the care of women and babies. This process would ideally be both local and national, and it would reflect the views of a broad cross-section of professionals

and interested groups in the community. Planning for the health of women and babies must go beyond an approach based on potential risks to the physical health of the woman, fetus and newborn infant; a positive effort is called for to involve the entire society in the promotion of health.

6. The allocation of health care resources to intensive life support systems for the newborn should be determined nationally. That decision must be informed by research findings, socioeconomic factors, and moral and ethical considerations. It should be based on consultation among care providers and representatives of parents and the community as a whole. It should include the establishment of minimum standards and requirements for staffing, equipment, and the location of units for the newborn.

7. Mothers are the primary and continuing human resource available to sustain optimum infant development. They must be given general and specific practical support so that they can carry out this primary role.

8. Every woman in employment should have an adequate period of paid maternity leave before and after childbirth. Social security systems should not penalise woman for motherhood. Women should also be relieved of unpaid work after childbirth, and home help services should be available. After birth, paid leave should be provided for the father so that he can foster a relationship with the baby and support the mother.

9. Self-help groups should be promoted and funded in local communities to enable parents to meet the responsibilities of infant care. Professionals have a duty to be knowledgeable about self-help groups in the community and they should inform parents about these groups. As one example, breastfeeding support groups in the community provide a valuable form of information exchange and support among women.

10. In any country or region existing cultural practices in the period following birth should be respected and maintained — unless they have been proven harmful. Better communication between women and health workers would improve opportunities to recognise strengths of local traditions, which could then be disseminated to other women.

Health and medical services

11. For healthy women and babies, support equivalent to that provided in hospital should be made available to all mothers and babies at home.

12. If the mother desires breastfeeding, it should be initiated within the first hour after birth. Practices concerning breastfeeding should follow the resolutions adopted at the Thirty-fourth World Health Assembly in 1981.

13. All parents and newborn infants have the right to be in close contact from the time of birth. Closeness between mother and infant should be promoted in all circumstances, including the period after caesarean birth or other medical interventions affecting the woman or infant. Women and babies should not be separated and should be together as much as the mother wishes. Rooming-in should be promoted; and thought should be given to abandoning central nurseries for normal babies. Furthermore, involvement of parents in the care of the unhealthy newborn should be promoted, including the actual care of the unhealthy infant and participation in decisions about treatment.

14. Mothers and babies should not be kept in hospital beyond the time when they can benefit from further hospital diagnostic or therapeutic measures. If rest or social or educational support are needed, they should be provided in the home.

15. Health care personnel should support efficacious and safe technologies, but they should not impose them on women and families. When the desire of parents is judged to go against the good of the infant, then a formal advisory system for solving these problems must be implemented in each health care facility.

16. Iatrogenesis (harm to the woman or her infant by diagnostic or therapeutic measures) should be avoided, for example harm from treatment of jaundice in the newborn. Jaundice affects many full-term newborn infants, but the vast majority of them are healthy and do not need diagnostic investigation or treatment.

17. Since hospital-acquired infections are a major threat to women and infants, hospitals should monitor their infection rates and introduce programs for the prevention of such infections. Rooming-in rather than a central nursery can be an important

part of such a program. Early discharge of women and infants would also be a part of such programs.

18. Every baby should have its own record from the moment of birth, which may include data about pregnancy and birth. This record, or at least a copy of it, should be kept at home by the women. It would include data about growth, development, nutrition, immunisation and medical history. It can form a basis for communication among givers of health care and with the woman. The woman should also have her own health record in her home. Confidentiality of these records must be protected.

19. Resources should be allocated, both in hospital and in the community, to the follow-up of the health of the newborn infant and the woman. Ideally, personnel involved in the birth and in hospital aftercare would make the first home contact with the woman and family to inquire about their wellbeing. Every woman and baby should have the opportunity to receive community-based health care. Home-based care givers should encourage the promotion of health in the woman and her baby.

20. Home-based alternative technologies for women and babies, such as portable phototherapy for neonatal jaundice, should be developed to allow expansion of coverage to the population that lacks access to hospital care. Such innovations should be evaluated just as rigorously as complex hospital technology.

Prevention and screening

21. All women and newborn infants should receive immunisation and screening tests in accordance with the recommendations of their own countries, whether at home, in a clinic or in a hospital. Before screening of women or babies is contemplated, it must be evaluated by random controlled trials, examining not only efficacy and safety but also psychosocial costs and benefits. Each country should evaluate the relevance of particular screening procedures to its own particular needs or resources. The means of administration of vitamin K and the type of eye prophylaxis in the newborn infant need further evaluation. When indicated, immunisation with anti-D is recommended for the woman.

22. The period following birth may be an important time for making family planning advice and services available to both parents. The person giving such information to women should be

someone in whom they have confidence. In many contexts, the best person will be a nurse or midwife. Information should be given on a variety of contraceptive techniques, so that women can make informed choices.

23. The eradication of neonatal tetanus is a high priority.

24. Low birth weight, which correlates strongly with both perinatal mortality and morbidity, should receive high priority for research into causes and prevention. Meanwhile, however, some actions seem to reduce the incidence of low birth weight and other causes of perinatal mortality and morbidity. Services should be developed with such actions in mind and the public should be fully informed of the reasons for and importance of these actions, which include: family planning (to avoid a large number of children and too short intervals between children); prenatal care to identify possible risks to the fetus and women and treat any diseases or conditions developing during pregnancy; nutritional and social support during pregnancy; avoidance of cigarettes, alcohol and drugs during pregnancy; and appropriate care during labour and delivery.

Routine care

25. Every woman and infant should have access to a basic level of care regardless of whether the birth takes place at home or in a primary or secondary health care setting. At every birth, wherever it takes place, one attendant should take overall responsibility for the woman and infant.

26. Government agencies should support the provision of health care by alternative providers, such as empirical midwives. The role and efficacy of these alternative providers should be systematically evaluated.

27. Every woman should receive basic care immediately following birth. In those parts of the world where haemorrhage, infection and pregnancy-induced hypertension are important causes of maternal mortality and morbidity, every effort should be made to provide effective treatment and to prevent long-term sequelae. An effective referral system is necessary for the woman when complications arise during pregnancy, birth, or the period following birth. Such a system must include free transport where necessary.

28. A first priority is that every newborn baby, whether born at home or in hospital, should be assessed for breathing difficulties and be given the necessary support to initiate and sustain respiration. Every birth attendant should be trained in and equipped to deal with immediate care and resuscitation of the newborn, including identification of the need for consultation or referral to more specialised care.

29. Every newborn baby should be evaluated initially for vital signs and gross congenital abnormalities. Evaluations should take place next to the mother if possible, in a room at the right temperature and without hazard to baby or woman.

30. Discharge from hospital should depend on the wellbeing of the mother and infant, the wishes of the parents, and the availability of home support. In particular, discharge policies should not be based on the single criterion of weight and should concentrate on earliest possible discharge.

Unhealthy infants

31. Staff in every special care unit for the newborn must be aware of the wishes and attitudes of the community it serves. Communication with the community is vital. Policies of special care units must be consistent with the community's values.

32. Parents have the right to early active involvement in the care of their unhealthy infant: early and free visits to the special infant care unit; encouragement of feeding and skin-to-skin contact, whether or not the infant is connected to monitoring systems; facilities where parents can live while the infant is in special care; and participation in decisions regarding diagnosis and treatment.

33. Low birth weight is both a risk factor and a social indicator. A decision to refer a low birth weight infant for care in another unit should take account not only of the infant's condition and the ability to care for him or her locally, but also the need to avoid separation of families.

34. A woman who becomes seriously ill during pregnancy or labour or whose fetus is endangered should be provided with an appropriate level of care, ideally before birth. Transport must also be available for every unhealthy infant who needs care elsewhere. Vehicles for the transport of infants should be equipped

with the basic means of maintaining body temperature and supporting respiration. If she wishes, the woman should be able to accompany her infant. A referral network must be established and understood by all concerned. The infant should be accompanied by the record prepared by the primary care provider. Communication between the different levels of care is important.

35. All countries should develop criteria by which to determine whether or not certain treatments for the newborn should be regarded as experimental. Examples of 'experimental' treatment, in present circumstances, include the management of extremely premature infants and serious congenital defects. Guidelines should be formulated for the selection of infants for whom maximum intensive care and surgery are justified. The possibility of short- and long-term negative consequences of such treatment should be fully communicated to the parents.

36. Ideally, unhealthy infants requiring intensive care receive it in special units within maternity hospitals. In these units, paediatric and specialised nursing staff should be on duty 24 hours a day. The minimum acceptable facilities for life support, including biochemical tests and radiology, should be available. No institution providing tertiary care should be permitted to refuse to accept a case presenting at their facility, at least for assessment, stabilisation and referral.

Research

37. Most research on women following birth and on infants has focused on clinical management. Priority should now be given to research on: the organisation and overall content of services; preventative services; assessing the appropriate use of technologies; and the long-term future of women and infants. This research should include surveys of the view of parents and the community.

38. Any technology used in care following birth should undergo evaluation before its introduction for general use. Such evaluation should include efficacy and safety, economic implications, and cultural acceptability. The results of technology assessment should be widely disseminated to professionals and the general public. WHO should continue to promote and expand a network

of technology assessment centres to assist countries in selecting new technologies and assessing them. This network will constitute a focal point for the dissemination of information.

39. All research should use the strongest possible design. In the assessment of any technology, this design is a randomised controlled trial, probably a multi-centre collaborative trial that can achieve adequate sample size. Community-based research, organised by community groups and assisted by relevant experts, should be encouraged.

40. In improving care following birth research on the services themselves, including relevant social science research, can help to change both individual practices and policy. This type of research lacks funding and institutional support now enjoyed by biomedical research. Health workers should be encourage to inquire into their own performance with the support of a competent team with expertise in study design, analysis of data, and dissemination of results.

41. Two areas of research needing high priority are: fetal growth and its retardation and the prevention of low birth weight infants; and health problems in the woman following birth, including postpartum depression.

42. Care following birth should be evaluated on a population as well as in an institution. The basic requirements are knowledge of: the population for whom care is being provided; the services available for unhealthy women and unhealthy newborn infants; which women and which infants receive what kinds of service and their outcomes, including mortality and short- and long-term morbidity; the satisfaction of the parents with the services and the satisfaction of those who work in the services; and the financial costs. This evaluation should be done in the context of overall evaluation of perinatal care.

43. All governments should appoint a broad-based representative committee, including health care providers and the users of health care, to establish guidelines and recommendations for the care of mothers and infants. These guidelines should be based on a continuing evaluation system and should be widely distributed and frequently revised. Such guidelines should include minimum standards for equipment and care practices following birth.

44. All countries should make an effort to improve perinatal records. Birth and death certificates should include birth weight, and they should be linked whenever possible. A good statistical system is essential, beginning with registration of all births and deaths. Permanent perinatal surveillance systems are needed at the national level.

Education and training

45. For staff working in hospitals or home health services, initial and inservice training should be based on the needs of women and babies and be linked to local services, so that training is realistic and relevant. Training should include that ability to conduct research and/or interpret research findings. All professionals should receive the lists of relevant random controlled studies. Training of all health care staff should make them aware of the stresses and anxieties that both care receivers and givers may undergo.

46. Those working in special care units face infants with severe illness, handicap, and often death, so they must be oriented to the implications of such stresses and how to cope with them, and they should receive emotional support. Regarding breastfeeding, special attention must be given to the training and practices of health professionals who come in contract with women in the postpartum period. Contradictory advice must be avoided. The practice of giving food other than milk during the first months is to be discouraged.

47. WHO should be active in ensuring that appropriate courses in public health, with special emphasis on maternal and child health, are taught at universities and schools of medicine, nursing and midwifery.

Public information and the media

48. In societies where young people have little opportunity to learn about childbirth, infant care and the responsibilities of parenthood, education is need to prepare them for these experiences.

49. Information about the period following birth which is accurate, clear, attractively presented, of high quality and consistent

should be disseminated widely to parents, schoolchildren, teachers, health professionals and politicians.

50. WHO and its regional offices should institute a regular programme of meetings with journalists, media and public relations leaders, and editors of professional journals to familiarise them with the recommendations of WHO meetings and other issues affecting maternal and child health. WHO should promote the implementation of the recommendations of the Trieste meeting and the two earlier meetings.

WHO report on health promotion and birth

Prepared by the North American and European consulting groups (combined consensus, 1986)

Introduction

In September 1985, the European Regional Office of the World Health Organisation held a four-day meeting to attempt to apply the principles of health promotion to the field of childbearing in North America. A year later a similar meeting was held in Berlin, West, Federal Republic Germany, to explore the applicability of these strategies to the European situation.

Many of the participants at the two conferences were or had been childbirth practitioners or maternity care activists in North America or Europe. Others were experienced Health Promotion professionals. While acknowledging some difficulties, all were convinced that maternity care represented a nearly ideal issue with which to test health promotion theory.

Making childbearing a priority will challenge health promotion strategists, who have tended to focus on preventing such problems as drunken driving or smoking. Childbearing, as a normal physiological process which (past a certain point) no-one would want to prevent, is a much more complex area. The consulting groups could have applied a more traditional approach, concentrating on individual risk reduction behaviours. They could have recommended merely intensifying present strategies through more pre-conception care, for example, or increasing technical screening techniques in pregnancy, and the further enhancement of anti-smoking, anti-drinking and rubella immunisation programs for pregnant women. However, it was precisely the limitations and potential dangers of such conventional strategies which prompted a critique of health education, and provoked development of the more comprehensive analysis of health promotion.

Based on these analysis, the issue of childbearing will demand particularly ingenious and far-reaching strategies. Indeed, current cornerstones of modern maternity care are incompatible with a health promotive approach, specifically:

- the suppression, subordination or elimination of the midwifery profession;
- reliance on routine (yet highly variable) medically directed ante-natal care;
- increasing fragmentation of care (from one phase of childbearing, or from one part of the maternity service to another);
- encouragement of women's dependency on the medical profession;
- nearly total hospitalisation for birth itself;
- escalation of screening technologies during pregnancy, and technological/surgical interventions during pregnancy and birth.

Giving birth represents a special form of initiation into a society's beliefs and practices surrounding health and illness, life and death. Since women are the health care providers for more than three quarters of family illnesses, their perceptions and experiences affect everyone powerfully. An undermining experience of birth contributes to a woman's dependence on doctors, hospitals, and pharmacological remedies, both for herself and her family.

Women's dependence on doctors and the increase in interventions have further defined childbearing as a medical event. This medicalisation of childbirth has been an effective means to a more pervasive medicalisation of society as a whole. By now, North American society and much of Europe have invested heavily in this belief system.

Since such powerful rituals are associated with birth, death and mating in all societies, any efforts to alter the accustomed way of birth may represent a profound threat to the established order.

For these and other reasons, there is likely to be powerful opposition to health promotion approaches to childbearing; doctors in general and obstetricians in particular may become vigorous opponents of most of the fundamental tactics which the consulting groups believe to be essential to the success of these strategies.

Despite these difficulties, the centrality of childbearing also means that strategies which affect it may alter society's overall health beliefs and behaviours, in the direction of health promotion, in the long run. For example, an affirming childbirth experience may so strengthen a woman's confidence that she is better able to question invasive interventions when coping with a child's, or another family member's illnesses. Reliance on drugs as a means of dealing with life's normal stresses may seem less attractive, and may therefore be less likely to become part of her child's repertoire of coping behaviours.

The recommendations which follow represent the combined consensus of the two consulting groups. They are designed to be applied as an integrated whole, not selectively.

Statement of intent

Childbearing issues involve fundamental human and civil rights, which should be inviolable. Specifically, these are women's rights to:

- Complete information regarding all aspects of care, both self-care and health and medical care options;
- Choice of place of birth, as well as of caregiver and birth attendants, including supportive friends and/or relatives;
- Privacy during all caregiving activities;
- Choice about which, if any, interventions to accept;
- Experience birth as a highly personal, sexual, family event;
- Sustain the mother-child relationship throughout the post-birth period, without fear of separation.

We urge all governmental and private bodies concerned with human rights in all countries to include an examination of the conditions under which childbearing takes place as one index of any nation's, or indigenous people's, civil and human rights.

The following fundamental principles intend to locate autonomy, authority, and the definition of the need in the childbearing woman and her family, and in their community, rather than in the professional community or in the state. At the same time the state will have a key role in enabling and strengthening the initiative of communities by making certain that the needed resources are available, whether it be technical support, national data or funding.

Thus the overall strategy is to work both from the bottom up and the top down, pincer- fashion.

Fundamental principles of health promotion in childbearing

1. Certain rights and supports for women are indispensable in any health promotive approach to childbearing: adequate housing; nutrition; health care and medical services; job security; safe working conditions; and maternity leave. Protection of such rights for women must also be acknowledged as one dimension of the rights of children.
2. Implicit in the health promotion approach is the adoption of a social model of childbearing, which recognises birth as a healthy life event. This model would replace the medical or risk model which emphasises the pathological, separating women into isolated categories, and may quite often become counterproductive through iatrogenesis, creating the very problems the medical profession hoped to avoid.
3. A further dimension of the replacement of the medical model with the social model of childbearing involves a new understanding of death and disability as possible outcomes of any pregnancy in any setting. Specific recognition, discussion and acceptance of these facts are an integral part of the health promotion approach.
4. The social model of childbearing also gives equal value to both personal experience and more quantitative information as the

basis for education, decision-making and practice. A social model recognises the interplay between society, individuals and their environment, and consequently gives priority to prevention over intervention and to community action over routine medical initiatives.

5. Childbearing women in each local community are the best resource to develop programs which will meet their own needs. Governments should secure the necessary funding, technical support and data for planning groups at the community level.

6. Midwives are the most cost effective and appropriate primary care givers for all childbearing women in all instances and in all settings. Member states should aim for full utilisation of midwifery care for all women, throughout pregnancy, labour and delivery, and the postpartum period. Continuity of care should be sustained.

7. Home is the most appropriate birth setting for most childbearing women. Women (and their birth attendant) choosing this options must be provided with necessary diagnostic, consultative, emergency and other services as required, regardless of the place of birth.

8. Member states are also encouraged to develop community-controlled, out-of- hospital birth centres where midwives may offer comparable services to women seeking an alternative to the home setting. Such centres would also be provided with the appropriate supports described above.

General Recommendations

Basic Strategies

COALITION BUILDING AND INTERNATIONAL NETWORKING

Making the childbearing experience an empowering one requires health promotion policies which provide resources for citizen groups, for public interest initiatives and for coalition-building among organisations working in this field. Member states also need to support the development of national and international networks of such organisations for the purposes of information sharing and dissemination, as well as mutual support.

To reach this goal an established percentage of a country's public resources should be assigned to the development of health promotion programs, giving specific attention to childbearing.

PUBLIC HEALTH INTEREST GROUPS AND SPECIAL TASKS

1. A proportion of funds thus allocated should be used for the development and technical support of a public interest council on childbearing, to be composed of groups and individuals with relevant skills and a commitment to improving childbearing for all women. A majority of the council's members should be women with no financial, professional or personal interest in the medical profession or health industries. Council members would be drawn representatively from all ethnic, racial and economic strata. Among the Council's functions would be public advocacy, networking, and the collection and dissemination of all information relevant to childbearing. This would include:

    *   comparative information regarding birthing services and procedures in different areas (from medical and surgical intervention rates to the quality and continuity of care);
    *   information about side effects of medical procedures from the viewpoint of both morbidity and mortality, both short and long term.

2. Also included in this policy would be the identification and funding of certain other new or existing national or international organisations, which may carry out specific tasks required by this approach to birthing. (Specific data collection or communication tasks, for example.)

    The councils would be, in effect, forums for policy promulgation. They would commission studies designed to examine and verify the assumptions underlying conventional practices or proposed new policies, and would also assist the community to identify its needs or raise issues of concern to it.

    Ideally, a member state's council would be representative in the sense that it would also reflect regional public interest councils organised for similar purposes. Given the local nature of the health promotion approach in general, and the frequently highly regional nature of birthing practices in particular, some mechanism of this kind would be ideal and perhaps should be stressed, even though it is understood that member states must develop their own techniques for implementation.

Other national or international organisations would take on specialised tasks suited to their missions or capabilities in order to facilitate, for example, communication among midwives, information-sharing about community groups, or reporting on the impact of Western birth technology on women in the Third World.

Public education and information

MEDIA

Broad-based media councils should be established to monitor the mass media's portrayal of pregnancy and birth, and for generating timely, high quality information on pregnancy and birth. This information would be disseminated to all science and general programming media writers and producers. Such councils would be made up primarily of individuals who can reflect a public interest perspective, as specified above, and would be accountable to public interest councils as well as to the general public.

Radio and television producers, and even science and medical writers are often, on questions of childbearing, frequently unaware of the often biased nature of information presented by some health professionals, or of the scientific validity of much information presented by community and public interest groups. As a result of the creation of media councils, the media would no longer be as dependent on existing special interest group information from professional medical organisations and could become more accurate in its portrayals of birth.

Currently, health organisations in may countries have established media committees with a common intent to influence current media programming.

PUBLIC EDUCATION

Educational programs for the general public which highlight birth as a normal life event are the primary component of the health promotion approach to childbearing. Comprehensive national and local data on childbearing medical procedures and practices, and women's experiences of these, as collected by the public interest councils described in the previous section, should be freely accessible to childbearing women and community planning groups.

Organisations creating such education programs should receive generous financial and technical support from public resources.

DEATH AWARENESS

Comprehensive health promotion programs for the general public, for children and young people, and for pregnant women and their families, will include a new attitude toward death and disability, namely, the recognition that they are possible outcomes of any pregnancy in any setting.

Included in this awareness is the knowledge that the fear of death may also lead to the inappropriate use of technology, which may both distort the birthing experience and also contribute to iatrogenic damage.

Public education programs are designed to bring a much higher level of awareness about childbearing to every level of society. In general, information about rates of medical interventions, the nature of the birth process, the skills of different practitioners, and the factors associated with specific birth outcomes have not been accessible to the average childbearing woman or her family. Public knowledge on these issues has been almost totally controlled and dominated by professional medical societies, who have selectively presented biased information to news media, departments of public health, and the general public, virtually without challenge.

Their information has focused on mortality, and the risk of death — to either the mother or the baby. In the public imagination, the type of conventional, high-technology care now available is seen as a necessary price to pay in order to avoid death, and any questioning or criticism evokes the suggestion that a woman is either negligent or foolhardy. She is thus willing to undergo any intervention in order not to be seen as willing to risk her infant's life. The fear of death has thus taken on a paramount importance, not only as a reality, but as a moral and legal issue.

Most biologists acknowledge that about 3% of any population group will have unpreventable death associated with reproduction. There are many other situations where no intervention could have prevented a fetal or newborn death. At the same time, doctors, women and families are virtually without preparation for death as one possible complication of any childbirth. Faith in the modern hospital is so great that a death in this setting is usually assumed to be inevitable, whereas in other settings deaths at birth immediately are assumed to be due to negligence or incompetence.

Medical personnel in general have distorted notions about death and their role in relation to it; and although many training programs do now make token efforts to address the issue, this work has focused almost entirely around terminally ill and aging adults with chronic diseases, and hardly at all on birthing.

CHILDBEARING EDUCATION FOR CHILDREN AND YOUTH

Educational programs for children and young people which emphasise and integrate and human childbirth experience as a healthy life event must be developed. Member states should provide long term financial and other support to those groups initiating such curricula.

Education of children on the subject of birth and sexuality is not widespread in public schools, despite the existence of a few excellent human sexuality programs, most of which focus on sexuality alone or as a context for birth control, and not on childbirth itself. While it is currently very fashionable in some countries to teach children about birth through exposing them to the birthing processes of animals, these efforts are not substitutes for discussions of human birth.

While in many communities childbirth reform groups have been able to present lectures or programs about birth to schoolchildren, in some communities they have been absolutely prevented from doing so, either by pressure from the local medical community, or from school authorities fearful of criticism for allowing the viewpoint of a 'pressure group', or from other groups who disapprove of nakedness or other exposure of the reality of a normal birth.

Thus most women, by the time they come to their own birthing experience are poorly prepared to raise the necessary questions or to challenge medical authority. Preparation for this moment must begin much earlier in life.

CHILDBEARING EDUCATION FOR PREGNANT WOMEN

Community-based development of public-interest programs of education and preparation for pregnancy for women and their partners, as desired, should be encourage, and the incentives and resources provided to bring such programs about. They would be designed to liberate women's potential for mutual support and information sharing as well as to reinforce and enhance the validity of self-help ante-natal care.

There is a history of efforts by both parents and professionals to change childbearing practices in many countries. This history and these issues need to be part of every form of preparation of pregnant women, couples and families for birth. Such childbirth programs would draw upon the work of the public interest councils for information and resources in assisting women planning their births to make fully informed decisions. Such childbearing education programs could also include self-help/mutual support forms of education and care during the pregnancy period, in the form of drop-in centres or study groups, but with the principles of outreach built in, so that pregnant women, who are sometimes the least able to do so, are not always forced to reach out themselves to seek information or caring and supportive concern but may expect it will come to them.

People who have a public interest perspective, who are drawn by and from the community and trained by local public interest groups, in the spirit of the basic principles, need only be available as guides and facilitators for the spontaneous initiative of most childbearing women. They will also know how to draw out those women who need support but have difficulty asking for it.

Public policy

INTERSECTORAL CO-ORDINATION

Thorough intersectoral co-ordination among all relevant social resources and benefits, such as housing, income maintenance, home-making services, parental leave, education, etc. — and between these types of social services and essential health, medical and dental care services — is essential for any effective health promotion program focusing on childbearing.

If the intersectoral challenge were fully met, governments should guarantee full nutritional supports to every woman, and benefits for each pregnancy. Health benefits, such as free dental and medical care would cover all pregnant women and their children from the beginning of pregnancy to the child's first birthday, including medical care for at least the childbearing year (three months postpartum) and the nine months following (the infant's first year of life).

Since education is the single investment most likely to guarantee better birth outcomes, and also job security, any programs which provide educational support are likely to be worth it, for pregnant teenagers or women with children who are receiving various forms of unemployment/social benefits.

REMOVING BARRIERS TO ACCESS TO: INFORMED CHOICE OF PLACE OF BIRTH AND BIRTH ATTENDANT

As a cornerstone of the health promotion approach, women must be guaranteed that all legislative, regulatory, professional and institutional supports necessary will be available to ensure that a woman can choose her preferred birth setting — home, birth centre or institution. This guarantee also implies her free choice of the primary care attendant she desires, who will provide the needed continuity.

The rights of women and families to make these choices freely also implies that the concept of ultimate medical responsibility will be redefined in the health promotion approach as a shared commitment between the woman and her primary care attendant. Medical responsibility means that physicians and institutional back-up must be provided on request of the women and/or her primary care attendant.

In order to protect the rights of women and families to make these choices freely, all criminal penalties to either the families or birth attendants resulting from the exercise to these rights and choices must be removed.

To insure the choice of attendant, every midwife shall be paid in a equitable manner consistent with the skills and responsibility demanded by her services.

Barriers to choice of place of birth and primary care attendants vary from country to country. Current laws against midwifery in North America represent a legacy of prejudice from earlier generations of lawmakers, a prejudice which was fomented by prominent physicians who claimed to represent 'scientific medicine'. Without scientific evidence, they lobbied successfully for the outlawing of midwifery. As a result, midwives currently practising in North America are often subjected to entrapment, lawsuits and criminal proceedings, and in some cases, prison. Midwives may lose their licences if they perform home births, and may be denied hospital privileges. Women having home births are often denied obstetric or paediatric services if they need them.

In other countries, such as the United Kingdom, midwives are accepted, but women still have no choice as to who their midwife will be, as they are often on rotation systems of more than ten midwives. Home birth, while a legal choice, it made almost impossible.

While these impediments to choice still exist, it is impossible to determine the extent of women's and families' needs. No such program as the consulting groups are proposing could begin until these barriers are removed. Similarly, we have no reliable index of how high the demands for midwifery training programs would go if these barriers did not exist.

HOME BIRTH BENEFIT PACKAGE

The notion of birth as a healthy life event should lead to recognition of the childbearing woman's home as the most appropriate birthing setting.

For those women who choose birth at home or in a birth centre, new service benefits should be provided which are comparable with those who choose or require hospital birth. These services should include: midwifery with adequate medical and institutional back-up; education and care throughout pregnancy, intrapartum and postpartum periods, and additional social supports as may be needed, for example, home and family support services during the perinatal period.

The Netherlands, with perinatal mortality and morbidity statistics comparable to their neighbouring countries, has never had fewer than one third of all births at home, and the percent of home births has increased steadily the past seven years to the percent level of 40%. In some areas of Denmark, close to ten percent of births are at home and the 1986 revised national perinatal guidelines promote increasing numbers of home births. The evidence in Western Europe suggests that the trend to hospital birth has probably peaked and a counter-trend to out-of-hospital birth is beginning.

PERSONNEL POLITICS

Obstetricians should not be responsible for primary care in child-bearing. This means that in some countries there should be a significant reduction in the production of obstetricians and a comparable rise in the number of midwives trained and/or employed, so that the midwives are fully available to the entire population of child-bearing women.

DE-LICENSING/CERTIFICATION, AND REDRESS OF GRIEVANCES

Member states are urged to abandon conventional procedures giving exclusive rights to practice (such as licensing). In its place there should be peer-directed programs which certify a certain level of competency. Periodic review and evaluation of the qualifications of these practitioners by their own professional members must be a mandatory feature of all certification programs. Information about these qualifications and limitations would be available to the community and to individuals seeking the services of a given practitioner.

Member states are also urged to build in non-adversarial mechanisms for the redress of grievances by clients of certified practitioners.

We urge the abandonment of existing structures of professional licensure since the present system apparently serves primarily to protect the economic interests of professionals, and offers little to the public in the way of accountability.

Certification, on the other hand, may create a place for public accountability, if quality review is built in at the same time, and if, in line with the principles of community control outlines in the basic principles above, members of the community participate actively in the process of certification and review.

A central feature of the new certification programs would become grievance procedures, whereby clients of certified health workers may present complains, receive a fair hearing and expect redress where appropriate. Community representatives will also assist in the development of equitable grievance procedures designed to deal openly and fairly with complaints and malpractice, as the case may be.

Professional and higher eduction

PROFESSIONAL TRAINING

The curricula for the education of all health professionals should reflect the role of the midwife as primary caregiver in maternity care, and the preferred location for most births as settings outside the hospital, either home or birthing centre.

The present systems of professional training for health workers involved with birthing has established medical knowledge and philosophy, and the hospital milieu, as the standard by which all care in childbirth should be judged. As a result, students in the health professions do not have any sense of how to value appropriately the training and unique skills of midwives; nor are they adequately informed about the advantages of out-of-hospital settings for birth.

To remedy this situation, future medical education programs should require full understanding of the breadth and depth of midwifery as an art in its own right in the provision of primary care services, and the recognition that maternity care is ideally a form of primary care.

Special training is needed for health workers to realise why the tertiary care setting is the least appropriate for the basic training of midwives, and why the hospital is therefore an equally inappropriate setting for physicians to learn about normal childbirth.

MIDWIFERY TRAINING AND CONTINUING EDUCATION

Out-of-hospital birth settings should be implemented and maintained as the basic standard for all midwifery education and training programs, whether primary or continuing education. These programs must also equip the midwife to provide appropriate care in a hospital setting.

Midwifery training in hospitals has significantly eroded the confidence and skills of many midwives to manage normal births. This type of training has also eroded the confidence of women who give birth in hospitals, who often feel that their bodies are not to be trusted.

Many midwives are now as dependent on hospital technology as their physician counterparts, and in fact may feel that they best demonstrate their competence through managing births according to physician standards. Only out-of-hospital birth attending can sharpen midwives' much needed skills so as to give women the confidence they need.

Knowledge building

KNOWLEDGE REVIEW

A research approach whose results will be made available fully to the public must be developed. The data available from such research must be of sufficient quantity and quality that valid and equitable policies and regulations concerning childbearing women and their families can be promulgated; and that this research approach will correct existing biases in research priorities and strategies of data collection, including the almost total lack of qualitative and interdisciplinary information.

INTERNATIONAL STANDARDS

An internationally comparable standard childbirth data classification system should be established as a basis for monitoring and comparing national experience with the major medical intervention rates and the major iatrogenic diseases associated with childbearing, both short and long term.

Member states should begin reporting regularly these data, as an integral part of their national health status reports.

As part of a larger strategy to begin shifting the balance toward the health promotion approach to birth, it will become necessary to change the character of the flow of information available to both professionals and to the general public. Nothing less than a complete review and re-examination of existing research priorities will reveal the extent to which changes will be needed.

For too many years public health researchers have been satisfied with crude health indicators like mortality, yet even these have not been kept in a way that is internationally comparable. At the very least, these data should be reorganised to serve not only the efforts to locate serious problems, but also how to identify those practices which are clearly health promoting. Specifically, we need a whole new index of morbidity, so that we do not congratulate ourselves on short terms gains at the expense of long-term problems.

Chief among the lacunae are those reports which have been labelled increasingly by medicine as 'anecdotal', and rejected out of hand. Specifically, significant efforts need to be made to bring personal experience into the mainstream, as one method for acknowledging that these experiences are, in fact, 'data', and a rich source of legitimate knowledge on which to base action, policy and plans for the future.

Glossary

Accountability   The notion that taking on a particular responsibility involving the needs and welfare of the general public or of certain individuals, particularly (but not only) when public funds are involved in providing the services, also requires a more or less public report or accounting of how that responsibility is being discharged, apart from the reporting that would be expected normally to superiors, colleagues or professional societies. Many people believe that the very large public expenditures for medical care and medical education require accountability.

Advocacy   Active, supportive representation of the interests, issues and/or needs of an individual or specific group by another, usually private, individual or group before the public or before a particular agency or organisation. This is not to be confused with legal representation, and is not necessarily the same activity carried out by publicly elected representatives.

Childbearing   Refers to the continuum of experience and activity which begins with pregnancy and ends, roughly, at the end of the first three months of the infant's life, sometimes called the 'childbearing year' (may refer to women or families). In some contexts the term 'birthing' may be used to refer to childbearing but may in fact be confused with the process of labour and birth.

Coalition A formal or informal, temporary or permanent linkage of separate organisations which have different identities, purposes or memberships, who have come together into a single entity for one or more common purposes.

Continuity of care Refers to the concept that, ideally, childbearing women and their families should be cared for by the same person, or small team of persons, throughout pregnancy, labour, birth and the post-birth period. The origin of this concept is the conviction that fragmented care, given by different practitioners in different settings during these four medically defined intervals during the childbearing year, contributes to women's inability to obtain the cumulative, sustained psychological support recognised as necessary to sustain optimum well-being and the best outcomes during this sensitive period; and that such fragmentation may actually increase the likelihood of complications being overlooked or even induced through gaps in observation or communication by caregivers.

Family Refers to an irreducible unit of mother and baby, which may also include a chosen family of friends, or other family members such as siblings, father, grandparents and other extended family members.

Iatrogenesis The causation of unintended illness (short- or long-term) or death, either directly — through the application of health and medical care by practitioners — or indirectly — through the organisation, functioning or requirements of established health programs or practices.

Medicalisation Describes the process by which everyday life events or normal conditions of life and being are transformed into medical problems, subjected to medical controls and definitions, which an emphasis on risk, pathology and therapeutic intervention or management.

Networking Generally, personal, informal passing on of contacts and resources (individuals, groups, services, campaigns, literature sources or other networks), to others to facilitate their efforts on a particular issue.

Outreach   Initiatives to locate and contact people in the community who may be in need of services or who have been recipients of services, in order to inquire about their well- being or needs, and if desired, to provide assistance. The classic origin of this concept is, in fact, the midwife who was located in a particular community or district and initiated visits to women of childbearing age to help then recognise pregnancy and plan for birth. Traditional midwives in developed countries and Western midwives before the modern period also provided many other services concerned with fertility and reproduction.

Primary care   Refers to the concepts and practices derived from Alma Ata (WHO, 1978) which locate basic, essential, health and medical care services in the community, accessible to local residents and in co-operation with community representatives. Ideally, such care presumes a planned system, with a strong preventive component and practitioners with a generalist perspective, capable of treating simple illnesses or conditions and able to recognise and refer more complex problems. In this context primary care does *not* refer to the first provider in the caregiving system to see the client, regardless of training or setting.

Public interest   A specific perspective developed from the expressed needs and interests of both:

- citizens and taxpayers who contribute to and/or support the deployment of public funds for health and medical care services, education or research; and
- users, clients or consumers of direct health and medical care services (whether or not they actually pay for such services).

Special interest   A specific perspective developed from the expressed needs and interests of:

- providers of direct services who derive their income from the delivery of health and medical care;
- commercial and industrial interests whose products or services are used by consumers and/or providers;
- non-profit, private societies whose purpose is to promote the interests, income or political control of providers or commercial entities.

Resolution on a Charter on the rights of women in childbirth

The European Parliament,

- having regard to the motion for a resolution by Mrs Squarcial-upi, Mrs Cinciari Rodano and Mrs Trupia (Doc. B2–712/86),
- having regard to the motion for a resolution by Ms Tongue and Mr Loman (Doc B2–23/86),
- having regard to the Council Directive of 11 December 1986 on the application of the principle of equal treatment between men and women engaged in . . . a self-employed capacity and on the protection of self-employed women during pregnancy and motherhood (OJ No L 395, 19.12.1986),
- having regard to the proposal for a Council Directive on the approximation of the laws of the Member States relating to infant formulae and follow-up milks of 4 January 1985 (OJ No C 28/3, 30.1.1985)
- having regard to the communication from the Commission on toxic substances in breast milk (COM(86) 197 final),
- having regard to the resolution of the European Parliament of 16 April 1986 (OJ No C 120/49-51, 20.5.1986) embodying the opinion and closing the procedures for consultation of the European Parliament on the above proposal for a directive,
- having regard to ILO Convention NO 103 of 7 September 1955 on the protection of women during motherhood,
- having regard to the study by Mrs Dagmar Coester-Waltjen on the protection of working women during pregnancy and motherhood in the Member States (V–1829/84),
- having regard to the report by the Committee on Women's Rights (Doc. A2–38/88),

a. aware of the efforts made by the Commission of the European Communities to help women lead their lives under the best possible conditions,

b. whereas the ways of approaching childbirth and the method used are being discussed in many Member States,

c. considering that maternity should be entered into the basis of free will,

d. whereas one of the major reasons for the decrease in perinatal mortality of babies and mothers in Europe is ante and post-natal care, the treatment given in childbirth and the case received by new-born babies, thanks to medical progress, the growing specialisation of doctors and the proper training of midwives,

e. concerned, nonetheless, that the high and, in certain Member States, increasing incidence of Sudden Infant Death Syndrome (SIDS), particularly in babies of 2 to 6 months, is a considerable cause of concern, not least because its causes are still little understood by doctors and because most parents are totally ignorant about it, even though it is the main cause of post-natal infant mortality,

f. whereas psychological factors play an important part in the way childbirth is dealt with, creating various degrees of stress, depending on the country and the professional, economic and social status of the woman and her family,

g. whereas cultural factors play a major part in childbirth, especially in so far as forms of childbirth are a reflection of the way in which society receives the child as a new member,

h. demanding that women receive appropriate treatment during pregnancy and childbirth in accordance with their needs and personal characteristics,

i. whereas, although society has made considerable efforts to remove the worries of women before childbirth, a psychological state of ancestral fear still seems to persist, the explanation for which is the fact that risks during pregnancy and childbirth also persist,

j. whereas it is in the interests of both women and society in general that the problems surrounding pregnancy and confinement should be solved and that women should be given adequate and comprehensive information so as to enable them to take their own decisions in whatever situation they may find themselves in,

k. whereas no surgical operation (caesarean section) should be performed in the case of hospital confinements except in cases of absolute need,

1. Considers that a woman can give birth without anxiety only if she is given appropriate assistance by specialised personnel, whether she chooses to give birth in a hospital or clinic or at home, if the future parents are given full information and if ante-natal care of a preventive, medical, psychological and social nature is made available to all free of charge;

2. Calls for adequate and comprehensive information on the social assistance available to mothers-to-be with problems to be made available in health centres and hospitals;

3. Calls on the Commission to take steps towards drawing up a directive designed to bring all national regulations and provisions regarding pregnancy, childbirth and parenthood into line as far as possible with the regulations and provisions in force in the most advanced Member State;

4. Believes that the Member States should also undertake a thorough review and reorganisation of all legislation concerning women in pregnancy and childbirth, with regard to both the social services and equipping of medical centres and the care of new-born babies;

5. Considers that the Commission's plan to draw up a code of conduct for social protection during motherhood is unsatisfactory, and calls for a directive to be drawn up on this subject;

6. Regrets the ever-increasing number of caesarean sections performed in the Community;

7. Regrets the low rate of breast-feeding in certain Member States of the Community;

8. Emphasises the necessity of women's health centres (e.g. Well Women Centres) to ensure all women access to consultations and counselling and preventative medicine;

9. Also calls upon the Commission to draw up a proposal for a charter on the rights of women in childbirth applicable to all Community countries, enabling any pregnant women to obtain a medical card which allows her to choose the country, district and institution where she wishes to receive care. This card, on

which the rights of women in childbirth should be reproduced, should also guarantee women access to the following facilities, services and rights:

- to a personal obstetric file containing data on the pregnancy, to be made available to the woman concerned and to those attending her during and after pregnancy,
- ante-natal diagnostic testing, such as the flocculation test, ultrasound scanning or an amniocentesis test, free of charge and carried out on a voluntary basis, by agreement with the woman concerned and on the advice of her doctor,
- to attendance, together with the woman's partner, at pre-natal classes covering the physical and psychological aspects of the sequence of events during pregnancy and after the birth,
- to be informed, prior to maternity, of the risks, symptoms, precautions and remedies, particularly those available free of charge from the health services, of the most significant causes of post-natal infant mortality, and in particular Sudden Infant Death Syndrome (SIDS),
- to a free choice of hospital and how (in what position) to give birth and how to feed and rear the baby,
- to proper health care if the woman concerned chooses to give birth at home, depending on her psychological and physical condition, the condition of the unborn baby and the suitability of the home environment,
- to natural childbirth, meaning that the moment of childbirth should neither be brought forward nor delayed unless this is made strictly necessary by the condition of the mother or of the child about to be born,
- to giving birth by caesarean section only if this is absolutely necessary,
- to the presence, if the woman so wishes, of a person, either her partner, a relative or a friend, before, during and after the birth,
- to decide, together with the doctor, after having been fully informed about the options available, what forms of treatment are to be used,

- to keep her baby with her throughout her stay in hospital and to feed it according to its needs rather than according to hospital schedules,
- to freedom to choose whether their milk should be used to feed other babies,
- the right for members of the family to visit the mother and her baby, provided this does not interfere with the care required by the baby,
- to an appropriate period of absence from work during the breast-feeding period and the formal introduction of flexible working hours,
- to adequately equipped and competently staffed wards for premature babies located within the maternity clinics,
- to a medical card enabling a pregnant woman to receive care and treatment in any Community country,
- to facilities, such as the services of an interpreter, for women who are nationals of other countries, so that they too may exercise the rights listed above;

10. Calls on the Member Sates to make it possible for women to give birth anonymously and, where necessary, to register the newborn child without stating its parentage or whilst ensuring that its parentage is kept secret;

11. Calls on the Member States to protect mothers by making the seizure or other implementing measures with regard to property, furniture or personal possessions unenforceable from 8 weeks before to 8 weeks after the birth;

12. Calls further on the Member States:
    a. to adopt appropriate measures to enable more women to quality as doctors and midwives to provide care for women during pregnancy and during and after birth of their children,
    b. to promote and fund research on the causes of infertility in women and men, including environmental and industrial causes,
    c. to organise publicity campaigns to inform the general public about the dangers of using drugs during pregnancy,
    d. to implement the AIM Programme (advanced information on medicine in Europe), in which connection it would be desir-

able for doctors' and patients' organisations, as the users and consumers, to be consulted,

e. to give publicity to all community legislation and all proposals put forward by the Community institutions, and notably to the resolutions voted by the European Parliament, concerning the harmonisation of legislation on preparations for nursing mothers and breast-milk substitutes,

f. to draw attention of the social partners to the need to comply strictly in the field of employment with ILO Convention 103 on the protection of women during motherhood, in particular with regard to dismissal and the provision of appropriate work for pregnant and nursing employees;

13. Calls on the Commission to carry out an in-depth study on the causes of infant and maternal mortality in the Community, including for example, poverty, bad health and poor housing, and in this respect, to pay particular attention to the incidence of Sudden Infant Death Syndrome (SIDS) and the research that is currently being undertaken into its causes and to report back to Parliament with its findings, in particular, its proposals as to how it can best support such research;

14. Instructs its President to forward this resolution to the Commission, the Council, the WHO, the Council of Europe and the governments of the Member States.

Index

E

early discharge 250, 259, 278, 284
    cost 260
Eastern Europe 36, 52, 79, 118, 121, 152, 166, 249, 279, 306, 327
education 104, 232, 267
    of adults 232
    of children 232
    WHO recommendation 233
EFM, see electronic fetal monitoring
electromyographic perineometry 169
electronic fetal monitoring 15, 17, 46, 68, 93, 116, 130, 135, 141, 158–165, 193, 316, 347
    brain damage 159
    efficacy 159, 160
    interpretation 161
    popularity 163
    randomised controlled trial 159, 160, 161, 162
    risks 162
    WHO recommendation 165
EMG, see electromyographic perineometry
empirical midwives 111, 112, 124, 126, 127, 129, 223, 288, 308, 346
    WHO recommendation 288
endorphin 158
enema 140, 141
England 146, 190, 194, 196, 216, 259, 261, 262, 309, 330
    see also United Kingdom
epidemiology 13, 22, 38, 46, 49, 80, 99, 101, 103, 104, 117, 129, 133, 215, 264, 272, 305, 310, 324
epidural anaesthesia, see epidural block
epidural block 22, 117, 154, 155, 167, 315, 324, 326
    combining with oxytocin 156
    effectiveness 156
    position during birth and labour 157
    randomised controlled trial 324
    rates 117
    risks 156, 157
episiotomy 112, 116, 141, 165–174, 214, 347
    cerebral palsy 169, 170
    complications 171
    findings 172
    infection 172
    pelvic floor 169
    perineal trauma 168
    randomised controlled trial 168, 171, 174
    rates 117, 166, 167, 173
    risks 170, 172
    special management 168
    types 166

    WHO recommendation 174
Esalen 308
Eskimos 223, 228
ethics committees 284
Ethiopia 259, 276
Europe 48, 49, 53, 57, 59, 74, 80, 81, 97, 104, 111, 112, 121, 122, 131, 152, 154, 155, 219, 220, 235, 238, 247, 282, 283, 307, 308
European Economic Community 178
European Perinatal Society 134, 310
European Society of Obstetricians and Gynaecologists 317
evaluation at birth 250
    WHO recommendation 251
experimental treatment 279
    WHO recommendation 279

F

family allowance 235
family planning 287
    WHO recommendation 288
Femme Sage Femme 46
fetal distress 144, 181
fetal heartrate monitoring, see electronic fetal monitoring
fetal malformation 95
fetal mortality, see perinatal mortality
fetal movement monitoring 93
fetoscopy 15
FIGO, see International Federation of Gynaecology and Obstetrics
financial support 225
    WHO recommendation 225
Finland 6, 14, 75, 104, 147, 175, 177, 189, 262, 312, 323
First World War 11
Food and Drug Administration 140
Forældre og Fødsel 46
forceps 9, 112, 117, 131, 162, 167, 188–194, 315, 330
    findings 191
    rates 117
    risks 190
Fortaleza 56, 58, 59, 60, 61, 105, 111, 112, 115, 126, 130, 131, 164, 196, 197, 310, 328, 345
France 6, 46, 83, 92, 166, 220, 255, 275, 312, 318, 325
From Research to Decision Making 315

G

gastroenteritis 226

New Zealand 14, 155, 190, 191, 312, 325, 330, 331
nipple stimulation 16, 149
nitrous oxide 155
North America 52, 53, 57, 59, 74, 79, 80, 81, 97, 98,
   104, 111, 124, 126, 128, 131, 154, 166, 175,
   182, 223, 238, 282, 307, 308
Norway 87
nosocomial infection 119

O

O'Driscoll 144
obstetrics 121
Office of Technology Assessment 133, 137
Ontario 124, 314
opiates 155
Oregon 281, 330
Oxford 80
Oxford University 146
oxytocin 16, 147, 148, 156, 159
  risks 148

P

paid maternity leave 234
paid parental leave 234
participants in consensus meetings
  Fortaleza 338
  Trieste 341
  Washington 52, 335
peer review 319
pelvic floor 169
perinatal care 44, 58
  policy 128, 129
  policy on personnel 128
perinatal mortality 38, 71, 178
  rates 117
  see also fetal mortality
perinatal surveillance system 101, 293
perineal trauma 168
Peru 262
pethidine 155
phototherapy 256
placenta praevia 181
pneumonia 226
positioning during labour and birth 116, 130, 150
  changes in practice 152
  criteria 150
  effects 151
  WHO recommendation 153

post-natal care
  depression, see post-natal depression
  financial support 225
  health care 225
  protection from abuse 225
  social equity 226
  support 230, 234
  warmth, food and shelter 224
post-natal depression 184, 251, 252
  medicalisation of 253
  WHO recommendation 253
postpartum depression, see post-natal depression
post-term pregnancy 146, 147
pre-eclampsia 147, 181
prematurity 71, 93, 148, 159, 160, 184, 185, 224, 235,
  258, 294
  WHO recommendation 280
prenatal bonding, see bonding
prenatal care 8, 10, 11, 12, 13, 15, 20, 45, 52, 54, 56, 58,
   63, 64, 65, 66, 67, 68, 71, 72, 73, 74, 75, 76,
   77, 79, 80, 97, 99, 103, 104, 125, 135, 164,
   165, 179, 258, 263, 267, 305, 307, 308, 309,
   322, 323
  location 75
  scientific basis 80, 100
prenatal education 72, 77
  see also education
prenatal visits 65, 100
preterm delivery, see prematurity
privacy 223, 224, 246
  WHO recommendation 223
progestagens 68

Q

Quebec 124, 166, 189, 228, 314

R

randomised controlled trial 14, 21, 22, 7t, 81, 84, 85,
   86, 87, 89, 90, 91, 93, 102, 103, 116, 119,
   142, 143, 150, 151, 159, 160, 161, 162, 164,
   168, 169, 171, 172, 174, 216, 245, 260, 261,
   262, 274, 287, 289, 294, 324, 328, 329
  WHO recommendation 294
research 103, 290–296
  design 294
  ethics 103
  priority 290
  quality of 293

doppler 84
  efficacy 83, 91
  exposure conditions 88
  long-term effects 81
  perinatal outcome 91
  randomised controlled trial 84, 87, 91, 93
  routine screening 91
  routine use 84
  safety 87, 88, 91
  selective use 83
  sensitivity 85
  specificity 85
UNICEF 227, 243, 261
United Kingdom 5, 6, 11, 13, 14, 15, 35, 36, 46, 47, 79,
        88, 89, 90, 101, 117, 133, 147, 155, 175, 176,
        177, 182, 187, 189, 220, 232, 260, 266, 282,
        303, 310, 312, 317, 318, 320, 321, 324, 325,
        331, 332
United Nations 5, 43, 46, 235
United Nations Centre 312
United Nations Children's Emergency Fund, see
        UNICEF
United States 5, 6, 11, 13, 14, 17, 22, 35, 51, 64, 71, 73,
        83, 89, 92, 93, 111, 117, 118, 120, 122, 124,
        125, 128, 133, 137, 139, 140, 146, 147, 152,
        155, 165, 166, 167, 172, 175, 176, 177, 178,
        181, 182, 183, 186, 187, 189, 190, 196, 220,
        222, 227, 232, 248, 259, 260, 262, 268, 275,
        281, 306, 312, 316, 317, 318, 319, 322, 325,
        327, 330, 332
  Consensus Conference 182
  Consensus Statement 90
  Federal Government 125
  Food and Drug Administration 16, 17
  Institute of Medicine 73
Uruguay 102
USSR 313
uterine rupture 148

V

vacuum extraction 162, 188–194, 315
  findings 191
  rates 117
  risks 190
vaginal birth after caesarean 182, 183, 196
  rates 196
value judgements 37
VBAC, see vaginal birth after caesarean
Victoria 147, 191
Vienna 19

Director of Maternal and Child Health 19
vitamin K 287
Vologda 314

W

Wales 146, 190
Washington 52, 55, 60, 64, 105, 181, 187, 189
Western Australia 191
Western Europe 36, 46, 52, 79, 118, 120, 158, 166, 175,
        306
WIC 71
World Health Assembly 314
World Health Organisation 5, 6, 7, 8, 14, 18, 19, 36,
        43, 44, 45, 48, 50, 53, 55, 62, 63, 75, 77, 80,
        81, 87, 89, 90, 93, 125, 126, 147, 155, 175,
        182, 187, 190, 192, 222, 228, 231, 232, 243,
        275, 276, 283, 285, 287, 295, 303, 304, 306,
        307, 310, 311, 314, 317, 318, 322, 332, 333
  Consensus Conference 210
  Director General 126, 322, 325
  European Perinatal Study Group 49, 50, 54, 79,
        102, 114, 175, 229, 263, 275
  European Region 46, 235
  Headquarters 333
  International Code of Marketing of Breast-
        milk Substitutes 231
  Perinatal Study Group 49
  Regional Director for Europe 60, 321, 322, 325
  Regional Director for the Americas 55
  Regional Office for Europe 6, 41, 46, 49, 50, 51,
        54, 94, 125, 175, 178, 181, 194, 295,
        303, 304, 305, 307, 310, 311, 315, 328,
        332, 345, 349
  Regional Office for the Americas 51, 52, 54,
        345, 349

X

x-rays 12, 15, 19, 65, 82, 86
  childhood cancer 86
  safety 86

Z

Zimbabwe 259